T0229672

# Dermal Drug Delivery
From Innovation to Production

# Dermal Drug Delivery

## From Innovation to Production

EDITED BY
Tapash K. Ghosh

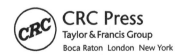

CRC Press
Taylor & Francis Group
Boca Raton  London  New York

CRC Press is an imprint of the
Taylor & Francis Group, an **informa** business

CRC Press
Taylor & Francis Group
6000 Broken Sound Parkway NW, Suite 300
Boca Raton, FL 33487-2742

First issued in paperback 2022

ISBN-13: 978-1-466-58270-5 (hbk)
ISBN-13: 978-1-03-233741-8 (pbk)
DOI: 10.1201/9781315374215

**Visit the Taylor & Francis Web site at**
**http://www.taylorandfrancis.com**

**and the CRC Press Web site at**
**http://www.crcpress.com**

# Contents

# Preface

With the continued advancement of better-quality control and patient outcome reporting systems, changes in the development, control and regulation of all pharmaceutical delivery systems including transdermal and topical products have been happening on a continuous basis. In light of various quality issues that have been reported by patients and practitioners resulting in the recall or removal of products from the market, both the pharmaceutical industries and regulatory agencies have been adopting new measures to address these issues. With chapters written by experts in this field, this book takes a 21st century multidisciplinary and cross-functional look at these dosage forms to improve the development, design, manufacturing, quality, clinical performance, safety, and regulation of these products.

This book offers a wealth of up-to-date information organized in a logical sequence corresponding to various stages of research, development, and commercialization of dermal drug delivery products. The authors have been carefully selected from different sectors of pharmaceutical science for their expertise in their selected areas to present objectively a balanced view of the current state of these products' development and commercialization via regulatory approval. Their insights will provide useful information to others to ensure the successful development of the next generation dermal drug products.

Key features include:

- Presents current advancements including new technologies of transdermal and topical dosage forms.
- Presents challenges in the development of the new generation of transdermal and topical dosage forms.
- Introduces new technologies and QbD (quality by design) aspects of manufacturing and control strategies.
- Includes new perspectives on pre-clinical and clinical development, regulatory considerations, safety and quality.
- Discusses regulatory challenges, gaps and future considerations for dermal drug delivery systems.

# The Editor

**Tapash K. Ghosh, PhD** is currently employed at the Office of Pharmaceutical Quality (OPQ), at Center for Drug Evaluation and Research of the U.S. Food and Drug Administration (CDER, FDA). Before working at OPQ, he was at the Office of Clinical Pharmacology (OCP) at CDER, FDA. This book is the fourth one in his credit, all published by the CRC Press in their pharmaceutical science series. Before joining the FDA, he held faculty positions in two academic institutions and also worked briefly in pharmaceutical industries. He is also in the expert panel of the United States Pharmacopeia (USP). He is the author of numerous scientific publications and has delivered scientific speeches nationally and internationally on different scientific topics related to drug development.

# Contributors

**Dina W. Ameen**
Department of Pharmaceutics
Center for Dermal Research
Rutgers University
Piscataway, New Jersey

**Muralikrishnan Angamuthu**
Department of Pharmaceutics and Drug
    Delivery
The University of Mississippi
Starkville, Mississippi

**Ajay K. Banga**
Department of Pharmaceutical Sciences
Mercer University
Atlanta, Georgia

**Tony Bennett**
Global Manufacturing and Supply
GSK, UK

**April C. Braddy**
Division of Bioequivalence III
Center for Drug Evaluation and
    Research (CDER)
Food and Drug Administration (FDA)
Silver Spring, Maryland

**Scott A. Burton**
3M Drug Delivery Systems Division
St. Paul, Minnesota

**Dale P. Conner**
Division of Bioequivalence III
Center for Drug Evaluation and
    Research (CDER)
Food and Drug Administration (FDA)
Silver Spring, Maryland

**Lisa A. Dick**
3M Drug Delivery Systems Division
St. Paul, Minnesota

**Shulin Ding**
Silver Spring, Maryland

**Daniel M. Dohmeier**
3M Drug Delivery Systems Division
St. Paul, Minnesota

**John T. Farrar**
Departments of Epidemiology,
    Anesthesia, and Neurology
Center for Clinical Epidemiology and
    Biostatistics
University of Pennsylvania
Philadelphia, Pennsylvania

**Gregory Fieldson**
Tolmar Inc.
Ft. Collins, Colorado

**Tapash K. Ghosh**
Silver Spring, Maryland

**Anushree Herwadkar**
Department of Pharmaceutical
    Sciences
Mercer University
Atlanta, Georgia

**Sarah A. Ibrahim**
Center for Drug Evaluation and
    Research (CDER)
Food and Drug Administration
    (FDA)
Silver Spring, Maryland

**Shamir N. Kalaria**
Center for Translational Medicine
University of Maryland
Baltimore, Maryland

**Chan Ko**
3M Drug Delivery Systems Division
St. Paul, Minnesota

**Majella E. Lane**
School of Pharmacy
University College of London
London, UK

**Howard I. Maibach**
Department of Dermatology
University of California
San Francisco, California

**Margareth R.C. Marques**
United States Pharmacopeia
 (USP)
Rockville, Maryland

**Nathaly Martos**
Department of Pharmaceutics
Center for Dermal Research
Rutgers University
Piscataway, New Jersey

**Bozena Michniak-Kohn**
Department of Pharmaceutics
Center for Dermal Research
New Jersey Center for
 Biomaterials
Rutgers University
Piscataway, New Jersey

**Amit Mitra**
Center for Drug Evaluation and
 Research (CDER)
Food and Drug Administration
 (FDA)
Silver Spring, Maryland

**S. Narasimha Murthy**
Department of Pharmaceutics and Drug
 Delivery
The University of Mississippi
Starkville, Mississippi
and
Institute for Drug Delivery and
 Biomedical Research (IDBR)
Bengaluru, India

**Timothy A. Peterson**
3M Drug Delivery Systems Division
St. Paul, Minnesota

**Ann M. Purrington**
3M Drug Delivery Systems Division
St. Paul, Minnesota

**Tannaz Ramezanli**
Department of Pharmaceutics
Center for Dermal Research
Rutgers University
Piscataway, New Jersey

**H.N. Shivakumar**
Institute for Drug Delivery and
 Biomedical Research (IDBR)
KLE College of Pharmacy
Bengaluru, India

**Neha Singh**
Recipharm Laboratories Inc.
Morrisville, North Carolina

**Caroline Strasinger**
Center for Drug Evaluation and
 Research (CDER)
Food and Drug Administration (FDA)
Silver Spring, Maryland

**Sonia Trehan**
Center for Dermal Research
Rutgers University
Piscataway, New Jersey

**Pei-Chin Tsai**
Department of Pharmaceutics
Center for Dermal Research
Rutgers University
Piscataway, New Jersey

**Rashmi Upasani**
Purdue Pharma L.P.,
Durham, North Carolina

**Kenneth A. Walters**
An-eX Analytical Services Ltd.
Cardiff, UK

**Steven M. Wick**
3M Drug Delivery Systems Division
St. Paul, Minnesota

**Lindsey C. Yeh**
Icahn School of Medicine at
   Mount Sinai
Foster City, California

**Zheng Zhang**
Center for Dermal Research
New Jersey Center for Biomaterials
Rutgers University
Piscataway, New Jersey

# 1 Dermal and Transdermal Drug Delivery Systems
## *An Overview and Recent Advancements*

*Kenneth A. Walters and Majella E. Lane*

## CONTENTS

## 1.1   INTRODUCTION

The first edition of this book was published in 1997 and became a standard reference text in the field of dermal and transdermal drug delivery systems (Ghosh et al., 1997). In Chapter 2 of the original edition, Bill Pfister gave a comprehensive description of the current status of transdermal and dermal therapeutic systems. Following his review, Pfister concluded:

> Since the introduction of the first [transdermal delivery system] ... 15 years ago, there have been dozens of new [transdermal and dermatological delivery systems] introduced into the market. The future outlook is bright for the development of new and improved [systems] for passive or active delivery of drugs to or through the skin. The current product successes represent only the "tip of the iceberg" of the technologies and products yet to emerge from the depths of ongoing, innovative, controlled drug delivery R&D activities in pharmaceutical, biotechnology, and ... medical device companies.

The purpose of this current chapter is to review progress in this field over the past 22 years. Have we successfully extracted and developed products from the metaphorical *"iceberg"* or has it succumbed to global warming? In 1997 most of us researching and developing pharmaceutical drug delivery systems for the skin, and for systemic delivery via the skin, considered that tremendous progress had been made in the 43 years since the publication of Frazier and Blank's (1954) *A Formulary for External Therapy of the Skin*. Our improved understanding of the physicochemical properties of dermal and transdermal formulation systems and their ingredients had resulted in the development of physically, chemically and biologically stable products, which remained potent after two or three years on the shelf. The regulatory process of product approval for marketing did guarantee that the drug in an approved formulation was relatively safe and was effective when applied to a diseased tissue. However, formulators would always ask the questions: (a) Is the formulation optimized? (b) Could it be safer? (c) Could it be more effective therapeutically?

In 1997 our knowledge of the skin and the processes that control percutaneous absorption were well understood. The seminal work of Scheuplein and Blank in the late 1960s and early 1970s (reviewed in Scheuplein and Blank, 1971) had laid down the ground rules and these had been reviewed and updated on a reasonably regular basis (see e.g., Barry, 1983; Walters, 2002; Hwa et al., 2011). Thus we knew, for example, that permeation of compounds across the skin was, in most cases, controlled by the stratum corneum, and that the chemical composition and morphology of this layer determined the rate and extent of absorption

(Elias, 1981). We knew how to modify the skin barrier, by chemical or physical means, to alter the rate of diffusion of many permeating molecules (Walters and Hadgraft, 1993).

This chapter will review progress in the development of dermal and transdermal delivery systems over the past 15 years. Skin permeation and enhancement technologies, together with delivery systems, have been the regular subject of updates and reviews (see e.g., Roberts et al., 2002; Smith and Maibach, 2005; Elias and Feingold, 2006; Roberts and Walters, 2008; Williams and Walters, 2008; Benson and Watkinson, 2012; Wiedersberg and Guy, 2014; Pastore et al., 2015; Dragicevic and Maibach, 2015; Brown and Williams, 2019), as have the differences between diseased and normal stratum corneum (Bouwstra and Ponec, 2006; Jakasa et al., 2006; Cork et al., 2009; Ortiz et al., 2009; Gattu and Maibach, 2011; Malikou et al., 2018). Since much of the recent advances in skin transport mechanisms has been reviewed elsewhere (including this volume) we have limited our review to recent advances in the product development and use of drug delivery systems for dermal and transdermal therapy.

## 1.2 STRUCTURE OF THE SKIN BARRIER

Both dermal and transdermal drug therapy for local and systemic effect require the active agent to be delivered to the site of action. Thus the potential for successful therapeutic outcome is that the drug be capable of penetrating into and permeating across the various membranes that constitute the skin. The relationships between the structure of human skin and its transport properties have been the subject of extensive research for many years and there are many excellent and recent reviews covering these aspects (Hadgraft and Lane, 2011; Menon et al., 2012; Yang and Guy, 2015; Lundborg et al., 2018). Although it has been well established experimentally that it is the chemical morphology of the stratum corneum that controls the overall rate at which compounds can permeate across the skin, other factors can contribute to the extent of such permeation. Major secondary factors governing the extent of percutaneous absorption include temperature (Shahzad et al., 2015), permeant clearance from the skin (Trottet et al., 2004; Anissimov et al., 2013) and desquamation (Simon and Goyal, 2009; Simon et al., 2011).

The cells of the epidermis originate in the basal lamina between the dermis and viable epidermis (Figure 1.1). In this layer there are melanocytes, Langerhans cells, Merkel cells and keratinocytes. A secure link between the basal keratinocytes and the basal matrix is essential for skin integrity, but these cells must also be capable of detaching and dividing to begin the process of terminal differentiation that will form the stratum corneum. The development of the stratum corneum from the keratinocytes of the basal layer involves several steps of cell differentiation. The cells progress through the stratum spinosum, the stratum granulosum, the stratum lucidium to the stratum corneum (Baroni et al., 2012). Cell turnover, from stratum basale to stratum corneum, is estimated to be on the order of about three weeks. In the stratum granulosum many granules containing lamellar subunits appear (Figure 1.2). These are the precursors of the intercellular lipid lamellae of

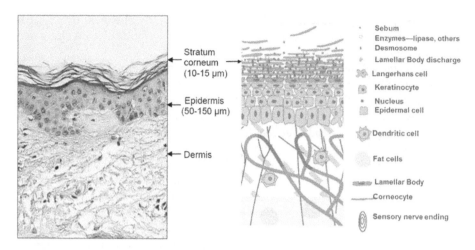

**FIGURE 1.1** Structure of the skin. (Courtesy of Sean Cleary; reproduced with permission from Menon et al. 2010.)

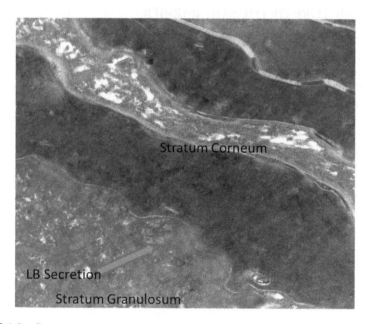

**FIGURE 1.2** Stratum corneum – stratum granulosum interface. (Reproduced with permission from Menon et al. 2012.)

the stratum corneum (Menon et al., 2012). In the outermost layers of the stratum granulosum the lamellar granules migrate to the apical cell surface where they fuse and eventually extrude their contents into the intercellular space. At this stage in the differentiation process the keratinocytes lose their nuclei and other cytoplasmic organelles, become flattened and compacted to form the stratum lucidum, which eventually becomes the stratum corneum. The extrusion of the contents of lamellar granules is a fundamental requirement for the formation of the epidermal permeability barrier (Nishifuji and Yoon, 2013). The cornified cell envelopes of the stratum corneum keratinocytes are comprised of crosslinked protein complexes that are very insoluble and chemically resistant. These complexes play an important role in the structural assembly of the intercellular lipid lamellae of the stratum corneum. The composition of the stratum corneum intercellular lipids is unique in biological systems; a remarkable feature being the lack of phospholipids and preponderance of cholesterol and ceramides. The intercellular lipid lamellae are highly structured, very stable and provide a highly effective barrier to chemical penetration and permeation.

## 1.3 THE RELATIONSHIP BETWEEN SKIN STRUCTURE AND PERMEATION

It has been known for some time that permeation across the skin is controlled mainly by the tortuous but continuous intercellular lipid of the stratum corneum (Figure 1.3; Hadgraft and Lane, 2011). As such, the rate at which permeation occurs is largely dependent on the physicochemical characteristics of the penetrant, the most important being the relative ability to partition into the intercellular lamellae. Three

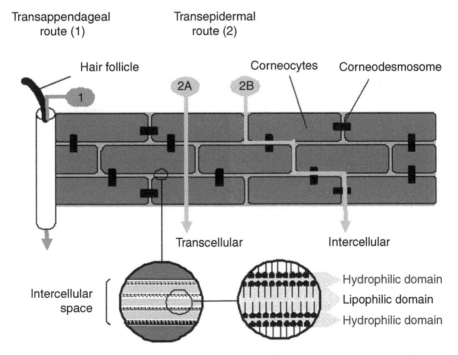

**FIGURE 1.3** "Brick and mortar" model of the stratum corneum and routes of permeation. (Reproduced from Physical Chemistry Chemical Physics, 2011, 5216, with permission of the Royal Society of Chemistry.)

major variables account for differences in the rate at which different compounds permeate the skin: the concentration of permeant applied, the partition coefficient of the permeant between the stratum corneum and the vehicle, and the diffusivity of the compound within the stratum corneum. As has been shown, however, the stratum corneum is not a pure lipid membrane and the relationship between the permeability rate and permeant lipophilicity is sigmoidal, which reflects the existence of hydrophilic barriers. Relatively polar permeants would preferentially partition into and diffuse through these hydrophilic regions. There is a further loss of direct partitioning sensitivity in permeation when the permeant is more lipophilic. This is often attributed to the more aqueous viable epidermis, which can present a significant resistance to the permeation of highly lipophilic compounds. This suggests, therefore, that compounds with partition coefficients of between logP 1 and 3 would permeate the skin comparatively rapidly. It is clear that such physicochemical requirements will limit the number of candidates for transdermal drug delivery.

## 1.4 TRANSDERMAL DRUG DELIVERY FOR SYSTEMIC EFFECT

In 1997 the number of therapeutic drugs that were successfully delivered to the systemic circulation via the transdermal route worldwide was limited to ten. Of these, seven were marketed in the USA (Pfister, 1997). Since then, in the USA a further ten therapeutic systems have been added to the list of approved transdermally delivered systemic drugs (Table 1.1).

**TABLE 1.1**
**Systemic Transdermal Patch Medications**

| Drug | Indication | FDA Approval |
|---|---|---|
| Scopolamine | Travel sickness | 1979 |
| Nitroglycerin | Angina | 1982 |
| Clonidine | Hypertension | 1984 |
| Estradiol | Female HRT | 1986 |
| Fentanyl | Chronic pain | 1990 |
| Testosterone | Hypogonadism | 1995 |
| Nicotine | Smoking cessation | 1996 |
| Estradiol/norethindrone acetate | Female HRT | 1998 |
| Ethinyl estradiol/norelgestromin | Female contraception | 2001 |
| Oxybutynin | Enuresis | 2003 |
| Methylphenidate | ADD/ADHD | 2006 |
| Selegiline | Depression | 2006 |
| Rivastigmine | Alzheimer's disease | 2007 |
| Rotigotine | Parkinson's disease | 2007/2012 |
| Granisetron | Chemotherapy-induced emesis | 2008 |
| Buprenorphine | Moderate to severe pain | 2010 |
| Sumatriptan | Migraine | 2013* |

* Withdrawn from the market by Teva Pharmaceuticals in June 2016.

### 1.4.1 COMBINATION PRODUCTS FOR FEMALE CONTRACEPTION

The introduction of a hormonal patch for female contraception was seen as a significant advance in the avoidance of unwanted pregnancies, especially in younger women where there was a risk of missing the daily oral dose (Graziottin, 2008). Ortho-Evra® is a combination transdermal contraceptive patch containing 6 mg norelgestromin and 0.75 mg ethinyl estradiol. The patch is a 20 cm² drug-in-adhesive matrix with a standard backing membrane of polyethylene and polyester. The adhesive is polyisobutylene/polybutene and this carries the two active ingredients together with crospovidone and lauryl lactate, the adhesive layer being protected during storage by a release liner of polyethylene terephthalate with a polydimethylsiloxane coating. The patch is designed to deliver 150 µg norelgestromin and 20 µg ethinyl estradiol daily and is applied to the buttocks, lower abdomen, upper torso (excluding breasts) or the upper arm on the first day of menstruation and left in place for a week. The patch is removed and replaced with a new patch on a weekly basis for a further two weeks. The fourth week is patch free.

The pharmacokinetics of the Ortho-Evra® patch were evaluated under a series of conditions and described in a series of articles by Abrams et al. (Abrams et al., 2001a;b;c; 2002a), reviewed in Abrams et al. (2002b). Based on studies of oral norgestimate (250 µg) and ethinyl estradiol (35 µg), the serum concentration reference ranges for norelgestromin and ethinyl estradiol are 0.6–1.2 ng/mL and 25–75 pg/mL, respectively. In the first study, 12 healthy females applied the patch to the abdomen for seven days and, following removal of the initial patch, wore a second patch for ten days. Blood samples were collected for nineteen days after application of the first patch. Following application of the initial patch, serum levels of both ethinyl estradiol and norelgestromin reached a plateau by about 48 hours. Serum concentrations of ethinyl estradiol remained within the reference range described on p. 8, as did those for norelgestromin, over the period of study (Abrams et al., 2001a). These data were confirmed in a multiple-dose study over three cycles, although there was evidence of minimal accumulation between week one of cycle one and week three of cycle three (Abrams et al., 2001b). The conditions of heat, humidity and exercise had no effect on patch pharmacokinetics and adhesion (although one patch of 87 applied became detached) (Abrams et al., 2001c). The influence of application site was evaluated by determining serum levels of the two active agents following application of patches to the abdomen, upper torso (excluding the breasts), buttock and upper arm (Abrams et al., 2002a). The data indicated that the ability to maintain serum levels within the reference values was unaffected by the site of application, although following application to the abdomen absorption was approximately 20% lower than that observed for the other sites (Figure 1.4).

Clinical studies involving the Ortho-Evra® contraceptive patch have been reviewed (Creasy et al., 2001). The patch was found to provide ovulation inhibition by suppression of gonadotropins, cycle control similar to that of oral norgestimate and ethinyl estradiol, and decreased mean maximum follicular diameter. Efficacy, safety and compliance of patch use were also demonstrated (Smallwood et al, 2001). The patch was not associated with phototoxicity or photoallergy. By 2006,

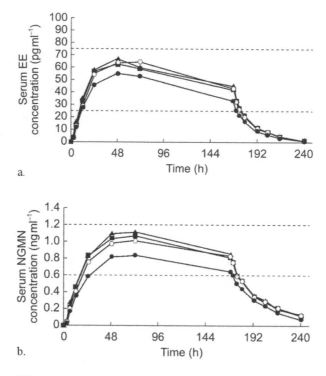

a.

b.

**FIGURE 1.4** Mean serum concentration versus time profile of (a) ethinyl estradiol (EE) and (b) norelgestromin following successive applications of the contraceptive patch for seven days at each of four anatomical sites (● abdomen; ▲ arm; ■ buttock; ○ torso). Dashed horizontal lines indicate reference range. (Reproduced from Abrams et al. 2002a, by permission from Blackwell Science Ltd.)

the contraceptive patch was widely accepted as being an efficacious and safe regimen, with the successful completion of three phase III trials, two of which were randomized comparisons with an oral contraceptive. Although the likelihood of pregnancy was similar between the patch and the pill, compliance with the patch was notably better, particularly in younger women, and the safety and tolerability of the patch was similar to that of oral contraception (Graziottin, 2006). In the same year the increased risk of nonfatal venous thromboembolism, linked to the oral use of the progestin, norgestromate and ethinyl estradiol, was shown to be similar in those subjects using the contraceptive patch (Jick et al., 2006; Jick et al., 2007). However, a later study suggested that the increased risk of venous thromboembolism associated with the use of the contraceptive patch was two-fold greater than that associated with norgestimate-containing oral contraceptives (Dore et al., 2010). These and other studies (Jick et al., 2010) led to a safety update and an FDA requested change to the labeling of Ortho-Evra® in 2011. Nonetheless, an evaluation by Bodner et al. (2011, p. 525) of 80 adolescents and 178 adult users concluded that there was "an overall positive impression of Evra with good compliance…".

Other combination transdermal contraceptive patches under development include those containing gestodene and ethinyl estradiol (Gao et al., 2009), ethinyl estradiol and medroxyprogesterone acetate (Agrawal and Pruthi, 2011), and ethinyl estradiol and levonorgestrel (Archer et al, 2012; Archer et al, 2013). Of these three combination patch systems under development, the later (code name AG200-15; Agile Therapeutics) is in phase III development. The AG200-15 transdermal system is designed to deliver 100–120 µg of levonorgestrel and 25–30 µg ethinyl estradiol per day. The phase III trials for AG200-15 enrolled nearly 2,000 women and formed the basis for the Company's application to the U.S. Food and Drug Administration in 2012. The pharmacokinetic profiles for AG200-15 were established in an open-label, single center study in 36 healthy women, which compared the patch profiles to those obtained using a combination oral contraceptive containing ethinyl estradiol (35 µg) and norgestimate (250 µg). The study was conducted over three cycles with a randomized crossover design. After a run-in cycle of 21 days on and seven days off using AG200-15, participants were randomized to receive one of two treatments: a 21/7-day cycle of AG200-15 either followed or preceded by one cycle of the oral contraceptive. During the third week of AG200-15 use, the mean maximum serum concentration ($C_{max}$) and steady-state concentration for ethinyl estradiol were 51.3 ± 17.3 pg/mL and 35.7 ± 14.5 pg/mL, respectively; and for levonorgestrel, the corresponding values were 2400 ± 1140 pg/mL, and 1847 ± 930 pg/mL, respectively. For AG200-15 the ethinyl estradiol $C_{max}$ was approximately 60% lower and the steady-state serum concentration was 15–20% lower than those obtained with the oral contraceptive (Archer et al., 2012). Safety and tolerability studies of low-dose levonorgestrel/ethinyl estradiol contraceptive patches indicated that the patch, and also combination oral contraceptives, were well tolerated in both obese and non-obese women, serious adverse events occurring in less than 1% of participants in any treatment group (Kaunitz et al., 2015).

In addition to the combination contraceptive patches, the feasibility of a transdermal patch containing the progestogen (Figure 1.5) desogestrel as a single agent in an adhesive matrix has also been evaluated (Sachdeva et al., 2013). The authors investigated the comparative skin permeation (using hairless rat skin) and found that the permeation of desogestrel was significantly greater than that of levonorgestrel. Evaluation of different adhesives demonstrated that acrylic adhesives with and without functional groups (DuroTak™ 87–4098 and DuroTak 87-202A, Henkel) had a much greater solubility for the drug than a polyisobutylene adhesive (DuroTak 87-608A). Developments in transdermal contraceptive patches have been recently reviewed (Nelson, 2015).

### 1.4.2 INCONTINENCE: THE USE OF TRANSDERMAL OXYBUTYNIN

Overactive bladder syndrome is an extensive problem that blights the quality of life of a significant proportion of the American population (16–17%) (Stewart et al., 2003). The prevalence of urge incontinence increases with age in both women and men and can lead to impaired mobility and depression. Antimuscarinic agents have been the mainstay of therapy for overactive bladder for many years. These agents

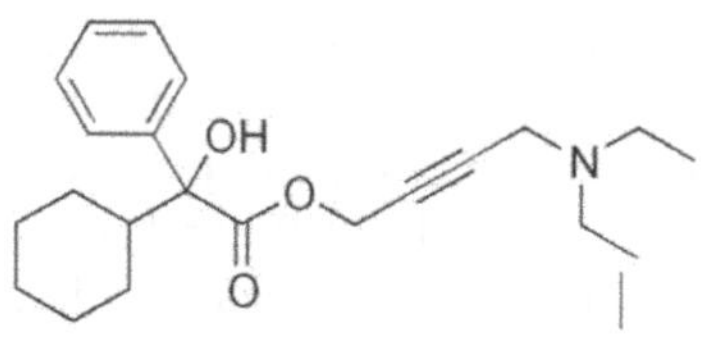

A) Oxybutynin

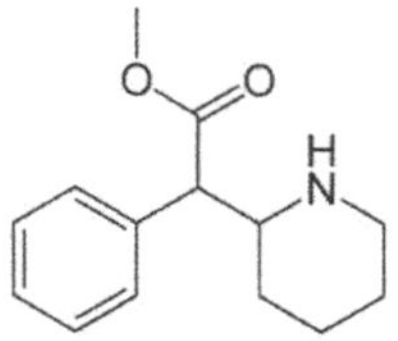

B) Methylphenidate

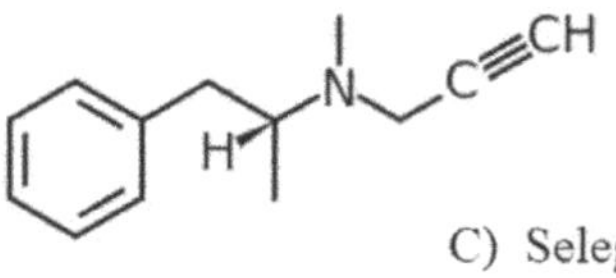

C) Selegiline

**FIGURE 1.5** Chemical structures of oxybutynin, methylphenidate and selegiline. For physicochemical data see Table 1.2.

lower intravesicular pressure and reduce the frequency of contractions by antagonizing parasympathetic control of the bladder. Several drug substances are indicated for therapy, including oxybutynin, tolterodine, darifenacin and fesoteradine, but their long-term use is often associated with antimuscarinic side effects and, to date, transdermal oxybutynin remains the first choice for treatment (Herbison and McKenzie, 2019). Oxybutynin (Figure 1.2), the oldest of the agents used for overactive bladder, has a very low oral bioavailability (~6%) because it undergoes extensive first-pass gut wall and hepatic metabolism. Although the primary hepatic metabolite, N-desethyloxybutynin, is active, it is responsible for the most prevalent side effect, dry mouth. Oral doses have been relatively high in both immediate and extended release preparations. On this basis, transdermal therapy was considered as a potentially beneficial means to improve drug delivery, reduce side effects and increase patient compliance. At present, there are two different transdermal formulations of oxybutynin, a patch system and a gel.

The first to market in 2003 was the patch (presently marketed as *Oxytrol*, Actavis; *Kentera*, UCB), which is a 39 cm² acrylic adhesive system containing 36 mg oxybutynin and triacetin within the acrylic adhesive. The patch is designed to provide a systemic dose of 3.9 mg of oxybutynin per day for three to four days. The adhesive matrix is supported on an occlusive polyester/ethylene-vinyl acetate backing membrane and protected in storage by a siliconized polyester release liner. Oxybutynin is a racemic mixture of R- and S-isomers (50:50), the R-enantiomer providing the majority of the antimuscarinic activity. The pharmacokinetics of oxybutynin were determined following oral and transdermal administration (Zobrist et al., 2001). Initial studies on the in vitro human skin permeation of the R- and S-enantiomers of oxybutynin showed that there was equal permeation of the two enantiomers. The drug was then applied as a single transdermal patch, worn for 96 hours or given as a single 5 mg immediate release tablet. Plasma concentrations of the R- and S-enantiomers of oxybutynin and the primary metabolite N-desethyloxybutynin were monitored for 108 hours after application of the transdermal system and for six hours following oral administration. The plasma concentrations of the R-enantiomers of both oxybutynin and N-desethyloxybutynin were slightly lower than the S-enantiomers following transdermal application (Figure 1.6). The AUC (area under the curve) ratios of N-desethyloxybutynin/oxybutynin were less than 1 for both the R- and S- enantiomers. Following oral dosing, as would be expected given the high first-pass metabolism, plasma N-desethyloxybutynin concentrations greatly exceeded oxybutynin. A later study confirmed the suitability of the transdermal route for delivery of oxybutynin, confirmed the suggested dosage regimen of two applications per week and demonstrated the bioequivalence of various anatomic application sites (abdomen, buttock and hip). Steady-state conditions are normally attained during the second application of the patch and average plasma levels are 3.1 ng/mL for oxybutynin and 3.8 ng/mL for N-desethyloxybutynin.

The safety and efficacy of the transdermal oxybutynin patch has been well established (Davila et al., 2001; Dmochowski et al., 2002; Dmochowski et al., 2005).

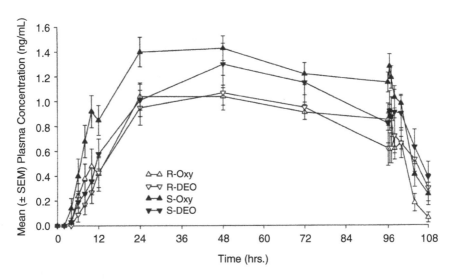

**FIGURE 1.6**  Plasma concentrations of R- and S-oxybutynin and R- and S-desethyloxybutynin following application of a single oxybutynin transdermal system. The patch was removed at 96 hours. (Reproduced from Zobrist et al., 2001 with permission.)

In order to determine an appropriate dose range, Dmochowski et al. (2002) randomized 520 adult patients to 12 weeks of double-blind daily treatment with 1.3, 2.6 or 3.9 mg oxybutynin transdermal delivery systems (TDS) or placebo administered twice weekly. This was followed by a 12-week open-label, dose titration period to assess efficacy and safety. At a dose of 3.9 mg oxybutynin daily, the number of weekly incontinence episodes was reduced over placebo. The average daily urinary frequency was also reduced and the quality of life significantly improved. Although the average voided volume increased in the 2.6 mg oxybutynin group, there were no further significant differences between 1.3 and 2.6 mg transdermal oxybutynin and placebo. In the open-label period a sustained reduction of nearly three incontinence episodes per day was reported for all groups. The investigators concluded that daily transdermal doses of 2.6 and 3.9 mg oxybutynin improved overactive bladder symptoms and quality of life, and were well tolerated. In a later analysis (Dmochowski et al., 2005), transdermal oxybutynin was shown to be significantly more effective than placebo in reducing median daily incontinence episodes and daily urinary frequency, and in increasing void volume. Dry mouth and constipation were the most frequent antimuscarinic related adverse events, and application site erythema occurred in 7.0% of participants who received oxybutynin with pruritus occurring in 16.1%. The overall conclusion was that transdermal oxybutynin was efficacious and safe, and could be considered as a treatment option that would enhance compliance in patients with overactive bladder. This conclusion was confirmed in a later study that also concluded that transdermal oxybutynin was a well-tolerated therapy for men with prostate conditions (Staskin et al., 2008).

An effective and safe hydroalcoholic gel transdermal system of oxybutynin is available in two strengths, 3% and 10% (*Gelnique*, Actavis) (Staskin et al., 2009). The indications are as for the patch type transdermal system. The 10% oxybutynin gel contains the following inactive ingredients: alcohol USP; glycerin USP; hydroxypropyl cellulose NF; sodium hydroxide NF; and purified water USP, whereas, in addition to the active, the 3% gel contains diethylene glycol monoethyl ether NF; alcohol USP; hydroxypropyl cellulose NF; propylene glycol NF; butylated hydroxytoluene NF; HCl 0.1 M NF; and purified water USP. The original gel formulation used in Gelnique 3% was designed by Antares Pharma AG and consisted of a combination of solvent systems and permeation enhancers that enabled systemic drug delivery (Alberti et al., 2005). The gel can be applied to the abdomen, thigh, shoulder or upper arm and it dries quickly leaving no residue. The dosage regimen for the 3% and 10% gels result in an application amount of 84 mg and 100 mg oxybutynin, respectively, daily. Steady-state blood levels of oxybutynin following repeated applications of the two gels are similar, with plasma concentrations of about 4–6 ng/mL, with $C_{max}$ ~8 ng/mL.

The effects of various parameters that may affect drug delivery from the 10% oxybutynin gel have been evaluated in healthy subjects. Factors investigated included application site effects on drug delivery, the effects of sunscreen application on oxybutynin absorption, the effects of post-application showering on steady-state pharmacokinetics, and person-to-person transfer of oxybutynin through skin-to-skin contact at the application site (Dmochowski et al., 2011). The AUCs from time 0 to

24h, following a single application of 1g *Gelnique* gel (100 mg oxybutynin) daily to the abdomen, upper arm/shoulder or thigh, were similar for the three application sites. Showering one hour after gel application did not affect the overall systemic levels of oxybutynin, and application of sunscreen 30 minutes before or after application, similarly, had no effect on oxybutynin availability. Active agents that are applied to the skin for systemic delivery are, for the most part, extremely potent drugs that have the requisite physicochemical properties to penetrate into and permeate across the skin. It is important, therefore, especially in instances where the application site is not protected, to evaluate the potential for dermal transfer from one individual to another. In Dmochowski et al.'s study (2011) abdomen-to-abdomen contact with vigorous movement for 15 minutes between treated and untreated partners, with and without clothing, was conducted one hour after application of the gel. The untreated partners not protected by clothing demonstrated detectable plasma concentrations of oxybutynin (mean $C_{max}$ of 0.94 ng/mL). Although two of 14 untreated subjects who participated in the clothing-to-skin contact regimen had measurable oxybutynin plasma concentrations ($C_{max} \leq 0.1$ ng/mL) over the 48 hours following contact with treated subjects, oxybutynin was not detectable in the plasma of the remaining 12 untreated subjects.

The efficacy and safety of a 3% oxybutynin topical gel in patients with urgency, and/or mixed urinary incontinence, was recently reported (Goldfischer at al., 2015). Treatment was well tolerated and effective.

Other investigational systems involving the transdermal delivery of oxybutynin include a bioadhesive film comprised of polyvinyl alcohol, a methacrylate and sorbitol as a plasticiser (Nicoli et al., 2006), metered dose spray formulations (Bakshi et al., 2008), and solvent systems including octyl salicylate and propylene glycol (Santos et al., 2010).

### 1.4.3 ATTENTION-DEFICIT HYPERACTIVITY DISORDER TREATMENT WITH TRANSDERMAL METHYLPHENIDATE

Methylphenidate (α-phenyl-2-piperidineacetic acid methyl ester, Figure 1.2) is a mild central nervous system stimulant used in the treatment of attention-deficit disorder (ADD) and attention-deficit hyperactivity disorder (ADHD) in children and adults (Ghuman et al., 2008; Wilens et al., 2011). The active agent exists both in a free base form and in an ionized form (most commonly as the hydrochloride). Methylphenidate hydrochloride and methylphenidate base have two stereogenic carbon atoms, which give rise to four stereoisomers. The four stereoisomers consist of two pairs of enantiomers, *d*- and *l*-threo-methylphenidate and *d*- and *l*-erythro-methylphenidate (Patrick et al., 1987). The most active stereoisomer is *d*-threo-methylphenidate and it is responsible for the therapeutic action of the drug. Methylphenidate is metabolized primarily by deesterification to ritalinic acid, which is pharmacologically inactive.

Several orally administered methylphenidate products are approved for the treatment of ADD and ADHD. These products include immediate-release and sustained-release methylphenidate tablets. Both of these products contain racemic threo-methylphenidate hydrochloride (i.e., a 1:1 mixture of $d$-threo-methyl-phenidate hydrochloride and $l$-threo-methylphenidate hydrochloride). Immediate-release methylphenidate is available in 5, 10 and 20 mg tablets. Sustained-release methylphenidate is available in 20 mg tablets. An average daily dose of oral methylphenidate of 20–30 mg may be sufficient to obtain therapeutic effect in adults. For children, daily oral doses in the range of 10–60 mg are appropriate for therapeutic effect, the exact optimal dose being determined by titration.

Methylphenidate undergoes extensive gut wall and hepatic first-pass metabolism resulting in low oral bioavailability (Srinivas et al., 1993). This observation, coupled with its attractive physicochemical properties (Table 1.2), suggested that the compound could be a suitable candidate for transdermal delivery (Singh et al., 1999). A passive transdermal system was subsequently developed by Noven and licensed to Shire Pharmaceuticals and was approved in the USA for the treatment of ADHD in children aged 6 to 12 years in 2006. FDA approval was further extended to the treatment of adolescents aged 13 to 17 years in 2009. The patch was temporarily recalled in 2009 following problems with removal of the release liner, possibly due to moisture ingress into the packaging system (see Wokovich et al., 2011). The product has been marketed by Noven Therapeutics since October 2010. The patch design is a drug-in-adhesive layer supported on a polyester/ethylene vinyl acetate laminate backing layer and protected by a fluoropolymer-coated polyester release liner. Within the adhesive layer, the methylphenidate is dispersed in acrylic adhesive

---

**TABLE 1.2**

**Physicochemical Characteristics and Estimated Maximum Fluxes of Selected Transdermal Drugs**

| Drug | MW | logP | Perm Coeff $k_p$* (cm/h x10³) | Aqueous Solubility (mg/mL) | Estimated Max Flux** (µg/cm²/h) |
|---|---|---|---|---|---|
| Scopolamine | 303 | 0.98 | 0.13 | - | - |
| Clonidine | 230 | 1.85 | 1.47 | 0.8 | 1.18 |
| Estradiol | 272 | 4.01 | 27.8 | 0.0036 | 0.10 |
| Fentanyl | 337 | 4.05 | 11.9 | 0.20 | 2.38 |
| Testosterone | 288 | 3.32 | 7.18 | 0.023 | 0.17 |
| Oxybutynin | 357 | 3.96 | 7.77 | 0.024 | 0.17 |
| Methylphenidate | 233 | 2.78 | 6.50 | 1.26 | 8.19 |
| Selegiline | 187 | 2.64 | 9.77 | 1.72 | 16.8 |
| Rivastigmine | 250 | 2.24 | 2.10 | 2.91 | 6.11 |
| Rotigotine | 315 | 5.39 | 145 | 0.01 | 1.45 |
| Granisetron | 312 | 3.00 | 3.04 | 0.028 | 0.085 |
| Buprenorphine | 468 | 4.90 | 7.59 | 0.0007 | 0.005 |

*Notes*: * All $k_p$'s calculated from Potts and Guy equation (Potts and Guy, 1992). ** Maximum flux calculated from predicted $k_p$ and aqueous solubilities (solubilities and logPs obtained from www.chemspider.com using EPISuite).

and this is dispersed in a silicone adhesive. Different dose levels are afforded by different patch sizes.

The methylphenidate patch (Daytrana) is available in patch strengths of 10, 15, 20 and 30 mg, representing the nominal dose delivered over a nine-hour wear time. It is recommended that the patch be applied to the hip area. In a study designed to determine the effect of skin site on methylphenidate absorption, González and colleagues applied patches, in an open-label, single-dose, randomized two-way crossover study, to either the hip area or the scapular region of pediatric subjects, and found that there was approximately 31% higher bioavailability following hip application (González et al., 2009). Several clinical studies have confirmed the value of transdermal delivery of methylphenidate as a therapy for patients with ADHD (Pelham et al., 2005a,b; Pierce et al., 2008). Although there have been reports of local adverse reactions, including irritant contact dermatitis, these are normally mild and easily overcome using simple strategies such as application site rotation and application of topical hydrocortisone following patch removal (Warshaw et al., 2008; 2010). More severe skin reactions are rare. Overall, transdermal therapy of ADHD offers several advantages over oral therapy including the fact that clinicians and parents/patients can determine the optimal clinical dose by controlling two variables, patch size and duration of patch wear (Arnold et al., 2007). However, a systematic monitoring of the safety of long-term therapy of ADHD in children has been suggested (Clavenna and Bonati, 2014), especially with the increased propensity for leukoderma following transdermal ADHD therapy (Cheng et al., 2017).

### 1.4.4 TRANSDERMAL THERAPY IN THE TREATMENT OF DEPRESSION

Selegilene (Figure 1.5) is a selective irreversible inhibitor of monoamine oxidases A and B and is used for the treatment of early-stage Parkinson's disease, depression and senile dementia. Although selegiline has a higher affinity for MAO-B, at antidepressant doses it inhibits both isoenzymes. The mechanism of antidepressant action is not fully understood but may be linked to enhancement of neurotransmitter activity (Wimbiscus et al., 2010; Magyar, 2011). Following oral administration, selegiline hydrochloride undergoes significant first-pass metabolism leading to a low and highly variable oral bioavailability (Barrett et al., 1996b), the active metabolites being amphetamine, methamphetamine and desmethylselegiline. The use of selegiline, orally, as an adjunct to L-DOPA in Parkinson's disease is limited by dietary restrictions because of the potential for hypertensive crises following the ingestion of foodstuffs containing high levels of tyramine. The dose regimen of 5 mg twice a day is defined by this limitation. Therefore, the higher doses of selegiline required for the treatment of depression via the inhibition of MAO-A precluded oral administration. The reduced level of presystemic metabolism of selegiline afforded by transdermal delivery suggested that this route could be beneficial and recent evidence indicates that brain MAO-A can be inhibited by delivery routes that avoid first-pass metabolism (Fowler et al., 2015).

The low molecular weight of selegiline (187.28) and its measured logP of 2.90 provided some level of comfort that transdermal delivery would be a viable alternative delivery route for the compound. Rohatagi and colleagues (Rohatagi et al., 1997) evaluated the absorption of selegiline through the skin of various species, including humans, using in vitro technology. Their results showed that penetration of selegiline through rat skin and hairless mouse skin was two-fold and three-fold higher than through human skin, respectively. The study also concluded that metabolism was negligible in human skin and that the cumulative 24 hours in vitro permeation from a drug-in-adhesive transdermal system containing 1.83 mg/cm$^2$ selegiline through human skin was 5.0 mg.

In an open-label crossover study the safety and pharmacokinetics of transdermal selegiline and oral selegiline hydrochloride were compared in elderly subjects (Barrett et al., 1996a). Plasma concentrations of selegiline and its metabolites were measured. Peak plasma levels of 1.19 ng/mL selegiline, 23.22 ng/mL N-desmethylselegiline, 4.78 ng/mL L-amphetamine and 14.08 ng/mL L-methamphetamine were observed following a single 10 mg oral dose, compared to peak plasma levels of 2.10 ng/mL selegiline, 0.85 ng/mL N-desmethylselegiline, 1.06 ng/mL L-amphetamine and 2.71 ng/mL L-methamphetamine after a single application of one transdermal system delivering 6.3 mg per 24 h. A comparison of dose-corrected AUCs suggested that selegiline exposure following transdermal application was > 50-fold greater than that obtained orally. Following application of the transdermal system there was a low level of dermal irritation as assessed by erythema and edema rating scales that were similar to the control arm.

Bodkin and Amsterdam (2002) randomly assigned 177 adult outpatients with major depressive disorder to receive transdermal selegiline (20 mg patch applied once daily) or placebo for six weeks. Diet was restricted to reduce the level of intake of tyramine. Greater improvement was observed after six weeks in patients treated with transdermal selegiline than in those given placebo. There were no differences in adverse events for the patients given selegiline and those given placebo, although application site reactions were more common with the selegiline transdermal system. Importantly, the side effects commonly seen with traditional monoamine oxidase inhibitor antidepressants were not observed. This was followed by a double-blind study that included younger patients with no dietary restrictions (Amsterdam, 2003). In this study, 289 patients (18 to 65 years old) were randomly assigned to receive either a 20 mg patch daily or placebo for up to eight weeks. The results demonstrated that transdermal selegiline had a statistically significant but modest antidepressant effect compared with placebo in the absence of a tyramine-restricted diet. Once again side effects were similar for treatment and placebo groups, with the exception of application site reaction, which was observed in 31.5% of treatment patients and 15.1% of placebo-treated patients.

The efficacy, safety and tolerability of the selegiline transdermal system was determined over a dose range of 6 mg/24 h to 12 mg/24 h in the treatment of major depressive disorder (Feiger et al., 2006). Patients were randomly assigned to blinded treatment with the active or placebo patch for eight weeks, with assessments at weeks 1, 2, 3, 5, 6 and 8. There was significantly greater improvement with the active patch compared to placebo. As in previous trials, the most prominent side effects were application site reactions and insomnia. Amsterdam and Bodkin (2006) presented data from a long-term study that assessed the safety and efficacy of initial and continuation selegiline transdermal therapy (6 mg/24 h) in patients with major depressive disorder.

After ten weeks of treatment, patients were randomly assigned to double-blind treatment with transdermal selegiline (6 mg/24 h) or placebo for a year. At the end of the study, significantly fewer treatment patients experienced relapse (16.8%) compared with placebo (30.7%). The early clinical studies on the use of transdermal selegiline in major depressive disorder were reviewed by Culpepper and Kovalick (2008).

In February 2006 the FDA approved the use of transdermal selegiline for the treatment of major depression (Emsam® Patch, manufactured by Mylan for Somerset Pharmaceuticals Inc). The patch is a drug in acrylic adhesive matrix that is supported on an occlusive backing membrane and protected by a silicone-coated release liner. The patch is available in different sizes (20 cm², 30 cm² and 40 cm²) but all contain 1 mg/cm² selegiline and deliver 0.3 mg/cm² selegiline over 24 hours (6 mg, 9 mg or 12 mg per 24 h). Relatively constant plasma levels of selegiline are achieved (Figure 1.7).

Between April 2006 and October 2010, a total of 3,155 adverse events in 1,516 patients were reported (Pae et al., 2012). This represented 5.2% of the total exposures and was independent of causality. The most frequently reported adverse events were application site reactions and insomnia. There were no confirmed reports of hypertensive crisis with food at any selegiline dose level. To date, transdermal selegiline is the only FDA-approved antidepressant for patients with significant problems ingesting, tolerating or absorbing oral medications. Furthermore, it remains the only MAOI (monoamine oxidase inhibitor) that can be initiated at a therapeutic dose without dietary restrictions and has a low incidence of side effects when compared to other MAOIs (Bied et al., 2015; Cristancho and Thase, 2016).

Although there are indications that oral selegiline may prove beneficial as an aid to smoking cessation when combined with transdermal nicotine (Biberman et al., 2003), studies with transdermal selegiline have suggested that this form of therapy is of little use for this indication (Kahn et al., 2012; Killen et al., 2010).

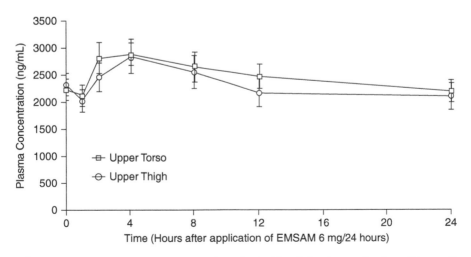

**FIGURE 1.7** Average plasma concentration of selegiline following application of Emsam® (6 mg/24 h) to healthy volunteers. (From Emsam® Prescription Notes.)

Alternative transdermal delivery systems for selegiline have been reported. Fang and colleagues (Fang et al., 2009) attempted to design a transdermal system using a hydrogel-based drug reservoir and a rate-controlling polyethylene membrane (Solupor). The skin permeation of the R- and S-forms of selegiline across pig skin in vitro was determined. R-selegiline gave a flux of 1.13 µg/cm²/h across porcine skin. There was an approximate two-fold reduction in the drug flux across the skin when Solupor was used as a rate-limiting membrane. The flux of R-selegiline from cellulose hydrogels was similar to that from an aqueous solution. There was equal absorption of R- and S-selegiline in the presence of the membrane and/or the hydrogel. The same group (Chen et al., 2011) evaluated a transdermal system for selegiline based on thermosensitive hydrogels. Copolymers of alginate and poloxamer (Pluronic F127) were used, either as physical blends or chemical grafting. Although the chemically grafted thermogels appeared to produce sustained selegiline release, they rapidly degraded whereas the physically mixed gels were relatively stable.

### 1.4.5 TRANSDERMAL RIVASTIGMINE IN THE TREATMENT OF ALZHEIMER'S DISEASE

Cholinesterase inhibitors are used for the treatment of mild to moderate Alzheimer's disease, where they act to delay the onset of more serious symptoms. Rivastimine (Figure 1.8) is an extremely potent drug that demonstrates inhibition of both butyrylcholinesterase and acetylcholinesterase. It has significant benefits on the cognitive, functional and behavioral problems that are symptomatic of the dementia associated with both Alzheimer's and Parkinson's diseases. The main side effects of oral rivastigmine are nausea and vomiting. Rivastigmine has a molecular weight of 250.3 and an estimated logP (ACD) of 2.055. Although rivastigmine is almost completely absorbed following oral administration, extensive first-pass metabolism reduces bioavailability to about 35% (Polinsky, 1998). Tse and Laplanche (1998)

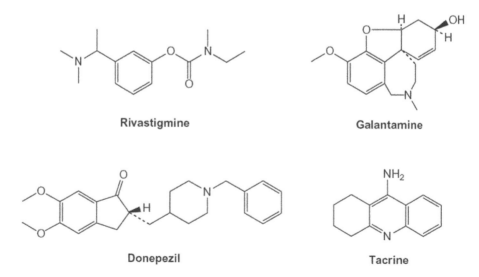

FIGURE 1.8 Anticholinesterase drugs used in Alzheimer's disease.

determined the pharmacokinetics of rivastigmine following oral, intravenous and dermal administration in minipigs. Dermal administration was via application of either one or three patches, each containing 18 mg rivastigmine, which were applied for 24 hours whereas the oral dose was 1 mg/kg, administered via gastric intubation. The dermal dose of either 18 mg or 54 mg was administered twice with a ten-day interval between doses, during which time placebo patches were placed on the application site. There was a very high level of first-pass metabolism following the oral dose resulting in a very low bioavailability of the parent drug (approximately 0.5%). Following the first transdermal dose, approximately 8% of the applied drug at both dose levels was absorbed. Following the second dose the absorption rate for both dose levels was increased about two-fold and the authors attributed this increase to hydration or abrasion of the application site.

The pharmacokinetics of transdermal rivastigmine was evaluated in a study that also determined patch adhesiveness following application to the upper back, chest, abdomen, thigh and upper arm (Lefèvre et al., 2007). This single-dose, open-label, crossover study in 40 healthy subjects used a 10 $cm^2$ patch containing 18 mg rivastigmine that was applied to each body site. Exposure levels and $C_{max}$ were highest at the upper back, chest and upper arm sites. Although adhesiveness varied with application site, there were no statistically significant correlations with pharmacokinetic parameters, except at the chest. The authors concluded that the pharmacokinetic profiles and adhesiveness, together with low rates of erythema at the upper back, chest and upper arm, indicated their suitability for clinical use. The same group subsequently demonstrated that the 10 $cm^2$ patch containing 18 mg rivastigmine was comparable in terms of average drug exposure to the highest capsule dose of 12 mg/day in patients with Alzheimer's disease (Lefèvre et al., 2008).

The efficacy, safety and tolerability of various dosage levels of the rivastigmine patch compared to oral dosage were evaluated in a 24-week, double-blind, double-dummy, placebo- and active-controlled trial, patients with Alzheimer's disease (Winblad et al., 2007). Therapeutic outcomes were similar between the 9.5 mg rivastigmine/24 h transdermal patch and oral dosage routes. However, adverse events such as nausea and vomiting were less frequent in the 10 $cm^2$ patch group compared to the capsule groups. A further analysis of the therapeutic outcome data from this study indicated that rivastigmine patch doses higher than 9.5 mg/24 h could offer additional benefits and suggested that the 13.3 mg/24 h patch was worthy of further investigation (Grossberg et al., 2011), a finding that was confirmed in later studies (Cummings et al., 2012; Grossberg et al., 2015). In the Cummings et al. study moderate or severe skin irritation occurred in less than 10% of patients across the four patch sizes that were evaluated (5, 10, 15 and 20 $cm^2$). This 24-week blinded trial was followed by a 28-week open-label extension. During both phases of this trial the condition of the patients' skin at the application site was evaluated (Cummings et al., 2010). In the first stage of the study 89.6% of patients in the target 10 $cm^2$ patch group (delivering 9.5 mg rivastigmine per 24 hours) recorded "no, slight or mild" skin reactions as their most severe application site reaction, erythema and pruritus being the most commonly reported reactions. During the following 28-week open-label study, the skin tolerability profile was similar to that seen in the double-blind phase. In Grossberg's later study (Grossberg et al., 2015), a 24-week randomized parallel-group double-blind investigation in patients with severe Alzheimer's disease, significant efficacy was observed with the 13.3 mg/24 h rivastigmine group compared to the 4.6 mg/24 h group.

Application site reactions occur in about 60% of patients following rivastigmine patch wear (Osada et al., 2018). The diagnosis and management of irritant contact dermatitis and allergic contact dermatitis secondary to transdermal rivastigmine have been reported (Greenspoon et al., 2011). Many of the reported reactions are of an irritant type and can be managed by patch application site rotation and emollient use. Allergic reactions can be managed using corticosteroids.

The rivastigmine patch (Exelon® Patch, Novartis) was approved for marketing by the FDA in June 2007, and is indicated for the treatment of mild to moderate dementia that is associated with Alzheimer's disease and Parkinson's disease. The patch is available in three sizes: 5 cm², containing 9 mg rivastigmine that delivers a nominal doses of 4.6 mg/24 h; a 10 cm² patch (containing 18 mg drug) nominally delivers 9.5 mg/24 h; and a 15 cm² patch (containing 27 mg drug) nominally delivers 13.3 mg/24 h (Figure 1.9). Each patch is replaced every 24 hours. Approximately 50% of the drug loading in the patch is released over the 24-hour wear period. The patch is made up of four layers: a backing layer that supports the drug-containing poly(butylmethacrylate, methylmethacrylate) matrix. The drug-containing layer is overlaid with a silicone adhesive that is protected by a release liner. Other excipients within the patch are silicone oil and vitamin E.

An alternative cholinesterase inhibitor that has been considered for transdermal delivery in Alzheimer's patients is donepezil (Figure 1.8, Table 1.3) (Choi et al., 2012; Sozio et al., 2012; Saluja et al., 2013; Galipoglu et al., 2015; Madan et al., 2015). With a maximum dose of 10 mg/day, a molecular weight of 380 and an estimated (EPISuite) logP of 4.86, donezipil is certainly a feasible candidate for

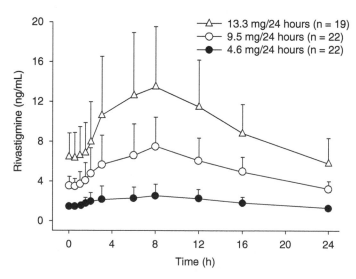

**FIGURE 1.9** Average plasma concentration of rivastigmine following application of different dose levels of the Exelon® patch to healthy volunteers. (From Exelon® Prescription Notes.)

**TABLE 1.3**
**Physicochemical Characteristics and Estimated Maximum Fluxes of Selected Transdermal Candidate Drugs**

| Drug | MW | logP | Perm Coeff $k_p$* (cm/h x10³) | Aqueous Solubility (mg/mL) | Estimated Max Flux** (µg/cm²/h) |
|---|---|---|---|---|---|
| Alprazolam | 308 | 3.87 | 13.3 | 0.013 | 0.018 |
| Apomine | 626 | 3.05 | - | - | - |
| Cannabidiol | 314 | 6.99 | - | - | - |
| Citalopram | 324 | 3.74 | 8.62 | 0.031 | 0.267 |
| Donepezil | 380 | 4.86 | 24.49 | 0.0005 | 0.012 |
| Doxazosin | 451 | 2.09 | .098 | 0.024 | 0.002 |
| Endoxifen | 374 | 5.61 | 90.78 | 0.003 | 0.272 |
| Finasteride | 373 | 3.20 | 1.79 | 0.012 | 0.021 |
| Fluoxetine | 309 | 4.65 | 47.09 | 0.038 | 1.79 |
| Huperzine A | 242 | 1.54 | 0.75 | 1.26 | 0.945 |
| Ketorolac | 376 | 2.45 | - | - | - |
| Lacidipine | 456 | 5.39 | 20.02 | 0.0005 | 0.010 |
| Letrozole | 285 | 2.22 | 1.24 | 0.103 | 0.127 |
| Levodopa | 197 | -2.24 | 0.003 | 320 | 0.0960 |
| Nortriptyline | 263 | 4.74 | 104.1 | 0.002 | 0.208 |
| Propranolol | 259 | 2.60 | 3.33 | 0.228 | 0.759 |
| Rasagiline | 171 | 2.60 | 11.5 | 3.73 | 42.9 |
| Sulfadiazine | 250 | -0.34 | 0.031 | 28.1 | 0.871 |
| Tolterodine | 326 | 5.73 | 216.8 | 0.004 | 0.862 |
| Vinpocetine | 351 | 4.30 | 14.73 | 0.013 | 0.191 |

*Notes*: * All $k_p$'s calculated from Potts and Guy equation (Potts and Guy, 1992). ** Maximum flux calculated from predicted $k_p$ and aqueous solubilities (solubilities and logPs obtained from www.chemspider.com using EPISuite).

the transdermal route. Kim et al. (2015) evaluated the single dose tolerability and pharmacokinetics of patches containing 43.75 mg, 87.5 mg or 175 mg donepezil in healthy volunteers. The patches were designed for three-day application periods. Sustained dose-dependent plasma concentrations were achieved over the wear period with $C_{max}$ varying between 5.24 ng/mL to 20.36 ng/mL for the low and high dose patches, respectively. Skin reactions were mild and the patches were well tolerated. This initial study confirmed the potential of transdermal donepezil as a candidate for the treatment of Alzheimer's disease.

### 1.4.6 ROTIGOTINE IN PARKINSON'S DISEASE

Rotigotine (Figure 1.10, Table 1.2) is a very potent and selective non-ergolinic dopamine D2 agonist that was first identified as a potential transdermal candidate drug in 1989. In their experiments on dopamine release in a rat's brain, Timmerman et al. (1989) noted that transdermal application induced a much longer duration of action of the drug (13 hours) compared to the oral route of delivery

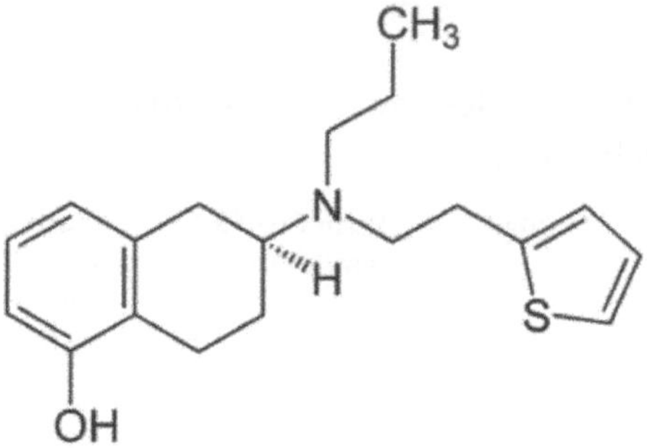

A) Rotigotine

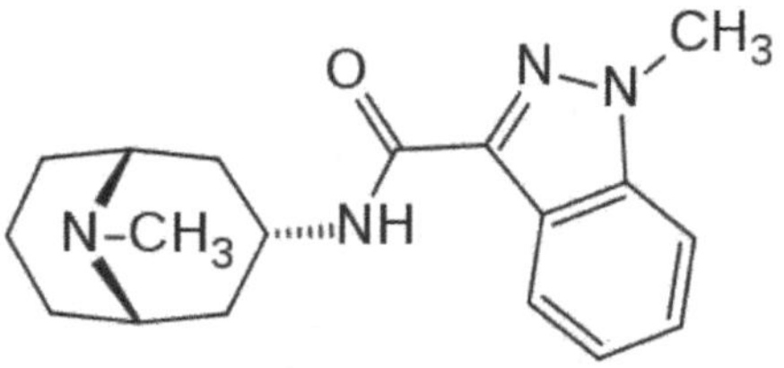

B) Graniterton

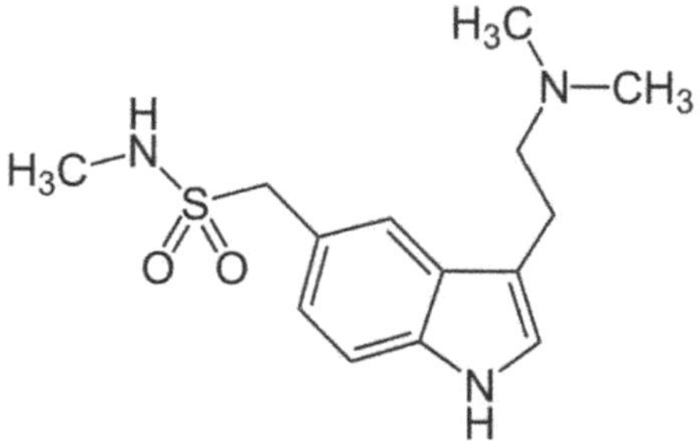

C) Sumatriptan

**FIGURE 1.10** Chemical structures of rotigotine, granisetron and sumatriptan. For physicochemical data see Table 1.2.

(five hours). This was confirmed by Löschmann et al. (1989), who determined that dermal application produced reversal of induced parkinsonism in the marmoset. Following oral delivery rotigotine is extensively metabolized in the gastrointestinal tract (Swart and De Zeeuw, 1992) and is presently only available for delivery by the transdermal route. Cawello et al. (2007) determined the mass balance of rotigotine in humans following administration of a silicone-based transdermal patch containing $^{14}$C-labeled rotigotine and quantified the pharmacokinetic profiles of total radioactivity and the corresponding rotigotine plasma concentrations. The patch was applied for 24 hours and contained 4.485 mg of unlabeled and 0.015 mg of $^{14}$C-labeled rotigotine. Radioactivity was monitored in unused patches, used patches, skin wash samples, plasma, urine and feces for 96 hours. Stratum corneum strip samples were taken at 96 hours post-application. A total of 94.6% of the administered dose was recovered within 96 hours after patch application. Over 24 hours, 46.1% of the total radioactivity was systemically absorbed. Total radioactivity recovered in urine and feces was approximately 40.3% of that applied, indicating that the majority of absorbed drug was cleared within 96 hours of application. Pharmacokinetic analysis from several clinical trials indicated that rotigotine exposure increased proportionally in the dose range of 2 mg/24 h to 8 mg/24 h; plasma concentrations at steady state were stable over the 24-hour wear period (Figure 1.11) and that bioavailability was variable depending on patch application site (hip, shoulder, abdomen, flank, thigh, upper arm); the respective mean ratios for AUC ranged between 0.87 (abdomen vs flank) and 1.46 (shoulder vs thigh) (Elshoff et al., 2012). Furthermore, there were no pharmacokinetic issues associated with renal insufficiency (Cawello et al., 2012).

A phase II clinical trial evaluated the effectiveness of various doses of transdermal rotigotine at replacing levodopa (Hutton et al., 2001). In this trial, 85 Parkinson's disease patients were randomized to placebo or one of four doses of rotigotine for 21 days. Significantly greater reductions in levodopa dose were achieved compared to placebo for the two highest doses of rotigotine. The transdermal system was found to be safe and well tolerated. In a later clinical study the safety and efficacy of rotigotine in patients with early-stage Parkinson's disease was evaluated. In the open-label study, 31 patients in the early stages of Parkinson's disease received rotigotine

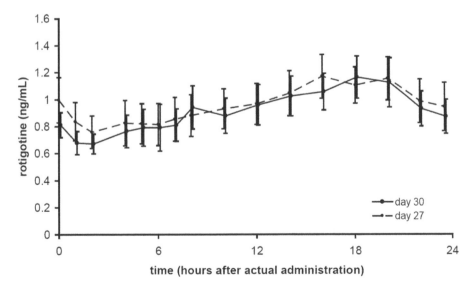

**FIGURE 1.11** Average (±95% CI) plasma concentrations of rotigotine in patients with early-stage Parkinson's disease following application of 8 mg/24 h on two different days during the maintenance phase. (From Neupro® Prescription Information.)

up to a maximum of 18.0 mg/day. Significant improvements were seen for patients achieving the maximum dose. Overall, the data suggest that rotigotine is safe, well tolerated and effective treatment for early-stage Parkinson's disease (Güldenpfennig et al., 2005). These data were confirmed in multicenter, randomized, double-blind studies (Watts et al., 2007; Jankovic et al., 2007), where it was concluded that transdermal rotigotine, titrated to a dosage of 6 mg/day, was effective for the treatment of early-stage Parkinson's disease. The long-term effectiveness and safety of the rotigotine patch has been established (Lewitt et al., 2013; Giladi et al., 2013). The most common side effects were somnolence (18–25%), application site reactions (12–15%) and nausea (9%).

Many patients with Parkinson's disease suffer gastrointestinal disturbances and dysphagia when the symptoms are treated with oral medication. Recent studies have indicated that such gastrointestinal symptoms can be improved by switching from oral medication to transdermal therapy (Hirano et al., 2015; Woitalla et al., 2015).

Transdermal rotigotine has also been evaluated for efficacy in restless leg syndrome (Stiasny-Kolster et al., 2004; Hening et al., 2010; Högl et al., 2010; Trenkwalder et al., 2015). Rotigotine transdermal patches that released 2–3 mg/24 h were found to significantly reduce the severity of restless leg symptoms, and follow-up studies demonstrated sustained efficacy for patients with moderate-to-severe restless legs syndrome for up to five years (Oertel et al., 2011). The pharmacological and pharmacokinetic properties of the rotigotine transdermal system in both Parkinson's disease and restless leg syndrome have recently been comprehensively reviewed by Elshoff and colleagues (Elshoff et al., 2015).

The only marketed rotigotine patch (Neupro®, UCB Inc) was approved in the USA in 2007. It is available at six dose levels, nominally delivering from 1 mg to 8 mg/24 h. Dose level is determined by patch size (5 cm²–40 cm²). The patch is a drug-in-adhesive patch composed of a flexible, tan-colored backing membrane, consisting of an aluminized polyester film coated with a pigment-layer on the outer side. The silicone-based adhesive layer contains the active component and the following excipients: ascorbyl palmitate, povidone, sodium metabisulfite and dl-á-tocopherol. The release liner is a fluoropolymer-coated polyester film.

Alternative means of delivering rotigotine across the skin have been evaluated and include entrapment within elastic vesicles (Honeywell-Nguyen et al., 2003), iontophoretic transport (Nugroho et al., 2004; Ackaert et al., 2010) and microemulsion-based hydrogels (Wang et al., 2015). Although all three methods appear promising, no other transdermal system containing rotigotine has been marketed to date.

### 1.4.7 TRANSDERMAL GRANISETRON FOR ANTI-EMESIS DURING CHEMOTHERAPY

Granisetron (Figure 1.10, Table 1.2) is a serotonin 5-HT$_3$ receptor antagonist that is used as an anti-emetic to treat nausea and vomiting during and following chemotherapy. The drug was approved for use in the USA in 1994 and a transdermal system (Sancuso®, ProStrakan Inc) was approved in September 2008. Sancuso® is a drug-in-adhesive matrix patch that contains 34.3 mg granisetron in a 52 cm² patch. The patch nominally delivers 3.1 mg/24 h and is worn for up to seven days. The pharmacokinetics of transdermal granisetron were described by Howell et al. (2009) using data from a phase I study in healthy volunteers and from phase II and III studies (a total of over 800 subjects). Following a 2 mg oral dose, plasma $C_{max}$ was reached two hours after dosing and $C_{ave}$ was 2.6 ng/mL. Following application of a 52 cm² patch plasma $C_{ave}$ was 2.2 ng/mL over six days. Clearance was not affected by age, gender, weight or renal function.

In a double-blind phase III study, the efficacy and tolerability of the granisetron transdermal system was compared to daily oral granisetron for the control of chemotherapy-induced nausea and vomiting. It was concluded that the transdermal system offered an alternative route for delivering granisetron for up to seven days that is was as effective as oral granisetron (Boccia et al., 2011).

The granisetron transdermal patch was found to be moderately effective in alleviating the refractory symptoms of gastroparesis – delayed stomach emptying (Simmons and Parkman, 2014).

Another $5\text{-}HT_3$ receptor antagonist that may be useful as a transdermal anti-emetic to treat nausea and vomiting during and following chemotherapy is ondansetron. Patel and colleagues (2015) evaluated the in vitro and in vivo skin permeation rates of ondansetron from a gel formulation. While permeation of ondansetron through pig skin from a base gel was low, the addition of isopropyl myristate or camphor improved delivery. Microporation further enhanced transdermal delivery. Permeation through human skin from these gels remains to be determined.

### 1.4.8 TRANSDERMAL OPIOIDS FOR PAIN RELIEF

The ability of the opioid fentanyl (Figure 1.12, Table 1.2) to cross the skin was recognized in the mid-1970s (Michaels et al., 1975) and subsequently measured and reported by Sebel et al. in 1987. A transdermal fentanyl product was approved in the USA in 1990 and has been widely and successfully used for pain relief (Skaer, 2014). The first fentanyl patch comprised a reservoir design where drug delivery was limited by a rate controlling membrane that was placed between the reservoir and the skin (Durogesic®, Janssen). Although a reservoir patch is still available, more recent fentanyl patch products have been of the drug-in-adhesive matrix design (Table 1.4) and the redesigned products have been shown to be bioequivalent to the original reservoir patch (Marier et al., 2006; Hair et al., 2008; Moore et al., 2011) and to each other (Kress et al., 2010). Recently, the development and evaluation of a tamper resistant fentanyl patch has been described (Cai et al., 2015). In this patch, fentanyl loaded geopolymeric granules are incorporated into an adhesive layer.

Fentanyl transdermal patches are designed to deliver the drug across the skin over a 72-hour period (Figure 1.13). The Duragesic® patch is available in five dose levels (graded by patch area) ranging in nominal hourly dose levels of 12.5 µg/h to 100 µg/h, the largest patch being 42 cm².

Chronic pain and hyperalgesia may sometimes be difficult to treat with classical opioids, such as fentanyl, that act predominately at the µ-opioid receptor. On the other hand, buprenorphine (Figure 1.12, Table 1.2) and its active metabolite are

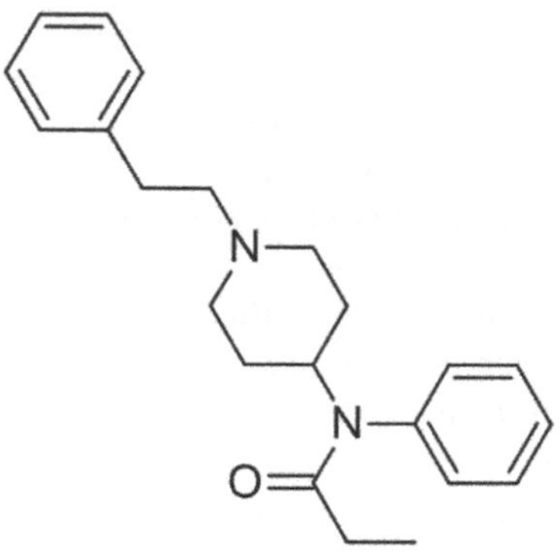

A) Fentanyl

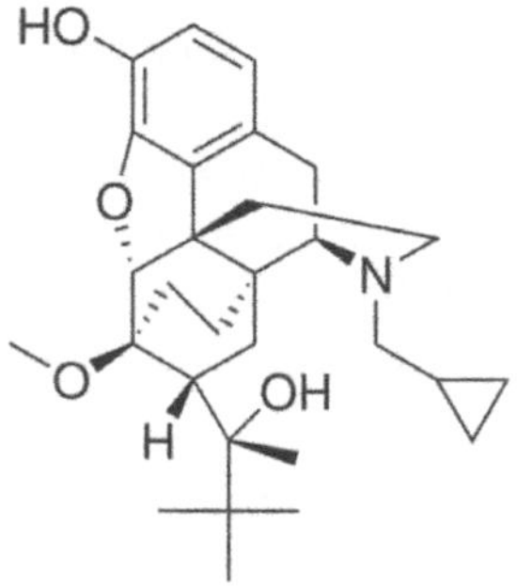

B) Buprenorphine

**FIGURE 1.12** Chemical structures of fentanyl and buprenorphine. For physicochemical data see Table 1.2.

**TABLE 1.4**
**Examples of Marketed Transdermal Fentanyl Patches**

| Product Name | Available Dosage (µg/h) | Patch Design |
|---|---|---|
| Durogesic DTRANS® | 12/25/50/75/100 | Matrix |
| Fencino® | 25/50/75/100 | Matrix |
| Fentalis® | 25/50/75/100 | Reservoir |
| Matrifen® | 12/25/50/75/100 | Matrix/RCM |
| Tilofyl® | 25/50/75/100 | Matrix |

*Source*: Lane, 2013a

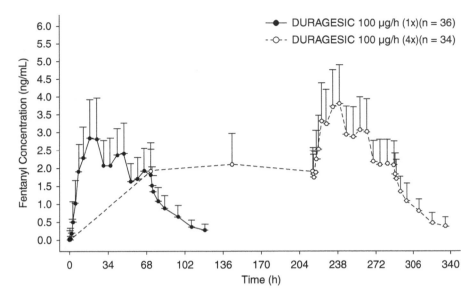

**FIGURE 1.13**  Fentanyl serum concentrations following single and multiple applications of Duragesic® 100 µg/h. (From Duragesic® Prescribing Information.)

thought to act through $\mu$-, $\kappa$- and $\delta$-receptors and may possess different analgesic and anti-hyperalgesic effects compared with pure $\mu$-receptor agonists (Andresen et al., 2011). Buprenorphine was first launched in the clinic in 1979. The ability of buprenorphine to cross the skin was evaluated by Roy and colleagues (Roy et al., 1994) who concluded that their in vitro data suggested that transdermal delivery of buprenorphine was sufficient to achieve systemic analgesic effect. Investigations of the permeations 3-alkyl-ester prodrugs of buprenorphine through human skin in vitro showed that they were completely hydrolyzed on passing through the skin yielding the parent compound, but also demonstrated that buprenorphine flux through skin from a prodrug solution did not exceed the flux of buprenorphine base itself (Stinchcomb et al., 1996). A transdermal version of buprenorphine was approved for marketing in Europe and has been available since 2001 (Transtec®, Grunenthal; delivering 35, 52.5 and 70 µg/h over 96h). The product Butrans® (Purdue Pharma) was approved by the FDA in June 2010 and launched in the USA in early 2011. Butrans® patches are designed to deliver 5, 10 or 20 µg/h buprenorphine over seven days and are drug-in-adhesive matrix design. The inactive ingredients in Butrans® are levulinic acid, oleyl oleate, povidone and a polyacrylate cross-liked with aluminum. Transdermal buprenorphine is prescribed for chronic non-cancer and cancer pain treatment.

The clinical effectiveness of transdermal buprenorphine over 72 hours was evaluated in 445 patients with chronic malignant or non-malignant pain requiring long-term treatment with potent opioid analgesics. Patients were treated with either systems delivering 35, 52.5 or 70 µg/h active or with placebo in a randomized double-blind setting. More effective pain relief was reported in patients treated with buprenorphine over those treated with placebo. In an open follow-up study 239 patients continued treatment with transdermal buprenorphine. The author concluded that the clinical benefit, high level of patient compliance and improved quality of life confirmed the usefulness of transdermal buprenorphine (Böhme, 2002). Similarly, in a population of 157 patients, transdermal buprenorphine (35.0, 52.5 or 70.0 µg/h) was shown to be an effective analgesic against chronic, severe pain at all dose levels. Patients treated with buprenorphine experienced a 56.7% reduction in use of sublingual rescue analgesic during the study compared with an 8% reduction with the placebo patch (Sittl et al., 2003).

In a post-marketing surveillance study, effectiveness and safety data on the use of transdermal buprenorphine (Transtec®) under routine clinical conditions was evaluated in a total of 13,179 patients (3,690 with cancer pain and 9,489 with non-cancer pain). In the majority of patients, the initial dose of 35 µg/h only needed to be increased in about 18% of subjects. Transdermal buprenorphine was found to provide effective, sustained and dose-dependent analgesia in patients regardless of their age or pain syndromes. Fewer than 5% of patients discontinued treatment because of unsatisfactory pain relief. The tolerability profile was as expected for an opioid and there was no clinically relevant development of tolerance (Griessinger et al., 2005). Treatment was generally well tolerated (Likar et al., 2006) and, provided patients were assessed on an individual basis, cognitive and psychomotor performance appeared relatively normal following long-term use of transdermal buprenorphine (Dagtekin et al., 2007). Further evaluations have confirmed the suitability and effectiveness of the 72 h transdermal buprenorphine patch for the control of pain (Deandrea et al., 2009; Hans and Robert, 2009; Pergolizzi et al., 2009; Skaer, 2014; Kitzmiller et al., 2015).

Buprenorphine lower-dose (Butrans®, 5, 10 and 20 µg/h) transdermal patches, administered once every seven days, are indicated in the management of chronic non-malignant pain. In a pivotal phase III study that assessed the new seven-day transdermal treatment for use in the management of chronic low back pain, patients who tolerated and responded to transdermal buprenorphine (10 or 20 µg/h) during an open-label run-in period were randomized to continue active treatment or receive matching placebo. Patients receiving buprenorphine reported statistically significantly lower pain scores following a 12-week treatment period compared with placebo. The buprenorphine transdermal system was found to be efficacious and generally well tolerated (Steiner et al., 2011).

Pharmacokinetic studies with the seven-day buprenorphine patch have shown that no dosage alterations were required between young and elderly patients (Al-Tawil et al., 2013). Three consecutive once-weekly applications of the 10 µg/h dose level provided consistent and sustained delivery of buprenorphine. Steady-state plasma concentrations were reached within 48 hours of the first application and patch adhesion analysis confirmed the appropriateness of the seven-day application period (Kapil et al., 2013).

Semisolid topical opioid formulations have also been evaluated as potential therapeutic modalities for local pain relief including peripheral inflammation (Smith et al., 2015) and post-herpetic neuralgia (Musazzi et al., 2015). Other modalities for local transdermal pain relief include capsaicin for neuropathic pain and osteoarthritis (Guedes et al., 2018; Tenreiro-Pinto et al., 2018) and tizanidine hydrochloride for the relief of muscle pain, although the latter remains speculative (Shahid et al., 2018). Pain relief via the transdermal and dermal routes has been reviewed by Peptu et al. (2015) and more recently by Leppert and colleagues (Leppert et al., 2018).

### 1.4.9 TRANSDERMAL THERAPY FOR THE TREATMENT OF MIGRAINE

Sumatriptan (Table 1.2) is a synthetic analogue of naturally occurring neuro-active alkaloids such as dimethyltryptamine. It is a potent agonist of the 5-HT receptor and selectively activates types $5\text{-}HT_{1D}$ and $5\text{-}HT_{1B}$ subtypes that are present in cranial arteries (Razzaque et al., 1999). Activation of these receptors results in the vasoconstriction of dilated arteries. Sumatriptan has also been shown to inhibit the release of vasoactive neuropeptides from perivascular trigeminal axons in the dura mater following activation of the trigeminovascular system, which may account for its activity against cluster headaches. A number of double-blind clinical trials demonstrated that orally administered sumatriptan (100 mg) was superior to placebo in the acute treatment of migraine headaches and achieves significantly greater response rates than ergotamine or aspirin (Wilkinson et al., 1995).

In the mid-2000s, several reports on the skin permeation of sumatriptan and the effects of skin penetration enhancement strategies were reported. Pretreatment of porcine skin with ethanol, polyethylene glycol 600, sorbitan monolaurate, oleic acid, and terpenes limonene and 1,8-cineole produced an increase in sumatriptan flux (Femenía-Font et al., 2005a). The authors then went on to compare these results to data obtained using human skin and established that a linear relationship of flux through porcine and human skin although the flux through pig skin was double that through human skin (Femenía-Font et al., 2006a). It was found that a combination of chemical enhancement using 1-dodecyl-azacycloheptan-2-one (Azone, laurocapram) and iontophoresis (Femenía-Font et al., 2005b) was the most effective strategy to enhance transdermal absorption of sumatriptan through human skin in vitro. Further experiments aimed at developing a bioadhesive film containing sumatriptan demonstrated that diethylene glycol monoethyl ether (Transcutol) and 2-pyrrolidone decreased sumatriptan permeation when they were included in a film. Rendering the film occlusive was found to increase skin permeation (Femenía-Font et al., 2006b). This team achieved greater success with a sumatriptan succinate transdermal delivery system comprising (a) methylcellulose and propylene glycol (as a plasticiser), (b) polyvinyl pyrrolidone and sorbitol, and (c) polyvinyl pyrrolidone-polyvinyl alcohol plus sorbitol. All systems contained 5% Azone and methacrylate copolymer was used as an adhesive. The films were applied to an occlusive backing membrane. When evaluated on pig ear skin the methylcellulose film provided the greatest flux and this was further increased by iontophoresis (Balaguer-Fernández et al., 2008).

In 2007 scientists from NuPathe Inc and their collaborators reported on the pharmacokinetics and safety of their prototype novel iontophoretic sumatriptan delivery system (NP101) (Siegel et al., 2007) using a randomized, single-center, single-dose, six-period phase I study design. The study design compared application of patches delivering different currents (0.5 or 1.0 mA) for differing times and was designed to deliver doses ranging from 1.5 mg to 12 mg of sumatriptan over 1.5 h to 6 h with a fast-disintegrating oral tablet (50 mg sumatriptan succinate) and 6 mg subcutaneous injection of sumatriptan succinate. There was a linear relationship between total applied current and sumatriptan delivery. Patches delivering 6 mA and 12 mA per hour demonstrated favorable sumatriptan systemic profiles and maintained plasma levels above the target level ($\geq$ 10 ng/mL) for greater than seven hours. Although there was some erythema over the longer wear period, the patches were generally well tolerated. In a further phase I study, the pharmacokinetic properties of a single dose of sumatriptan delivered using an iontophoretic transdermal patch was compared to oral, injection and nasal delivery (Pierce et al., 2009). In this study, subjects received each of five treatments: sumatriptan 100 mg oral tablets, subcutaneous sumatriptan (6 mg), sumatriptan 20 mg nasal spray, a patch with 3 g of gel solution delivering 6 mg of sumatriptan transdermally (Zelrix I), or a transdermal patch containing 2.6 g of gel solution delivering 6 mg of sumatriptan (Zelrix II). Although $C_{max}$ for the two transdermal systems was approximately 70% less than that following the subcutaneous dose, plasma concentrations for the patches were intermediate between those for the oral and nasal sumatriptan doses, and reached 10 ng/mL within 30 minutes. Skin reactions at the patch site were mild and any erythema resolved in most subjects by 72 hours. The authors concluded that transdermal delivery of sumatriptan using iontophoresis may prove beneficial for many migraine sufferers because of the rapid and consistent delivery of the drug and the avoidance of common gastrointestinal disturbances that are associated with migraine. Over the longer term, the transdermal sumatriptan formulation (NP101) demonstrated tolerability and efficacy with successive uses over 12 months in 183 patients who applied 2,089 patches (Smith et al., 2012; Goldstein et al., 2012).

Following successful phase III trials, which enrolled a total of 800 patients with migraine, a transdermal sumatriptan patch was approved by the FDA in January 2013. The patch (tradename Zecuity®, NuPathe Inc) was approved for the acute treatment of migraine with or without aura in adults. The treatment safely and effectively relieves migraine pain, sonophobia and photophobia within two hours of patch activation. On activation the patch delivers 6.5 mg of sumatriptan through the skin over four hours. Zecuity contains 86 mg sumatriptan (base), as the succinate salt, in an aqueous formulation. The system is composed of an iontophoretic device and a drug reservoir card that contains two non-woven pads and two different gel formulations. The sumatriptan succinate gel formulation contains water, basic butylated methacrylate copolymer (polyamine), lauric acid, adipic acid and methylparaben with a non-woven viscose pad. The salt formulation contains water, hydroxypropylcellulose, sodium chloride and methylparaben with a non-woven viscose pad. The iontophoretic device consists of an adhesive fabric and foam and a plastic dome that contains an activation button, batteries and electronics (Figure 1.14). The use of the sumatriptan patch in patients with acute migraine has been the subject of several recent studies and reviews (Garnock-Jones, 2013; Meadows et al., 2014; Vikelis et al., 2014; Bigal et al., 2015; Vikelis et al., 2015).

However, despite the apparent clinical success of the Zecuity® patch system for the treatment of migraine, the number of adverse events related to scarring and

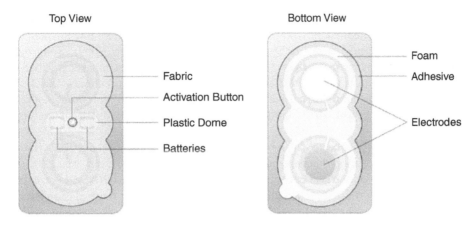

**FIGURE 1.14** The NuPathe Inc sumatriptan iontophoretic patch. (From Zecuity® Prescribing Information.)

burning led to its suspension from the market about ten months following launch (Loder et al., 2018). To date, no further applications to market are known.

Other skin delivery systems for sumatriptan that have been evaluated include elastic liposomes (Balaguer-Fernández et al., 2011), niosomes (González-Rodríguez et al., 2012) and dissolving microneedle arrays (Ronnander et al., 2018).

## 1.4.10 EARLY FEASIBILITY INVESTIGATIONS AND OTHER DEVELOPMENTS

Although there have been several variations, current patch type transdermal delivery systems continue to utilize basic design principles: drug-in-adhesive or drug in reservoir. Other systems include those that utilize small electrical currents (e.g., NuPathe's Zecuity® patch – now withdrawn from the market), sound or pressure waves (Mitragotri, 2013) or atmospheric microplasma irradiation (Shimizu et al., 2015) to increase drug delivery. Other systems completely bypass the stratum corneum by the use of microneedles (Ita, 2015; Quinn et al., 2015; Sharma et al., 2019) or ballistic delivery (Lahm and Lee, 2006; Guha et al., 2010). Research on skin permeability, the feasibility of transdermal drug delivery and the materials used in transdermal systems, however, remains buoyant. The scientific literature regularly publishes reports on new formulations to improve or enhance drug delivery through the skin. These range, for example, from descriptions of experiments on the incorporation of old drugs into new systems, such as formulating propranolol or sulfadiazine into liquid crystal-niosomal or other gel type formulations (Tavano et al., 2013; Zhou et al., 2015), through using silica and other nanoparticles (Nafisi et al., 2015; Zhang et al., 2015) or carbon nanotubes and electrospun fibers to control drug release (Majumder et al., 2010; Im et al., 2010; Schwengber et al., 2015), to using adhesives whose design was inspired from the hairs on the feet of the gecko (Tamelier et al., 2013).

Compounds that have yet to reach the market in transdermal delivery systems but have been evaluated for this route include pirfenidone for the treatment of idiopathic pulmonary fibrosis (Jose et al., 2015); zolmitriptan for migraine (Liu and Fang, 2015); apomine (Kuehl et al., 2009); diflunisal (Sallam et al., 2015); low molecular weight heparin (Lanke et al., 2009); nortriptyline (Melero et al., 2009); isoniazid (Caon et al., 2015); letrozole (Li et al., 2010) and anastrozole (Regenthal et al., 2018) as breast cancer therapies; endoxifen (Mah et al., 2013); deferoxamine (Duscher et al., 2015); an antihypertensive hydrochlorothiazide/carvedivol combination (Agrawal and Aggarwal, 2010) and lacidipine (Gannu et al., 2010); HIV inhibitors (Ham and Buckheit, 2015); galantamine (Park et al., 2012; Woo et al., 2015); the antidepressants fluoxetine and citalopram (Jung et al., 2013; Huang et al., 2013; Jung et al., 2015); the neuroprotectants cannabidiol and vinpocetine (Liput et al., 2013; Mao et al., 2013); levodopa (Lee et al., 2013); metformin (Yu et al., 2018); doxazosin and finasteride as a combination therapy for benign prostatic hyperplasia (Pupe et al., 2013); alprazolam (Soler et al., 2012); the muscle relaxant thiocolchicoside (Bigucci et al., 2015); the antipsychotic risperidone (Siafaka et al., 2015); tolterodine (Liu et al., 2012); and propranolol (Chantasart et al., 2013) (see Table 1.3 for the physicochemical properties of some of these compounds). Surprisingly, in patients with relapsing-remitting multiple sclerosis, treatment with an experimental patch containing a mixture of three myelin peptides (MBP85-99, MOG35-55 and PLP139-155) significantly reduced both magnetic resonance imaging and clinically defined measures of disease activity and was safe and well tolerated (Walczak et al., 2013).

Selective estrogen receptor modulators are used clinically for the prophylaxis and treatment of estrogen receptor positive breast cancer. Recently Güngör and colleagues (Güngör et al., 2013) have evaluated, theoretically and experimentally, the possibility of transdermal delivery of several selective estrogen receptor modulators. The maximum predicted flux of the compounds, which comprised clomiphene, droloxifene, endoxifen, 4-hydroxytamoxifen, tamoxifen and toremifene, was calculated from permeability coefficients derived from the equations developed by Potts and Guy (1992) and Cleek and Bunge (1993) and saturated aqueous solubilities of the compounds. The predicted values were compared to experimentally derived values obtained using porcine skin in vitro (Table 1.5). The authors concluded that there was good agreement between the predicted and the experimental values and that effective local tissue and tumor levels could be achieved from optimal formulations applied to the entire breast surface, with the added benefit of reduced systemic side effects.

Physical skin penetration enhancement technology has been at the forefront of recent research, with iontophoresis gaining renewed vigor following the development of the Zecuity® patch (Wong, 2014). For example, Kalaria and colleagues described the use of constant current anodal iontophoresis to evaluate the feasibility of delivering the acetylcholinesterase inhibitor Huperzine A, a compound that may be useful in Alzheimer's disease, with promising results (Kalaria et al., 2013). The same group had earlier reported similar promising results for rasagiline and selegiline (Kalaria et al., 2012). Djabri and colleagues (Djabri et al., 2012) considered iontophoresis as a means to deliver ranitidine hydrochloride through the skin of pediatric patients and concluded that therapeutic levels were achievable. Similarly, iontophoresis of the non-steroidal anti-inflammatory agent ketorolac enhanced local topical delivery to subcutaneous muscle from a hydroxymethylcellulose gel formulation (Gratieri et al., 2013).

**TABLE 1.5**
**Predicted Versus Experimental Skin Flux Values for Selective Estrogen Receptor Modulators**

| Drug | MW (Daltons) | Log P $_{(o/w)}$ | Predicted $J_{max}$ ($\mu g/cm^2/h$) | Measured $J_{exp}$ ($\mu g/cm^2/h$) |
|---|---|---|---|---|
| Clomiphene | 406 | 6.65 | 0.015 | $0.10 \pm 0.09$ |
| Droloxifene | 388 | 5.95 | 0.13 | $0.06 \pm 0.03$ |
| Endoxifen | 374 | 5.45 | 0.10 | $0.94 \pm 0.50$ |
| 4-Hydroxytamoxifen | 388 | 5.96 | 0.13 | $0.52 \pm 0.30$ |
| Tamoxifen | 372 | 6.39 | 0.042 | $0.14 \pm 0.08$ |
| Toremifene | 406 | 6.06 | 0.026 | $0.21 \pm 0.10$ |

*Source*: Güngör et al., 2013

Using magnetic fields to enhance transdermal drug delivery was proposed in 1999 (Murthy, 1999) when it was found that the influence of magnetic field strength on diffusion flux of benzoic acid across rat skin increased with increasing applied field strength. More recent experiments have shown that magnetophoretic influenced drug permeation enhancement of lidocaine across pig skin in vitro increased with increasing magnetic field strength. Mechanistic studies indicated that the magnetic field did not directly modulate permeability of the stratum corneum and that the predominant mechanism responsible for the enhancement was magnetokinesis (Murthy et al, 2010). Lidocaine flux across rat skin was also enhanced by combining magnetophoresis and chemical enhancement (menthol, dimethyl sulfoxide, sodium lauryl sulfate and urea, all at 5%w/v), the combination being additive but not synergistic (Sammeta et al., 2011). The feasibility of using magnetophoresis to enhance permeation across human skin is yet to be established.

Microneedle technology has been the focus of much attention in recent years and was the subject of a theme issue of the journal *Pharmaceutical Research* (Volume 28, Issue 1, January 2011). The guest editor, Gary Cleary, introduced "fifteen original papers from academia and industry [that covered] ... research and development of microneedles from concept to human clinical studies..." (Cleary, 2011, p. 1). Since the publication of this issue in early 2011 there have been almost 200 further papers published in the field, many of which concern the fabricating materials and their geometry. For example, Donnelly and colleagues described the use of blends of polyethyleneglycol 10,000 and poly(methylether/maleic anhydride) that, when inserted into skin, take up interstitial fluid and form continuous hydrogel conduits from attached drug reservoirs to the dermal microcirculation. The microneedles can be completely removed from the skin when necessary (Donnelly et al., 2012). The authors suggested that, using these microneedles, drug delivery through the skin could be "controlled by the crosslink density of the hydrogel system rather than the stratum corneum". Other materials that have been used for microneedle fabrication include maltose (Lanke et al., 2009), acrylate polymers (Gittard et al., 2013), silicon (Abla et al., 2013; Vučen et al., 2013), polyvinylpyrrolidone (Sun et al., 2013) and chitosan (Chen et al., 2013). Microneedle geometry can also have a substantial effect on their ability to penetrate skin. For example, Kochhar et al. (2013) found that there was an increase in percentage penetration of polyethyleneglycol-based microneedles into rat and pig skin in vitro with an increase in needle spacing. Increasing the aspect ratio and decreasing tip diameter reduced the tendency of acrylate-based microneedles to bend upon application to the skin (Gittard et al., 2013).

Using microneedles with other physical methods of skin penetration enhancement has also been evaluated (Han and Dab, 2015). Thus, a combination of sonophoresis and microneedles was found to increase the permeation of the model compound, bovine serum albumin, through pig ear skin by ten-fold, whereas the two enhancement methods individually enhanced permeation of the protein approximately four-fold (Han and Dab, 2013). The combination of iontophoresis with microneedles has been found to increase the skin permeation of ropinirole hydrochloride (Singh and Banga, 2013), prochlorperazine edisylate (Kolli et al., 2012), calcein and human growth hormone (Kumar and Banga, 2012) and leuprolide (Sachdeva et al., 2013).

More recently, Walsh and colleagues (Walsh et al., 2015) investigated the influence of nanotopography on the transdermal delivery of etanercept (a 150kD protein tumor necrosis factor inhibitor). A standard microneedle array was compared to a microneedle array with a nanostructured coating, the latter was found to deliver 10.6-fold more etanercept through rabbit skin than the uncoated arrays over a 72-hour period. The authors showed that nanotopography enhanced the delivery of the protein by remodeling the epidermal tight junction proteins via down regulation of claudins-1 and -4. Although it has yet to be evaluated on human skin, this technology may prove to be extremely useful for delivering large molecules through the skin for systemic effect.

## 1.5 TOPICAL THERAPEUTIC SYSTEMS: CURRENT STATUS

### 1.5.1 TOPICAL FORMULATIONS

Over the past two decades a myriad of new and improved topical drug delivery products have been introduced and are available for treatment of a wide variety of dermatological and nail conditions. In addition to conventional dermal formulations such as creams, gels, lotions and ointments, the number of dermal therapeutic patches (DTPs) available for local targeted delivery of drugs to the skin has increased markedly in this period. In this section the range of candidate molecules for dermal delivery is discussed. Representative examples of DTPs are provided and design characteristics of these dosage forms are provided. Other dermal and ungual formulations are also briefly reviewed with reference to their therapeutic applications. Conventional enhancement strategies as well as emerging formulation technologies are considered. Finally, challenges in the development and licensing of generic topical formulations are outlined.

### 1.5.2 DRUG CANDIDATES FOR DERMAL DELIVERY

The drugs that are currently available in dermal formulations include anaesthetics, antimicrobial agents, antibiotics, steroidal or nonsteroidal anti-inflammatory drugs

**TABLE 1.6**
**Physicochemical Properties of Selected Drugs Currently Formulated for Dermal Delivery**

| Drug | MW (Daltons) | M.P. (°C) | Log P $_{(o/w)}$ | Therapeutic classification |
|---|---|---|---|---|
| Betamethasone valerate | 476 | 190 | 4.1 | Steroid |
| Capsicum | 305 | 65 | 3.3 | Counter irritant |
| Clotrimazole | 345 | 147–149 | 6.3 | Antifungal |
| Erythromycin | 734 | 137 | 1.9 | Antimicrobial |
| Hydrocortisone | 363 | 214 | 1.6 | Steroid |
| Ibuprofen | 206 | 75–77 | 4.0 | NSAID |
| Lidocaine | 234 | 68–69 | 2.4 | Anaesthetic, analgesic |
| Methyl salicylate | 152 | -9.0 | 2.2 | Rubefacient |
| Salicylic acid | 138 | 158–161 | 2.0 | Keratolytic |
| Tretinoin | 300 | 180–190 | 6.8 | Retinoid |

(NSAIDs), keratolytic agents, topical analgesics, counterirritants and retinoids. The objective of these formulations is to achieve a localized therapeutic effect. Examples of the various therapeutic groups are provided in Table 1.6, which is by no means inclusive of all the classes currently available in dermal formulations. It will be evident from the molecular weight and melting point values cited that the limitations imposed by the skin for dermal delivery are not as narrow as for transdermal delivery. Rational formulation design must nonetheless be predicated on the selection of an active agent that will attain therapeutic levels at the target site. In vitro assays of potency coupled with an assessment of drug flux are therefore essential preformulation steps towards the development of efficacious and safe candidates for dermal delivery.

### 1.5.3 DERMAL THERAPEUTIC PATCHES – HISTORICAL DEVELOPMENT, MARKET AND PRODUCT CHARACTERISTICS

DTPs originated in Asia and were termed "cataplasms" or plasters. These plasters contained the active(s) in a gum rubber-based adhesive composition applied to a backing support. Although a number of these simple devices were listed in the USP and National Formulary for many years, today only salicylic acid plaster remains. These early DTPs have evolved into more sophisticated patches, manufactured by state-of-the-art adhesive coating technology. Lidocaine (as Lidoderm®) has been available as a proprietary prescription DTP for a number of years for the treatment of postherpetic neuralgia and generic versions were launched from 2013. A variety of other DTPs are currently available for treatment of muscle ache, back pain, calluses, corns, warts, skin abrasions, burns and infection and selected examples are provided in Table 1.7.

DTPs share many of the components of transdermal delivery systems and their design may normally include a backing film, a matrix formulated to contain the drug

**TABLE 1.7**
**Examples of Dermal Therapeutic Patches Currently Marketed in the USA and UK**

| Drug and strength | Indication | Product |
|---|---|---|
| Capsaicin 8% | Postherpetic neuralgia | Qutenza® |
| Diclofenac epolamine 1.3% | Acute pain due to minor strains, sprains, contusions | Flector® |
| Fluandrenolide 4 mg/cm$^2$ | Inflammatory and pruritic manifestations of dermatoses | Cordran® |
| Lidocaine 5.0% | Postherpetic neuralgia | Lidoderm® |
| Methyl salicylate 10.0% l-methol 3.0% | Relief of aches and pains | Salonpas® Pain Relief Patch |

and other excipients (permeation enhancers, plasticizers, antioxidants, etc.) and a pressure sensitive adhesive release liner. The design of some DTPs may also incorporate a rate-controlling membrane. The selection of the materials for the various components typically requires specialized and unique multidisciplinary skills. Some, but not all, of the considerations that will influence the design of the DTP include: the biopharmaceutic product profile, physical attributes of the dosage form, consumer preference, compliance and avoidance of side effects. Material science and processing technologies (solvent casting, hot melt coating, polymer extrusion, etc.) as well as slitting, die cutting, pouching, packaging and labelling are also required to complete the manufacture of a DTP which are also processes used in the formulation of transdermal delivery systems.

The backing film for a DTP will be selected from materials that are occlusive or nonocclusive, depending on the active to be delivered. An occlusive backing layer will result in hydration of the outer layers of the stratum corneum. Semi-occlusive films allow some water movement to occur. Nonocclusive materials allow free movement of water vapor from the skin surface. An occlusive backing layer is present in Cordran® which is used in the management of inflammation and dermatoses of the lower layers of the epidermis. Thicker nonocclusive backings are found in corn and callus removal products since the active needs to treat the outer layers of the stratum corneum. In these products the backing layer also serves to cushion the application site.

#### 1.5.4 CLASSIFICATION OF DERMAL FORMULATIONS BY THERAPEUTIC CATEGORY

#### 1.5.4.1 Treatment of Calluses, Corns and Warts

Calluses, corns and warts generally manifest as hyperkeratinization of the skin. It follows that actives which are keratolytic or which dissolve the intracellular keratin should be useful in the management of such conditions. The formulations currently available to treat these skin problems are predominantly topical solutions, gels or creams of salicylic acid or DTPs in the form of adhesive (rubber or karaya) matrices containing salicylic acid, which are applied as pads or disks to the affected area. Salicylic acid collodion preparations, which are nitrocellulose solutions that dry on the skin to leave a film, are also available. Salicylic acid may be formulated alone or with other components that also promote keratolysis (most commonly lactic acid). Podophyllotoxin is available as an alcohol-based topical solution or cream for warts affecting the genital areas. Imiquimod is also available in cream form for the same indication.

### 1.5.4.2 Pain

For the treatment of pain the active ingredient may have analgesic, anesthetic, antipruritic or counterirritant properties. The mechanism of action of analgesics, anesthetics or antipruritic agents relies on depression of cutaneous sensory receptors for pain, burning, stinging and itching. On the other hand, counterirritants work by producing a mild local inflammatory reaction. The main therapeutic ingredients employed for topical pain relief include ammonium salicylate, benzocaine, diethylamine salicylate, glycol salicylate, methyl salicylate, menthol, camphor, capsicum oleoresin, ethyl nicotinate, hexyl nicotinate, 2-hydroxyethyl salicylate, lidocaine, methyl nicotinate, methyl salicylate, sodium salicylate and tetrahydrofurfuryl salicylate. In most over-the-counter (OTC) preparations combinations of ingredients will be present. Formulations currently available include the DTPs discussed earlier, lotions, liniments, gels, creams, ointments and sprays.

### 1.5.4.3 Inflammation

The symptoms of pain associated with inflammation have been treated with both steroidal and nonsteroidal anti-inflammatory drugs (NSAIDs). The corticosteroids available for topical management of inflammation include alclometasone dipropionate, betametasone (dipropionate or valerate ester), clobetasone butyrate, fluandrenolide and hydrocortisone or its ester forms (acetate, butyrate) (Figure 1.15). Creams, foams, lotions, ointments and tapes (see Section 1.5.3 on DTP) have been used to administer these actives. Topical corticosteroid formulations are also applied under occlusive dressings to promote drug penetration and uptake into the skin in specific cases. The most commonly used NSAIDs include diclofenac diethylamine, diclofenac epolamine, diclofenac sodium, felbinac, ibuprofen, indomethacin, ketoprofen, naproxen and piroxicam. Preparations currently in use include creams, DTPs, foams, gels and sprays.

### 1.5.4.4 Anesthesia

EMLA cream (eutectic mixture of local anesthetics) is a 1:1 oil/water emulsion of a eutectic mixture of lidocaine and prilocaine bases (Figure 1.16). It provides local dermal analgesia when applied to the skin under an occlusive dressing. It is indicated for topical analgesia for intact skin including needle insertion, superficial skin procedures and laser treatment. Conventional o/w creams and ointments are also available for topical administration of lidocaine together with sprays. Tetracaine is available as a gel formulation for local anesthesia and has also been co-formulated with lidocaine in a cream preparation.

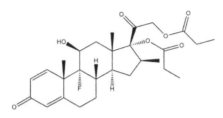

A) Alclometasone

A) Fluandrenolide

B) Betamethasone dipropionate

B) Hydrocortisone

C) Clobetasone

**FIGURE 1.15** Some topical anti-inflammatory steroids.

A) Lidocaine

B) Prilocaine

**FIGURE 1.16** Local anesthetics used for topical anesthesia and analgesia.

### 1.5.4.5 Antimicrobial Formulations

For the management of dry skin and atopic eczema, antimicrobials such as benzalkonium chloride are currently formulated in a range of conventional topical preparations including creams and ointments, as well as shower and bath emollients. Antimicrobials are also used in the management of acne in gel and cream formulations. For the management of dandruff, shampoos containing pyrithone zinc and selenium sulphide have been shown to have beneficial effects. Biopatch® is an antimicrobial dressing (in contrast to the DTPs described earlier) consisting of a hydrophilic polyurethane absorptive foam, which contains the broad spectrum antimicrobial agent chlorhexidine gluconate. In clinical use it is wrapped securely around vascular and nonvascular percutaneous devices to reduce the risk of infection and to inhibit microbial growth. It has been shown to inhibit bacterial growth for up to seven days, reducing the microbial population under the patch by an average of 100 times as compared to skin under nonmedicated patches.

### 1.5.5 PERMEATION ENHANCEMENT STRATEGIES FOR DERMAL FORMULATIONS

To promote drug delivery to or through the skin either chemical or physical enhancement approaches may be employed. Conventionally, the use of chemical penetration enhancers has been the most common approach for dermal formulations. These compounds may promote diffusion of the active through the skin or enhance transiently the solubility of the molecule in the skin; where both mechanisms of action are achieved there may be a synergistic effect. For a comprehensive review of this area the reader is referred to Lane (2013b).

With increasing interest in nanotechnology, the application of nanoemulsions or microemulsions (classified according to emulsion droplet size) to promote dermal delivery of actives has been explored. These systems are thermodynamically stable, colloidal drug delivery vehicles. Recent reviews on nanoemulsions and microemulsions have highlighted their favorable aesthetic and biophysical properties (Sonneville-Aubrun et al., 2004) as well as their potential to promote dermal delivery of actives (Schwarz et al., 2012). At the present time no commercial nanoemulsion or microemulsion for topical application is available. One reason for this is most likely the cost of the surfactants required for these formulations. Concerns have also been raised about the possible irritation potential of such formulations because of the high surfactant content compared with conventional formulations (Santos et al., 2008).

Nanotechnology has been the subject of intense speculation regarding its potential applications in the dermal and transdermal delivery field (Kilfoyle et al., 2012; Küchler et al., 2009; Kristi et al., 2010; Cevc and Vierl, 2010; Jensen et al., 2011). Nanoparticles themselves, however, are unlikely to penetrate or permeate intact human skin (Watkinson et al., 2013).

As briefly mentioned earlier, microneedles have received attention as a physical enhancement strategy for both dermal and transdermal applications. These devices consist of a plurality of micro-projections generally ranging from 25–2000 µm in height and which are attached to a base support (Figure 1.17). The application of such arrays to biological membranes creates transport pathways with dimensions of the order of microns. Microneedles have been shown to penetrate the skin across the

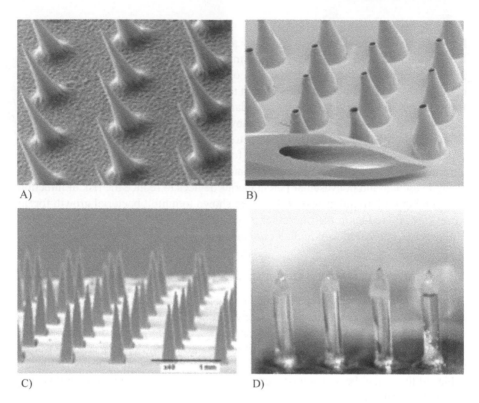

A) B)

C) D)

**FIGURE 1.17** Examples of microneedle arrays: (A) Silicone microneedle array, poke and patch design; (B) Stainless steel microneedle array, poke and patch. Needle length is 1000 μm; (C) Hollow metal microneedles, poke and flow design. Needle length is 500 μm; (D) Bevel-tip microneedles made of PLGA with calcein encapsulated in tips. Needle length 600 μm.

stratum corneum and into the viable epidermis avoiding contact with nerve fibers and blood vessels, which are located in the dermal layer. The early microneedles were fabricated with silicon but the major development in recent years has been the design of microneedles using biodegradable and biocompatible materials (Donnelly et al., 2010). Active agents can be loaded into the microneedle, or coated on to the microneedle, and a reservoir patch may also be adhered to the array. As well as effectively transporting conventional small actives into skin, promising results have been reported for macromolecular targeting ex vivo and vaccine delivery in humans, and a number of devices are currently in FDA-regulated phase II clinical trials (Cleary, 2011). The most straightforward of the microneedle protocols, the so-called "poke, press and patch" method, does have the perceived disadvantage that the lifetime of the created pores is relatively short (around two hours) and this precludes their use in longer-term transdermal delivery. Recently, however, Brogden et al. (2013) have reported that the application of diclofenac may extend pore lifetime, allowing drug delivery continuously for up to seven days.

### 1.5.6 Ungual Formulations

Topical treatment of skin and nail diseases is desirable in terms of patient acceptability and reduction of side effects associated with systemic drug delivery. This is particularly the case for nail diseases as they are frequently difficult to cure and require long periods of treatment compared with the skin. The nail plate is a highly keratinized tissue, which is characterized by low permeability to diffusing compounds, hence its barrier properties represent a significant challenge for formulation scientists. Currently, actives to treat nail fungal infections are available in lacquer form where the volatile formulation components evaporate to leave a residual film on the nail surface. Despite many literature reports employing chemical and physical enhancement strategies to enhance drug delivery to the nail, new formulation strategies have not impacted on this field to date (Walters et al., 2012).

### 1.5.7 Development and Licensing of Topical Formulations

The guidelines for developing a new chemical entity (NCE) to be administered by the topical route are rather straightforward. What appears to be less well understood are the pathways for development, and the regulatory routes for topical formulations of a known established active pharmaceutical ingredient (API) either in a new formulation, at a different concentration, or with APIs where topical administration is an alternative route of administration. For a more detailed discussion of this topic the reader is referred to Mugglestone et al. (2012), who provide guidance on the regulatory routes, which can help achieve marketing approval in Europe for topical formulations, with particular emphasis on clinical development.

For the marketing of generic formulations clinical endpoints are still required for the vast majority of formulations by a number of regulatory agencies in order to demonstrate bioequivalence to the reference listed formulation. Developments in recent years include the acceptance of tape-stripping by the Japanese regulatory agency and the increasing recognition of the utility and sensitivity of in vitro skin permeation testing for prediction of in vivo efficacy (Franz et al., 2009; Lehman et al., 2011).

## 1.6 CONCLUDING REMARKS

Considering the centuries over which the science of medicine has been developing, it is tempting to conclude that transdermal drug delivery for systemic effect is a relatively recent development. However, products such as ointments and balms were used by the ancients, often for systemic effect, and there is evidence that some Elizabethans of the sixteenth century were aware that particularly formulated ointments could be used for "stomack" complaints and for "any paine about the heart" (Figure 1.18). What has been achieved over the past 40 or so years is the ability to control, to some extent, the amount and the rate at which drugs cross the skin for systemic or local effect, despite the inherent barrier nature of the integument and its variability within individuals and across gender, ethnic groups and age (Farahmand and Maibach, 2009; Machado et al., 2010; Konda et al., 2012). Given these obstacles, extensive research over this time period has resulted in the bringing

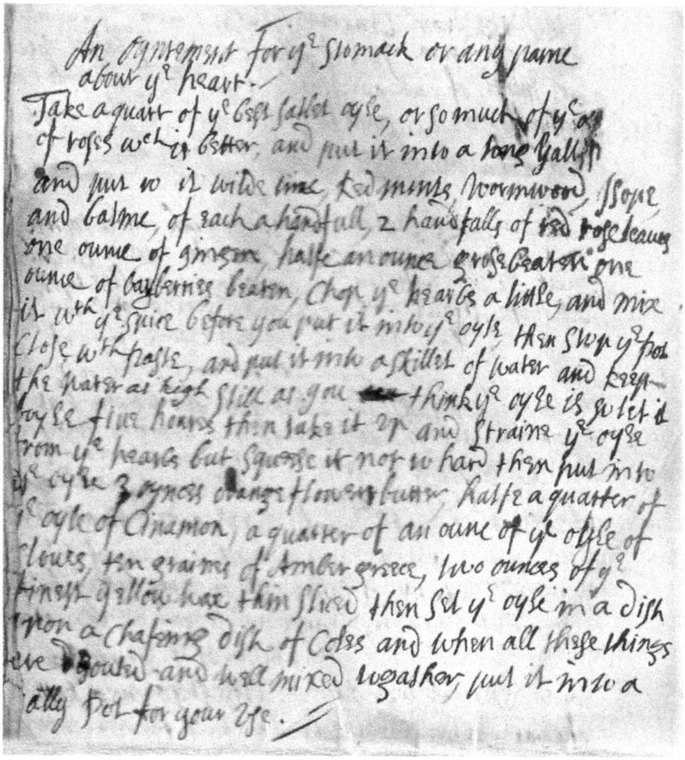

**FIGURE 1.18** Extract from the Sanford Archive that describes the preparation of an ointment for stomach and heart ailments (The Sanfords were a Somerset family who lived at Nynhead Court near Wellington, UK).

to market, as transdermal systemic medications, 19 individual drug substances in 17 separate drug products, and several more as locally acting transdermally delivered drugs. This has not come easy. A review of the number of publications that included the term "transdermal drug" reveals that between 1998 and 2012 the annual number of peer reviewed papers doubled (Figure 1.19). This amount of research mirrors, almost exactly, the doubling of the number of transdermal products launched over the same time period (eight products in 1998, 17 in 2013). This unscientific overview could suggest to the unwary that the more resources that are put into a problem the easier it will be solved. While in most scenarios this is definitely the case, Mother Nature has seen fit to protect our internal environment with a remarkable shield against the perils of the external environment, and this limits our ability to get therapeutic levels of many drugs delivered transdermally. As Watkinson recently concluded: "All of the drugs … that are now available as [transdermal] products meet the strict physicochemical and pharmacokinetic criteria that make a drug suitable for transdermal delivery" (Watkinson, 2013). We do, however, continue to come up with various means to overcome both the skin barrier and the strict criteria necessary to breach it. Microneedles, of course, will do both. Whether we can precisely define the

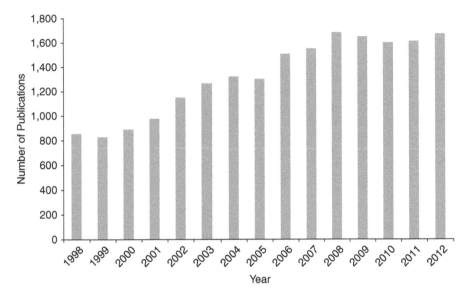

**FIGURE 1.19** Peer reviewed publications containing the term "transdermal drug" in the title and abstract 1998 through 2012. (Data derived from www.ncbi.nlm.nih.gov/pubmed.)

use of microneedles as transdermal therapy is questionable, but most transdermal scientists will claim it as one of their technologies. With this in mind we can conclude that Pfister's *"iceberg"* has not yet succumbed to global warming, the tip is certainly getting bigger, but there is a lot more mining to be done.

## REFERENCES

Abla MJ, Chaturvedula A, O'Mahony C, Banga AK. 2013. Transdermal delivery of methotrexate for pediatrics using silicon microneedles. *Ther Deliv* 4(5): 543–551.

Abrams LS, Skee DM, Wong FA, Anderson NJ, Leese PT. 2001a. Pharmacokinetics of norelgestromin and ethinyl estradiol from two consecutive contraceptive patches. *J Clin Pharmacol* 41: 1232–1237.

Abrams LS, Skee DM, Natarajan J, Wong FA, Leese PT Creasy GW, Shangold MM. 2001b. Pharmacokinetics of norelgestromin and ethinyl estradiol delivered by a contraceptive patch [Ortho Evra/Evra] under conditions of heat, humidity, and exercise. *J Clin Pharmacol* 41: 1301–1309.

Abrams LS, Skee DM, Natarajan J, Wong FA, Lasseter KC. 2001c. Multiple dose pharmacokinetics of a contraceptive patch in healthy women participants. *Contraception* 64: 287–294.

Abrams LS, Skee DM, Natarajan J, Wong FA, Anderson GD. 2002a. Pharmacokinetics of a contraceptive patch (Evra/Ortho Evra) containing norelgestromin and ethinyloestradiol at four application sites. *Br J Clin Pharmacol* 53(2): 141–146.

Abrams LS, Skee DM, Natarajan J, Wong FA. 2002b. Pharmacokinetic overview of Ortho Evra/Evra. *Fertil Steril* 77 (2 Suppl 2): S3–12.

Ackaert OW, Eikelenboom J, Wolff HM, Bouwstra JA. 2010. Comparing different salt forms of rotigotine to improve transdermal iontophoretic delivery. *Eur J Pharm Biopharm* 74(2): 304–310.

Agrawal SS, Aggarwal A. 2010. Randomised, cross-over, comparative bioavailability trial of matrix type transdermal drug delivery system (TDDS) of carvedilol and hydrochlorothiazide combination in healthy human volunteers: a pilot study. *Contemp Clin Trials* 31: 272–278.

Agrawal SS, Pruthi JK. 2011. Development and evaluation of matrix type transdermal patch of ethinylestradiol and medroxyprogesterone acetate for anti-implantation activity in female Wistar rats. *Contraception* 84(5): 533–538

Alberti I, Grenier A, Kraus H, Carrara DN. 2005. Pharmaceutical development and clinical effectiveness of a novel gel technology for transdermal drug delivery. *Expert Opin Drug Deliv* 2(5): 935–950.

Al-Tawil N, Odar-Cederlöf I, Berggren AC, Johnson HE, Persson J. 2013. Pharmacokinetics of transdermal buprenorphine patch in the elderly. *Eur J Clin Pharmacol* 69(2): 143–149.

Amsterdam JD. 2003. A double-blind, placebo-controlled trial of the safety and efficacy of selegiline transdermal system without dietary restrictions in patients with major depressive disorder. *J Clin Psychiatry* 64(2): 208–214.

Amsterdam JD, Bodkin JA. 2006. Selegiline transdermal system in the prevention of relapse of major depressive disorder: a 52-week, double-blind, placebo-substitution, parallel-group clinical trial. *J Clin Psychopharmacol* 26(6): 579–586.

Andresen T, Staahl C, Oksche A, Mansikka H, Arendt-Nielsen L, Drewes AM. 2011. Effect of transdermal opioids in experimentally induced superficial, deep and hyperalgesic pain. *Br J Pharmacol* 164(3): 934–945.

Anissimov YG, Jepps OG, Dancik Y, Roberts MS. 2013. Mathematical and pharmacokinetic modelling of epidermal and dermal transport processes. *Adv Drug Deliv Rev* 65(2): 169–190.

Archer DF, Stanczyk FZ, Rubin A, Foegh M. 2012. Ethinyl estradiol and levonorgestrel pharmacokinetics with a low-dose transdermal contraceptive delivery system, AG200-15: a randomized controlled trial. *Contraception* 85(6): 595–601.

Archer DF, Stanczyk FZ, Rubin A, Foegh M. 2013. Pharmacokinetics and adhesion of the Agile transdermal contraceptive patch (AG200-15) during daily exposure to external conditions of heat, humidity and exercise. *Contraception* 87(2): 212–219.

Arnold LE, Lindsay RL, López FA, Jacob SE, Biederman J, Findling RL, Ramadan Y. 2007. Treating attention-deficit/hyperactivity disorder with a stimulant transdermal patch: the clinical art. *Pediatrics* 120(5): 1100–1106.

Bakshi A, Bajaj A, Malhotra M, Amrutiya N. 2008. A novel metered dose transdermal spray formulation for oxybutynin. *Ind J Pharm Sci* 70: 733–739.

Balaguer-Fernández C, Femenía-Font A, Merino V, Córdoba-Díaz D, Elorza-Barroeta MA, López-Castellano A, Córdoba-Díaz M. 2011. Elastic vesicles of sumatriptan succinate for transdermal administration: characterization and in vitro permeation studies. *J Liposome Res* 21(1): 55–59.

Balaguer-Fernández C, Femenía-Font A, Del Rio-Sancho S, Merino V, López-Castellano A. 2008. Sumatriptan succinate transdermal delivery systems for the treatment of migraine. *J Pharm Sci* 97(6): 2102–2109.

Baroni A, Buommino E, De Gregorio V, Ruocco E, Ruocco V, Wolf R. 2012. Structure and function of the epidermis related to barrier properties. *Clin Dermatol* 30(3): 257–262.

Barrett JS, Hochadel TJ, Morales RJ, Rohatagi S, DeWitt KE, Watson SK, DiSanto AR. 1996a. Pharmacokinetics and safety of a selegiline transdermal system relative to single-dose oral administration in the elderly. *Am J Ther* 3(10): 688–698.

Barrett JS, Szego P, Rohatagi S, Morales RJ, De Witt KE, Rajewski G, Ireland J. 1996b. Absorption and presystemic metabolism of selegiline hydrochloride at different regions in the gastrointestinal tract in healthy males. *Pharm Res* 13(10): 1535–1540.

Barry BW. 1983. *Dermatological Formulations, Percutaneous Absorption.* New York: Marcel Dekker.

Benson HAE, Watkinson AC, eds. 2012. *Topical and Transdermal Drug Delivery.* Hoboken: Wiley.

Biberman R, Neumann R, Katzir I, Gerber Y. 2003. A randomized controlled trial of oral selegiline plus nicotine skin patch compared with placebo plus nicotine skin patch for smoking cessation. *Addiction* 98(10): 1403–1407.

Bied AM, Kim J, Schwartz TL. 2015. A critical appraisal of the selegiline transdermal system for major depressive disorder. *Expert Rev Clin Pharmacol* 8: 673–681.

Bigal ME, Lipton RB, Newman LC, Pierce MW, Silberstein SD. 2015. Sumatriptan iontophoretic transdermal system reduces treatment-emergent nausea and is effective in patients with and without nausea at baseline – results from a randomized controlled trial. *Headache* 55(8): 1124–1132.

Bigucci F, Abruzzo A, Saladini B, Gallucci MC, Cerchiara T, Luppi B. 2015. Development and characterization of chitosan/hyaluronan film for transdermal delivery of thiocolchicoside. *Carbohydr Polym* 130: 32–40.

Boccia RV, Gordan LN, Clark G, Howell JD, Grunberg SM. Sancuso Study Group. 2011. Efficacy and tolerability of transdermal granisetron for the control of chemotherapy-induced nausea and vomiting associated with moderately and highly emetogenic multi-day chemotherapy: a randomized, double-blind, phase III study. *Support Care Cancer* 19(10): 1609–1617.

Bodkin JA, Amsterdam JD. 2002. Transdermal selegiline in major depression: a double-blind, placebo-controlled, parallel-group study in outpatients. *Am J Psychiatry* 159(11): 1869–1875.

Bodner K, Bodner-Adler B, Grünberger W. 2011. Evaluation of the contraceptive efficacy, compliance, and satisfaction with the transdermal contraceptive patch system Evra: a comparison between adolescent and adult users. *Arch Gynecol Obstet* 283(3): 525–530.

Böhme K. 2002. Buprenorphine in a transdermal therapeutic system--a new option. *Clin Rheumatol* 21(Suppl 1): S13–16.

Bouwstra JA, Ponec M. 2006. The skin barrier in healthy and diseased state. *Biochim Biophys Acta* 1758: 2080–2095.

Brogden NK, Banks SL, Crofford LJ, Sinchcomb AL. 2013. Diclofenac enables unprecedented week-long microneedle-enhanced delivery of a skin impermeable medication in humans. *Pharm Res* 30: 1947–1955.

Brown MB, Williams AC. 2019. *The Art and Science of Dermal Formulation Development.* Boca Raton: CRC Press.

Cai B, Enqqvist H, Bredenberg S. 2015. Development and evaluation of a tampering resistant transdermal fentanyl patch. *Int J Pharm* 488(1–2): 102–107.

Caon T, Campos CE, Simoes CM, Silva MA. 2015. Novel perspectives in the tuberculosis treatment: administration of isoniazid through the skin. *Int J Pharm* 494(1): 463–470.

Cawello W, Ahrweiler S, Sulowicz W, Szymczakiewicz-Multanowska A, Braun M. 2012. Single dose pharmacokinetics of the transdermal rotigotine patch in patients with impaired renal function. *Br J Clin Pharmacol* 73(1): 46–54.

Cawello W, Wolff HM, Meuling WJ, Horstmann R, Braun M. 2007. Transdermal administration of radiolabelled [$^{14}$C]rotigotine by a patch formulation: a mass balance trial. *Clin Pharmacokinet* 46(10): 851–857.

Cevc G, Vierl U. 2010. Nanotechnology and the transdermal route. A state of the art review and critical appraisal. *J Contr Rel* 141: 277–299.

Chantasart D, Hao J, Li KS. 2013. Evaluation of skin permeation of B-blockers for topical drug delivery. *Pharm Res* 30: 866–877.

Chen CC, Fang CL, Al-Suwayeh SA, Leu YL, Fang JY. 2011. Transdermal delivery of selegiline from alginate-Pluronic composite thermogels. *Int J Pharm* 415(1–2): 119–128.

Chen MC, Huang SF, Lai KY, Ling MH. 2013. Fully embeddable chitosan microneedles as a sustained release depot for intradermal vaccination. *Biomaterials* 34(12): 3077–3086.

Cheng C, La Grenade L, Diak IL, Brinker A, Levin RL. 2017. Chemical leukoderma associated with methylphenidate transdermal system: data from the US Food and Drug Administration adverse event reporting system. *J Pediatr* 180: 241–246.

Choi J, Choi MK, Chong S, Chung SJ, Shim CK, Kim DD. 2012. Effect of fatty acids on the transdermal delivery of donepezil: in vitro and in vivo evaluation. *Int J Pharm* 422(1–2): 83–90.

Cork MJ, Danby SG, Vasilopoulos Y, Hadgraft J, Lane ME, Moustafa M, Guy RH, MacGowan AL, Tazi-Ahnini R, Ward SJ. 2009. Epidermal barrier function in atopic dermatitis. *J Invest Dermatol* 129: 1892–1908.

Clavenna A, Bonati M. 2014. Safety of medicines used for ADHD in children; a review of published prospective clinical trials. *Arch Dis Child* 99(9): 866–872.

Cleary GW. 2011. Microneedles for drug delivery. *Pharm Res* 28(1): 1–6.

Cleek RL, Bunge AL. 1993. A new method for estimating dermal absorption from chemical exposure. 1. General approach. *Pharm Res* 10: 497–506.

Creasy GW, Abrams LS, Fisher AC. 2001. Transdermal contraception. *Semin Reprod Med* 19: 373–380.

Cristancho MA, Thase ME. 2016. Critical appraisal of selegiline transdermal system for major depressive disorder. *Expert Opin Drug Deliv* 13: 659–665.

Culpepper L, Kovalick LJ. 2008. A review of the literature on the selegiline transdermal system: an effective and well-tolerated monoamine oxidase inhibitor for the treatment of depression. *Prim Care Companion J Clin Psychiatry* 10(1): 25–30.

Cummings JL, Farlow MR, Meng X, Tekin S, Olin JT. 2010. Rivastigmine transdermal patch skin tolerability: results of a 1-year clinical trial in patients with mild-to-moderate Alzheimer's disease. *Clin Drug Investig* 30(1): 41–49.

Cummings J, Froelich L, Black SE, Bakchine S, Bellelli G, Molinuevo JL, Kressig RW, Downs P, Caputo A, Strohmaier C. 2012. Randomized, double-blind, parallel-group, 48-week study for efficacy and safety of a higher-dose rivastigmine patch (15 vs. 10 cm²) in Alzheimer's disease. *Dement Geriatr Cogn Disord* 33(5): 341–353.

Dagtekin O, Gerbershagen HJ, Wagner W, Petzke F, Radbruch L, Sabatowski R. 2007. Assessing cognitive and psychomotor performance under long-term treatment with transdermal buprenorphine in chronic noncancer pain patients. *Anesth Analg* 105(5): 1442–1448.

Davila GW, Daugherty CA, Sanders SW. 2001. A short-term, multicenter, randomized double-blind dose titration study of the efficacy and anticholinergic side effects of transdermal compared to immediate release oral oxybutynin treatment of patients with urge urinary incontinence. *J Urol* 166(1): 140–145.

Deandrea S, Corli O, Moschetti I, Apolone G. 2009. Managing severe cancer pain: the role of transdermal buprenorphine: a systematic review. *Ther Clin Risk Manag* 5(5): 707–718.

Djabri A, Guy RH, Delgado-Charro MB. 2012. Transdermal iontophoresis of ranitidine: an opportunity in paediatric drug therapy. *Int J Pharm* 435: 27–32.

Dmochowski RR, Davila GW, Zinner NR, Gittelman MC, Saltzstein DR, Lyttle S, Sanders SW. 2002. Efficacy and safety of transdermal oxybutynin in patients with urge and mixed urinary incontinence. *J Urol* 168(2): 580–586.

Dmochowski RR, Newman DK, Sand PK, Rudy DC, Caramelli KE, Thomas H, Hoel G. 2011. Pharmacokinetics of oxybutynin chloride topical gel: effects of application site, baths, sunscreen and person-to-person transference. *Clin Drug Investig* 31(8): 559–571.

Dmochowski RR, Nitti V, Staskin D, Luber K, Appell R, Davila GW. 2005. Transdermal oxybutynin in the treatment of adults with overactive bladder: combined results of two randomized clinical trials. *World J Urol* 23(4): 263–270.

Donnelly RF, Garland MJ, Morrow DI, Migalska K, Singh TR, Majithiya R, Woolfson AD. 2010. Optical coherence tomography is a valuable tool in the study of the effects of microneedle geometry on skin penetration characteristics and in-skin dissolution. *J Control Release* 147: 333–341.

Donnelly RF, Singh TR, Garland MJ, Migalska K, Majithiya R, McCrudden CM, Kole PL, Mahmood TM, McCarthy HO, Woolfson AD. 2012. Hydrogel-forming microneedle arrays for enhanced transdermal drug delivery. *Adv Funct Mater* 22(23): 4879–4890.

Dore DD, Norman H, Loughlin J, Seeger JD. 2010. Extended case-control study results on thromboembolic outcomes among transdermal contraceptive users. *Contraception* 81: 408–413.

Dragicevic N, Maibach HI, eds. 2015. *Percutaneous Penetration Enhancers: Chemical Methods in Penetration Enhancement*. Berlin: Springer.

Duscher D, Neofytou E, Wong VW, Maan ZN, Rennert RC, Inayathullah M, Januszyk M, Rodrigues M, Malkovskiy AV, Whitmore AJ, Walmsley GG, Galvez MG, Whittam AJ, Brownlee M, Rajadas J, Gurtner GC. 2015. Transdermal deferoxamine prevents pressure-induced diabetic ulcers. *Proc Nat Acad Sci* 112(1): 94–99.

Elias PM. 1981. Lipids and the epidermal permeability barrier. *Arch Dermatol Res* 270: 95–117.

Elias PM, Feingold KR, eds. 2006. *Skin Barrier*. New York: Taylor & Francis.

Elshoff JP, Braun M, Andreas JO, Middle M, Cawello W. 2012. Steady-state plasma concentration profile of transdermal rotigotine: an integrated analysis of three, open-label, randomized, phase I multiple dose studies. *Clin Ther* 34(4): 966–978.

Elshoff JP, Cawello W, Andreas JO, Mathy FX, Braun M. 2015. An update on pharmacological, pharmacokinetic properties and drug-drug interactions of rotigotine transdermal system in Parkinson's disease and restless legs syndrome. *Drugs* 75(5): 487–501.

Fang JY, Hung CF, Chi CH, Chen CC. 2009. Transdermal permeation of selegiline from hydrogel-membrane drug delivery systems. *Int J Pharm* 380(1–2): 33–39.

Farahmand S, Maibach HI. 2009. Transdermal drug pharmacokinetics in man: interindividual variability and partial prediction. *Int J Pharm* 367: 1–15.

Feiger AD, Rickels K, Rynn MA, Zimbroff DL, Robinson DS. 2006. Selegiline transdermal system for the treatment of major depressive disorder: an 8-week, double-blind, placebo-controlled, flexible-dose titration trial. *J Clin Psychiatry* 67(9): 1354–1361.

Femenía-Font A, Balaguer-Fernández C, Merino V, Rodilla V, López-Castellano A. 2005a. Effect of chemical enhancers on the in vitro percutaneous absorption of sumatriptan succinate. *Eur J Pharm Biopharm* 61(1–2): 50–55.

Femenía-Font A, Balaguer-Fernández C, Merino V, López-Castellano A. 2005b. Iontophoretic transdermal delivery of sumatriptan: effect of current density and ionic strength. *J Pharm Sci* 94(10): 2183–2186.

Femenía-Font A, Balaguer-Fernández C, Merino V, López-Castellano A. 2006a. Combination strategies for enhancing transdermal absorption of sumatriptan through skin. *Int J Pharm* 323(1–2): 125–130.

Femenía-Font A, Padula C, Marra F, Balaguer-Fernández C, Merino V, López-Castellano A, Nicoli S, Santi P. 2006b. Bioadhesive monolayer film for the in vitro transdermal delivery of sumatriptan. *J Pharm Sci* 95(7): 1561–1569.

Fowler JS, Logan J, Volkow ND, Shumay E, Mc-Call-Perez F, Jayne M, Wang G-J, Alexoff DL, Apelskog-Torres K, Hubbard B, Carter P, King P, Fahn S, Gilmor M, Telang F, Shea C, Xu Y, Muench L. 2015. Evidence that formulations of the selective MAO-B inhibitor, selegiline, which bypass first-pass metabolism, also inhibit MAO-A in the human brain. *Neuropsychopharm* 40: 650–657.

Franz TJ, Lehman PA, Raney SG. 2009. Use of excised human skin to assess the bioequivalence of topical products. *Skin Pharmacol Physiol* 22(5): 276–286.

Frazier CN, Blank IH. 1954. *A Formulary for External Therapy of the Skin*. Springfield, IL: Thomas.

Galipoglu M, Erdal MS, Güngör S. 2015. Biopolymer-based transdermal films of donepezil as an alternative delivery approach in Alzheimer's disease treatment. *AAPS Pharm Sci Tech* 16(2): 284–292.

Gannu R, Palem CR, Yamsani VV, Yamsani SK, Yamsani MR. 2010. Enhanced bioavailability of lacidipine via microemulsion based transdermal gels: formulation optimization, ex vivo and in vivo characterization. *Int J Pharm* 388: 231–241.

Gao Y, Liang J, Liu J, Xiao Y. 2009. Double-layer weekly sustained release transdermal patch containing gestodene and ethinylestradiol. *Int J Pharm* 377(1–2): 128–134

Garnock-Jones KP. 2013. Sumatriptan iontophoretic transdermal system: A review of its use in patients with acute migraine. *Drugs* Aug 3. [Epub ahead of print]

Gattu S, Maibach HI. 2011. Modest but increased penetration through damaged skin: an over-view of the in vivo human model. *Skin Pharmacol Physiol* 24: 2–9.

Ghosh TK, Pfister WR, Yum SI [eds]. 1997. *Transdermal and Topical Drug Delivery Systems*. Buffalo Grove: Interpharm Press Inc.

Ghuman JK, Arnold LE, Anthony BJ. 2008. Psychopharmacological and other treatments in preschool children with attention-deficit/hyperactivity disorder: current evidence and practice. *J Child Adolesc Psychopharmacol* 18(5): 413–447.

Giladi N, Boroojerdi B, Surmann E. 2013. The safety and tolerability of rotigotine transdermal system over a 6-year period in patients with early-stage Parkinson's disease. *J Neural Transm* Mar 19. [Epub ahead of print].

Gittard SD, Chen B, Xu H, Ovsianikov A, Chichkov BN, Monteiro-Riviere NA, Narayan RJ. 2013. The effects of geometry on skin penetration and failure of polymer microneedles. *J Adhes Sci Technol* 27(3): 227–243.

Goldfischer ER, Sand PK, Thomas H, Peters-Gee J. 2015. Efficacy and safety of oxybutynin topical gel 3% in patients with urgency and/or mixed urinary incontinence: a randomized, double-blind, placebo-controlled study. *Neurourol Urodyn* 34(1): 37–43.

Goldstein J, Smith TR, Pugach N, Griesser J, Sebree T, Pierce M. 2012. A sumatriptan iontophoretic transdermal system for the acute treatment of migraine. *Headache* 52(9): 1402–1410.

González MA, Campbell D, Rubin J. 2009 Effects of application to two different skin sites on the pharmacokinetics of transdermal methylphenidate in pediatric patients with attention-deficit/hyperactivity disorder. *J Child Adolesc Psychopharmacol* 19(3): 227–232

González-Rodríguez ML, Mouram I, Cózar-Bernal MJ, Villasmil S, Rabasco AM. 2012. Applying the Taguchi method to optimize sumatriptan succinate niosomes as drug carriers for skin delivery. *J Pharm Sci* 101(10): 3845–3863.

Gratieri T, Pujol-Bello E, Gelfuso GM, de Souza JG, Lopez RF, Kalia YN. 2013. Iontophoretic transport kinetics of ketorolac in vitro and in vivo: Demonstrating local enhanced topical drug delivery to muscle. *Eur J Pharm Biopharm* Jun 19. pii: S0939–6411(13)00227-0. doi: 10.1016/j.ejpb.2013.06.009. [Epub ahead of print]

Graziottin A. 2006. A review of transdermal hormonal contraception, focus on the ethinylestradiol/norelgestromin contraceptive patch. *Treat Endocrinol* 5, 359–365.

Graziottin A. 2008. Safety, efficacy and patient acceptability of the combined estrogen and progestin transdermal contraceptive patch a review. *Patient Pref Adherence* 2, 357–367.

Greenspoon J, Herrmann N, Adam DN. 2011. Transdermal rivastigmine: management of cutaneous adverse events and review of the literature. *CNS Drugs* 25(7): 575–583.

Griessinger N, Sittl R, Likar R. 2005. Transdermal buprenorphine in clinical practice--a postmarketing surveillance study in 13,179 patients. *Curr Med Res Opin* 21(8): 1147–1156.

Grossberg GT, Farlow MR, Meng X, Velting DM. 2015. Evaluating high-dose rivastigmine patch in severe Alzheimer's disease: analyses with concomitant memantine usage as a factor. *Curr Alzheimer Res* 12(1): 53–60.

Grossberg GT, Olin JT, Somogyi M, Meng X. 2011. Dose effects associated with rivastigmine transdermal patch in patients with mild-to-moderate Alzheimer's disease. *Int J Clin Pract* 65(4): 465–471.

Guedes V, Castro JP, Brito I. 2018. Topical capsaicin for pain in osteoarthritis: a literature review. *Reumatol Clin* 14: 40–45.

Guha RA, Shear NH, Papini M. 2010. Ballistic impact of single particles into gelatin: experiments and modeling with application to transdermal pharmaceutical delivery. *J Biomech Eng* 132(10): 101003.

Güldenpfennig WM, Poole KH, Sommerville KW, Boroojerdi B. 2005. Safety, tolerability, and efficacy of continuous transdermal dopaminergic stimulation with rotigotine patch in early-stage idiopathic Parkinson disease. *Clin Neuropharmacol* 28(3): 106–110.

Güngör S, Delgado-Charro MB, Masini-Etévé V, Potts RO, Guy RH. 2013. Transdermal flux predictions for selected selective oestrogen receptor modulators (SERMs): comparison with experimental results. *J Contr Release* http://dx.doi.org/10.1016/j.jconrel.2013.09.017

Hadgraft J, Lane ME. 2011. Skin: the ultimate interface. *Phys Chem Phys* 13(12): 5215–5222.

Hair PI, Keating GM, McKeage K. 2008. Transdermal matrix fentanyl membrane patch (matrifen): in severe cancer-related chronic pain. *Drugs* 68(14): 2001–2009.

Ham AS, Buckheit RW. 2015. Current and emerging formulation strategies for the effective transdermal delivery of HIV inhibitors. *Ther Deliv* 6(2): 217–229.

Han T, Das DB. 2013. Permeability enhancement for transdermal delivery of large molecule using low-frequency sonophoresis combined with microneedles. *J Pharm Sci* 102(10): 3614–3622.

Han T, Das DB. 2015. Potential of combined ultrasound and microneedles for enhanced transdermal drug permeation: a review. *Eur J Pharm Biopharm* 89: 312–328.

Hans G, Robert D. 2009. Transdermal buprenorphine – a critical appraisal of its role in pain management. *J Pain Res* 15(2): 117–134.

Hening WA, Allen RP, Ondo WG, Walters AS, Winkelman JW, Becker P, Bogan R, Fry JM, Kudrow DB, Lesh KW, Fichtner A, Schollmayer E. 2010. Rotigotine improves restless legs syndrome: a 6-month randomized, double-blind, placebo-controlled trial in the United States. *Mov Disord* 25(11): 1675–1683.

Herbison P, McKenzie JE. 2019. Which anticholinergic is best for people with overactive bladders? A network meta-analysis. *Neurourol Urodyn* 38: 525–534.

Hirano M, Isono C, Sakamoto H, Ueno S, Kusunoki S, Nakamura Y. 2015. Rotigotine transdermal patch improves swallowing in dysphagic patients with Parkinson's disease. *Dysphagia* 30(4): 452–456.

Högl B, Oertel WH, Stiasny-Kolster K, Geisler P, Beneš H, García-Borreguero D, Trenkwalder C, Poewe W, Schollmayer E, Kohnen R. 2010. Treatment of moderate to severe restless legs syndrome: 2-year safety and efficacy of rotigotine transdermal patch. *BMC Neurol* Sep 28 10–86. doi: 10.1186/1471-2377-10-86.

Honeywell-Nguyen PL, Arenja S, Bouwstra JA. 2003. Skin penetration and mechanisms of action in the delivery of the D2-agonist rotigotine from surfactant-based elastic vesicle formulations. *Pharm Res* 20(10): 1619–1625.

Howell J, Smeets J, Drenth HJ, Gill D. 2009. Pharmacokinetics of a granisetron transdermal system for the treatment of chemotherapy-induced nausea and vomiting. *J Oncol Pharm Pract* 15(4): 223–231.

Huang CT, Tsai MJ, Lin YH, Fu YS, Huang YB, Tsai YH, Wu PC. 2013. Effect of microemulsions on transdermal delivery of citalopram: optimization studies using mixture design and response surface methodology. *Int J Nanomedicine* 8: 2295–2304.

Hutton JT, Metman LV, Chase TN, Juncos JL, Koller WC, Pahwa R, LeWitt PA, Samii A, Tsui JK, Calne DB, Waters CH, Calabrese VP, Bennett JP, Barrett R, Morris JL. 2001. Transdermal dopaminergic D(2) receptor agonist therapy in Parkinson's disease with N-0923 TDS: a double-blind, placebo-controlled study. *Mov Disord* 16(3): 459–463.

Hwa C, Bauer EA, Cohen DE. 2011. Skin biology. *Dermatol Ther* 24: 464–470.

Im JS, Bai BC, Lee Y-S. 2010. The effect of carbon nanotubes on drug delivery in an electro-sensitive transdermal drug delivery system. *Biomaterials* 31: 1414–1419.

Ita K. 2015. Transdermal delivery of drugs with microneedles – potential and challenges. *Pharmaceutics* 7: 90–105.

Jakasa I, Verbeck MW, Esposito M, Bos JD, Kezic S. 2006. Altered penetration of polyethylene glycols into uninvolved skin of atopic dermatitis patients. *J Invest Dermatol* 127: 129–134.

Jankovic J, Watts RL, Martin W, Boroojerdi B. 2007. Transdermal rotigotine: double-blind, placebo-controlled trial in Parkinson disease. *Arch Neurol* 64(5): 676–682.

Jensen LB, Petersson K, Nielsen HM. 2011. In vitro penetration properties of solid lipid nanoparticles in intact and barrier-impaired skin. *Eur J Pharm Biopharm* 79: 68–75.

Jick SS, Kaye JA, Russmann S, Jick H. 2006. Risk of nonfatal venous thromboembolism in women using a contraceptive transdermal patch and oral contraceptives containing norgestimate and 35 μg of ethinyl estradiol. *Contraception* 73: 223–228.

Jick SS, Kaye JA, Li L, Jick H. 2007. Further results on the risk of nonfatal venous thromboembolism in users of the contraceptive transdermal patch compared to users of oral contraceptives containing norgestimate and 35 μg of ethinyl estradiol. *Contraception* 76: 4–7.

Jick SS, Hagberg KW, Kaye JA. 2010. ORTHO EVRA and venous thromboembolism: an update. *Contraception* 81: 452–453.

Jose A, Mandapalli PK, Venuganti VV. 2015. Liposomal hydrogel formulation for transdermal delivery of pirfenidone. *J Liposome Res* 26: 1–9.

Jung E, Kang YP, Yoon IS, Kim JS, Kwon SW, Chung SJ, Shim CK, Kim DD. 2013. Effect of permeation enhancers on transdermal delivery of fluoxetine: in vitro and in vivo evaluation. *Int J Pharm* 456(2): 362–369.

Jung E, Lee EY, Choi HK, Ban SJ, Choi SH, Kim JS, Yoon IS, Kim DD. 2015. Development of drug-in-adhesive patch formulations for transdermal delivery of fluoxetine: in vitro and in vivo evaluations. *Int J Pharm* 487(1–2): 49–55.

Kahn R, Gorgon L, Jones K, McSherry F, Glover ED, Anthenelli RM, Jackson T, Williams J, Murtaugh C, Montoya I, Yu E, Elkashef A. 2012. Selegiline transdermal system (STS) as an aid for smoking cessation. *Nicotine Tob Res* 14(3): 377–382.

Kalaria DR, Patel P, Merino V, Patravale VB, Kalia YN. 2013. Controlled iontophoretic transport of Huperzine A across skin in vitro and in vivo: effect of delivery conditions and comparison of pharmacokinetic models. *Mol Pharm* Sep 13. [Epub ahead of print]

Kalaria DR, Patel P, Patravale V, Kalia YN. 2012. Comparison of the cutaneous iontophoretic delivery of rasagiline and selegiline across porcine and human skin in vitro. *Int J Pharm* 438(1–2): 202–208.

Kapil RP, Cipriano A, Friedman K, Michels G, Shet MS, Colucci SV, Apseloff G, Kitzmiller J, Harris SC. 2013. Once-weekly transdermal buprenorphine application results in sustained and consistent steady-state plasma levels. *J Pain Symptom Manage* 46(1): 65–75.

Kaunitz AM, Archer DF, Mishell DR, Foegh M. 2015. Safety and tolerability of a new low-dose contraceptive patch in obese and nonobese women. *Am J Obstet Gynecol* 212(3): 318. e1–8.

Kilfoyle BE, Sheihet L, Zhang Z, Laohoo M, Kohn J, Michniak-Kohn BB. 2012. Development of paclitaxel-TyroSpheres for topical skin treatment. *J Contr Rel* 163: 18–24.

Killen JD, Fortmann SP, Murphy GM Jr, Hayward C, Fong D, Lowenthal K, Bryson SW, Killen DT, Schatzberg AF. 2010. Failure to improve cigarette smoking abstinence with transdermal selegiline + cognitive behavior therapy. *Addiction* 105(9): 1660–1668.

Kim YH, Choi HY, Lim H-S, Lee SH, Jeon HS, Hong D, Kim SS, Choi YK, Bae K-S. 2015. Single dose pharmacokinetics of the novel transdermal donepezil patch in healthy volunteers. *Drug Des Dev Ther* 9: 1419–1426.

Kitzmiller JP, Barnett CJ, Steiner NS, Stoicea N, Kamar N, Luzum JA, Mikulik E, Bergese SD. 2015. Buprenorphine: revisiting the efficacy of transdermal delivery systems. *Ther Deliv* 6(4): 419–422.

Kochhar JS, Quek TC, Soon WJ, Choi J, Zou S, Kang L. 2013. Effect of microneedle geometry and supporting substrate on microneedle array penetration into skin. *J Pharm Sci* Sep 11. doi: 10.1002/jps.23724. [Epub ahead of print]

Kolli CS, Xiao J, Parsons DL, Babu RJ. 2012. Microneedle assisted iontophoretic transdermal delivery of prochlorperazine edisylate. *Drug Dev Ind Pharm* 38(5): 571–576.

Konda S, Meier-Davis SR, Cayme B, Shudo J, Maibach HI. 2012. Age-related percutaneous penetration part 2: effect of age on dermatopharmacokinetics and overvies of transdermal products. *Skin Ther Lett* 17(2): 5–7.

Kress HG, Boss H, Delvin T, Lahu G, Lophaven S, Marx M, Skorjanec S, Wagner T. 2010. Transdermal fentanyl matrix patches Matrifen and Durogesic DTrans are bioequivalent. *Eur J Pharm Biopharm* 75(2): 225–231.

Kristi J, Teskac K, Grabnar PA. 2010. Current view on nanosized solid lipid carriers for drug delivery to the skin. *J Biomed Nanotechnol* 6(5): 529–542.

Küchler S, Radowski MR, Blaschke T, Dathe M, Plendl J, Haag R, Schäfer-Korting M, Kramer KD. 2009. Nanoparticles for skin penetration enhancement – a comparison of a dendritic core-multishell-nanotransporter and solid lipid nanoparticles. *Eur J Pharm Biopharm* 71: 243–250.

Kuehl PJ, Stratton SP, Powell MB, Myrdal PB. 2009. Preformulation, formulation and in vivo efficacy of topically applied apomine. *Int J Pharm* 382: 104–110.

Kumar V, Banga AK. 2012. Modulated iontophoretic delivery of small and large molecules through microchannels. *Int J Pharm* 434(1–2): 106–114.

Lahm K, Lee G. 2006. Penetration of crystalline powder particles into excised human skin membranes and model gels from a supersonic powder injector. *J Pharm Sci* 95(7): 1511–1526.

Lane ME. 2013a. The transdermal delivery of fentanyl. *Eur J Pharm Biopharm* 84: 449–455.

Lane ME. 2013b. Skin penetration enhancers. *Int J Pharm* 447(1–2): 12–21.

Lanke SSS, Kolli CS, Strom JG, Banga AK. 2009. Enhanced transdermal delivery of low molecular weight heparin by barrier perturbation. *Int J Pharm* 365: 26–33.

Lee KE, Choi YJ, Oh BR, Chun IK, Gwak HS. 2013. Formulation and in vitro/in vivo evaluation of levodopa transdermal delivery systems. *Int J Pharm* Sep 2. pii: S0378–5173(13)00777-1. doi: 10.1016/j.ijpharm.2013.08.044. [Epub ahead of print]

Lefèvre G, Sedek G, Huang HL, Saltzman M, Rosenberg M, Kiese B, Fordham P. 2007. Pharmacokinetics of a rivastigmine transdermal patch formulation in healthy volunteers: relative effects of body site application. *J Clin Pharmacol* 47(4): 471–478.

Lefèvre G, Sedek G, Jhee SS, Leibowitz MT, Huang HL, Enz A, Maton S, Ereshefsky L, Pommier F, Schmidli H, Appel-Dingemanse S. 2008. Pharmacokinetics and pharmaco-dynamics of the novel daily rivastigmine transdermal patch compared with twice-daily capsules in Alzheimer's disease patients. *Clin Pharmacol Ther* 83(1): 106–114.

Lehman PA, Raney SG, Franz TJ. Percutaneous absorption in man: in vitro-in vivo correlation. 2011. *Skin Pharmacol Physiol* 24(4): 224–230

Leppert W, Malec-Milewska M, Zajaczkowska R, Wordliczek J. 2018. Transdermal and top-ical drug administration in the treatment of pain. *Molecules* 23: 681.

Lewitt PA, Boroojerdi B, Surmann E, Poewe W. 2013. Rotigotine transdermal system for long-term treatment of patients with advanced Parkinson's disease: results of two open-label extension studies, CLEOPATRA-PD and PREFER. *J Neural Transm* 120(7): 1069–1081.

Li L, Xu X, Fang L, Liu Y, Sun Y, Wang M, Zhao N, He Z. 2010. The transdermal patches for site-specific delivery of letrozole: a new option for breast cancer therapy. *AAPS PharmSciTech* 11(3): 1054–1057.

Likar R, Kayser H, Sittl R. 2006. Long-term management of chronic pain with transdermal buprenorphine: a multicenter, open-label, follow-up study in patients from three short-term clinical trials. *Clin Ther* 28(6): 943–952.

Liput DJ, Hammell DC, Stinchcomb AL, Nixon K. 2013. Transdermal delivery of cannabidiol attenuates binge alcohol-induced neurodegeneration in a rodent model of an alcohol use disorder. *Pharmacol Biochem Behav* Sep 5. pii: S0091–3057(13)00210-4. doi: 10.1016/j.pbb.2013.08.013. [Epub ahead of print]

Liu C, Fang L. 2015. Drug in adhesive patch of zolmitriptan: formulation and in vitro/in vivo correlation. *AAPS Pharm Sci Tech* Mar 14 [Epub ahead of print].

Liu J, Wang Z, Liu C, Xi H, Li C, Chen Y, Sun L, Mu L, Fang L. 2012. Silicone adhesive, a better matrix for tolterodine patches-a research based on in vitro/in vivo studies. *Drug Dev Ind Pharm* 38(8): 1008–1014.

Loder EW, Rayhill M, Burch RC. 2018. Safety problems with a transdermal patch for migraine: lessons from the development, approval, and marketing process. *Headache* 58: 1639–1657.

Löschmann PA, Chong PN, Nomoto M, Tepper PG, Horn AS, Jenner P, Marsden CD. 1989. Stereoselective reversal of MPTP-induced parkinsonism in the marmoset after dermal application of N-0437. *Eur J Pharmacol* 166(3): 373–380.

Lundborg M, Narangifard A, Wennberg CL, Lindahl E, Daneholt B, Norlen L. 2018. Human skin barrier structure and function analyzed by cryo-EM and molecular dynamics simu-lation. *J Structural Biol* 203: 149–161.

Machado M, Hadgraft J, Lane ME. 2010. Assessment of the variation of skin barrier function with anatomic site, age, gender and ethnicity. *Int J Cosmet Sci* 32: 397–409.

Madan JR, Argade NS, Dua K. 2015. Formulation and evaluation of transdermal patches of donepezil. *Recent Pat Drug Deliv Formul* 9(1): 95–103.

Magyar K. 2011. The pharmacology of selegiline. *Int Rev Neurobiol* 100: 65–84.

Mah CS, Kochhar JS, Ong PS, Kang L. 2013. A miniaturized flow-through cell to evaluate skin permeation of endoxifen. *Int J Pharm* 441(1–2): 433–440.

Majumder M, Stinchcomb A, Hinds BJ. 2010. Towards mimicking natural protein channels with aligned carbon nanotube membranes for active drug delivery. *Life Sci* 86: 563–568.

Malikou LS, Gargalionis AN, Piperi C, Papadavid E, Papavassiliou AG, Basdra EK. 2018. Molecular mechanisms of mechanotransduction in psoriasis. *Ann Transl Med* 6 (12): 245.

Mao YT, Hua HY, Zhang XG, Zhu DX, Li F, Gui ZH, Zhao YX. 2013. Ethosomes as delivery system for transdermal administration of vinpocetine. *Pharmazie* 68(5): 381–382.

Marier JF, Lor M, Potvin D, Dimarco M, Morelli G, Saedder EA. 2006. Pharmacokinetics, tolerability, and performance of a novel matrix transdermal delivery system of fentanyl relative to the commercially available reservoir formulation in healthy subjects. *J Clin Pharmacol* 46(6): 642–653.

Meadows KP, Pierce M, O'Neill C, Foster S, Jennings C. 2014. Samatriptan transdermal system can be correctly assembled and applied during migraine attacks. *Headache* 54(5): 850–860.

Melero A, Garrigues TM, Alós M, Kostka KH, Lehr CM, Schaefer UF. 2009. Nortriptyline for smoking cessation: release and human skin diffusion from patches. *Int J Pharm* 378(1–2): 101–107.

Menon GK, Cleary GW, Lane ME. 2012. The structure and function of the stratum corneum. *Int J Pharm* 435(1): 3–9.

Michaels AS, Chandrasekaran SK, Shaw JE. 1975. Drug permeation through human skin: theory and in vitro experimental measurement, *AIChE J* 21: 985–996.

Mitragotri S. 2013. Devices for overcoming biological barriers: the use of physical forces to disrupt the barriers. *Adv Drug Deliv Rev* 65(1): 100–103.

Moore KT, Adams HD, Natarajan J, Ariyawansa J, Richards HM. 2011. Bioequivalence and safety of a novel fentanyl transdermal matrix system compared with a transdermal reservoir system. *J Opioid Manag* 7(2): 99–107.

Mugglestone CJ, Mariz S, Lane ME. 2012. The development and registration of topical pharmaceuticals. *Int J Pharm* 435(1): 22–26.

Murthy SN. 1999. Magnetophoresis: an approach to enhance transdermal drug diffusion. *Pharmazie* 54: 377–379.

Murthy SN, Sammeta SM, Bowers C. 2010. Magnetophoresis for enhancing transdermal drug delivery: mechanistic studies and patch design. *J Control Rel* 148: 197–203.

Musazzi UM, Matera C, Dallanoce C, Vacondio F, De Amici M, Vistoli G, Cilurzo F, Minghetti P. 2015. On the selection of an opioid for local skin analgesia: structure-skin permeability relationships. *Int J Pharm* 489(1–2): 177–185.

Nafisi S, Schäfer-Korting M, Maibach HI. 2015. Perspectives on percutaneous penetration: silica nanoparticles. *Nanotox* 9: 643–657.

Nelson AL. 2015. Transdermal contraception methods: today's patches and new options on the horizon. *Expert Opin Pharmacother* 16(6): 863–873.

Nicoli S, Penna E, Padula C, Colombo P, Santi P. 2006. New transdermal bioadhesive film containing oxybutynin: in vitro permeation across rabbit ear skin. *Int J Pharm* 325(1–2): 2–7.

Nishifuji K, Yoon JS. 2013. The stratum corneum: the rampart of the mammalian body. *Vet Dermatol* 24(1): 60–72.

Nugroho AK, Li G, Grossklaus A, Danhof M, Bouwstra JA. 2004. Transdermal iontophoresis of rotigotine: influence of concentration, temperature and current density in human skin in vitro. *J Control Release* 96(1): 159–167.

Oertel W, Trenkwalder C, Beneš H, Ferini-Strambi L, Högl B, Poewe W, Stiasny-Kolster K, Fichtner A, Schollmayer E, Kohnen R, García-Borreguero D. 2011. Long-term safety and efficacy of rotigotine transdermal patch for moderate-to-severe idiopathic restless legs syndrome: a 5-year open-label extension study. *Lancet Neurol* 10(8): 710–720

Ortiz PG, Hansen SH, Shah VP, Menne T, Benfeldt E. 2009. Impact of adult atopic dermatitis on topical drug penetration: assessment by cutaneous microdialysis and tape stripping. *Acta Derm Venereol* 89: 33–38.

Osada T, Watanabe N, Asano N, Adachi Y, Yamamura K. 2018. Adverse drug events affecting medication persistence with rivastigmine patch application. *Patient Prefer Adherence* 12: 1247–1252.

Pae CU, Bodkin JA, Portland KB, Thase ME, Patkar AA. 2012. Safety of selegiline transdermal system in clinical practice: analysis of adverse events from postmarketing exposures. *J Clin Psychiatry* 73(5): 661–668.

Park CW, Son DD, Kim JY, Oh TO, Ha JM, Rhee YS, Park ES. 2012. Investigation of formulation factors affecting in vitro and in vivo characteristics of a galantamine transdermal system. *Int J Pharm* 436: 32–40.

Pastore MN, Kalia YN, Horstmann M, Roberts MS. 2015. Transdermal patches: history, development and pharmacology. *Br J Pharmacol* 172(9): 2179–2209.

Patel DR, Joshi A, Patel HH, Stagni G. 2015. Development and in-vivo evaluation of ondansetron gels for transdermal delivery. *Drug Dev Ind Pharm* 41(6): 1030–1036.

Patrick KS, Caldwell RW, Ferris RM, Breese GR. 1987. Pharmacology of the enantiomers of threo-methylphenidate. *J Pharmacol Exp Ther* 241(1): 152–158.

Pelham WE Jr, Manos MJ, Ezzell CE, Tresco KE, Gnagy EM, Hoffman MT, Onyango AN, Fabiano GA, Lopez-Williams A, Wymbs BT, Caserta D, Chronis AM, Burrows-Maclean L, Morse G. 2005a. A dose-ranging study of a methylphenidate transdermal system in children with ADHD. *J Am Acad Child Adolesc Psychiatry* 44(6): 522–529.

Pelham WE, Burrows-Maclean L, Gnagy EM, Fabiano GA, Coles EK, Tresco KE, Chacko A, Wymbs BT, Wienke AL, Walker KS, Hoffman MT. 2005b. Transdermal methylphenidate, behavioral, and combined treatment for children with ADHD. *Exp Clin Psychopharmacol* 13(2): 111–126.

Peptu C, Rotaru R, Ignat L, Hemelnicu AC, Harabagiu V, Peptu CA, Leon MM, Mitu F, Colocaru E, Boca A, Tamba BI. 2015. Nanotechnology approaches for pain therapy. *Curr Pharm Des* 21: 6125–6135.

Pergolizzi JV Jr, Mercadante S, Echaburu AV, Van den Eynden B, Fragoso RM, Mordarski S, Lybaert W, Beniak J, Orońska A, Slama O. 2009. The role of transdermal buprenorphine in the treatment of cancer pain: an expert panel consensus. *Curr Med Res Opin Curr Med Res Opin* 25(6): 1517–1528.

Pfister WR. 1997. Transdermal and dermal therapeutic systems: current status. In: Ghosh TK, Pfister WR, Yum SI (eds). *Transdermal and Topical Drug Delivery Systems*. Buffalo Grove: Interpharm Press Inc, pp. 33–112.

Pierce D, Dixon CM, Wigal SB, McGough JJ. 2008. Pharmacokinetics of methylphenidate transdermal system (MTS): results from a laboratory classroom study. *J Child Adolesc Psychopharmacol* 18(4): 355–364.

Pierce M, Marbury T, O'Neill C, Siegel S, Du W, Sebree T. 2009. Zelrix: a novel transdermal formulation of sumatriptan. *Headache* 49(6): 817–825.

Polinsky RJ. 1998. Clinical pharmacology of rivastigmine: a new-generation acetylcholinesterase inhibitor for the treatment of Alzheimer's disease. *Clin Ther* 20(4): 634–647.

Potts RO, Guy RH. 1992. Predicting skin permeability. *Pharm Res* 9: 663–669.

Pupe CG, Do Carmo FA, De Sousa VP, Lopes M, Abrahim-Vieira B, Ribeiro AJ, Veiga F, Rodrigues CR, Padula C, Santi P, Cabral LM. 2013. Development of a doxazosin and finasteride transdermal system for combination therapy of benign prostatic hyperplasia. *J Pharm Sci* 102: 4057–4064.

Quinn HL, Bonham L, Hughes CM, Donnelly RF. 2015. Design of a dissolving microneedle platform for transdermal delivery of a fixed-dose combination of cardiovascular drugs. *J Pharm Sci* 104: 3490–3500.

Razzaque Z, Heald MA, Pickard JD, Maskell L, Beer MS, Hill RG, Longmore J. 1999. Vasoconstriction in human isolated middle meningeal arteries: determining the contribution of 5-HT1B- and 5-HT1F-receptor activation. *Br J Clin Pharmacol* 47(1): 75–82.

Regenthal R, Voskanian M, Baumann F, Teichert J, Brätter C, Aigner A, Abraham G. 2018. Pharmacokinetic evaluation of a transdermal anastrozole-in-adhesive formulation. *Drug Des Dev Ther* 12: 3653–3664.

Roberts MS, Cross SE, Pellett MA. 2002. Skin transport. In Walters KA (ed.) *Dermatological and Transdermal Formulations*. New York: Marcel Dekker, pp. 89–195.

Roberts MS, Walters KA, eds. 2008. *Dermal Absorption and Toxicity Assessment*, 2nd Edition. New York: Informa Healthcare.

Rohatagi S, Barrett JS, McDonald LJ, Morris EM, Darnow J, DiSanto AR. 1997. Selegiline percutaneous absorption in various species and metabolism by human skin. *Pharm Res* 14(1): 50–55.

Ronnander P, Simon L, Spilgies H, Koch A, Scherr S. 2018. Dissolving polyvinylpyrrolidone-based microneedle systems for in-vitro delivery of sumitriptan succinate. *Eur J Pharm Sci* 114: 84–92.

Roy SD, Roos E, Sharma K. 1994. Transdermal delivery of buprenorphine through cadaver skin. *J Pharm Sci* 83(2): 126–130.

Sachdeva V, Zhou Y, Banga AK. 2013. In vivo transdermal delivery of leuprolide using microneedles and iontophoresis. *Curr Pharm Biotechnol* 14(2): 180–193.

Sallam MA, Motawaa AM, Mortada SM. 2015. An insight on human skin penetration of diflunisal: lipogel versus hydrogel microemulsion. *Drug Dev Ind Pharm* 41(1): 141–147.

Saluja S, Kasha PC, Paturi J, Anderson C, Morris R, Banga AK. 2013. A novel electronic skin patch for delivery and pharmacokinetic evaluation of donepezil following transdermal iontophoresis. *Int J Pharm* 453(2): 395–399.

Sammeta SM, Repka MA, Murthy SN. 2011. Magnetophoresis in combination with chemical enhancers for transdermal drug delivery. *Drug Dev Ind Pharm* 37: 1076–1082.

Santos P, Watkinson AC, Hadgraft J, Lane ME. 2008. Application of microemulsions in dermal and transdermal drug delivery. *Skin Pharmacol Physiol* 21(5): 246–529.

Santos P, Watkinson AC, Hadgraft J, Lane ME. 2010. Oxybutynin permeation in skin: the influence of drug and solvent activity. *Int J Pharm* 384(1–2): 67–72.

Scheuplein RJ, Blank IH. 1971. Permeability of the skin. *Physiol Rev* 51: 702–747.

Schwarz JC, Klang V, Hoppel M, Mahrhauser D, Valenta C. 2012. Natural microemulsions: formulation design and skin interaction. *Eur J Pharm Biopharm* 81(3): 557–562.

Schwengber A, Prado HJ, Zilli DA, Bonelli PR, Cukierman AL. 2015. Carbon nanotubes buckypapers for potential transdermal drug delivery. *Mater Sci Eng C Mater Biol Appl* 57: 7–13.

Sebel PS, Barrett CW, Kirk CJ, Heykants J. 1987. Transdermal absorption of fentanyl and sufentanil in man. *Eur J Clin Pharmacol* 32(5): 529–531.

Shahid N, Siddique MI, Razzaq Z, Katas H, Wagas MK, Rahman KU. 2018. Fabrication and characterization of matrix type transdermal patches loaded with tizanidine hydrochloride: potential sustained release delivery system. *Drug Dev Ind Pharm* 44: 2061–2070.

Shahzad Y, Louw R, Gerber M, du Plessis J. 2015. Breaching the skin barrier through temperature modulations. *J Contr Rel* 202: 1–13.

Sharma S, Howells O, Rajendran N, Mcintyre S, Amni-Asi S, Henri P, Liu Y, Guy O, Cass AEG, Morris MC. 2019. Microneedle array-based platforms for future theranostic applications. *Chembiochem* doi: 10.1002/cbic.201900112

Shimizu K, Hayashida K, Blajan M. 2015. Novel method to improve transdermal drug delivery by atmospheric microplasma irradiation. *Biointerphases* 10(2): 029516.

Siafaka PI, Barmpalexis P, Lazaridou M, Papageorgiou GZ, Koutris E, Karavas E, Kostoglou M, Bikiaris DN. 2015. Controlled release formulations of risperidone antipsychotic drug in novel aliphatic polyester carriers: data analysis and modeling. *Eur J Pharm Biopharm* 94: 473–484.

Siegel SJ, O'Neill C, Dubé LM, Kaldeway P, Morris R, Jackson D, Sebree T. 2007. A unique iontophoretic patch for optimal transdermal delivery of sumatriptan. *Pharm Res* 24(10): 1919–1926.

Simmons K, Parkman HP. 2014. Granisetron transdermal system improves refractory nausea and vomiting in gastroparesis. *Dig Dis Sci* 59(6): 1231–1234.

Simon L, Goyal A. 2009. Dynamics and control of percutaneous drug absorption in the presence of epidermal turnover. *J Pharm Sci* 98: 187–204.

Simon L, Kim KS, Kanneganti K. 2011. Effects of epidermal turnover on the dynamics of percutaneous drug absorption. *Math Biosci* 229(1): 16–21.

Singh ND, Banga AK. 2013. Controlled delivery of ropinirole hydrochloride through skin using modulated iontophoresis and microneedles. *J Drug Target* 21(4): 354–366.

Singh P, Boniello S, Liu P, Dinh S. 1999. Transdermal iontophoretic delivery of methylphenidate HCl in vitro. *Int J Pharm* 178(1): 121–128.

Sittl R, Griessinger N, Likar R. 2003. Analgesic efficacy and tolerability of transdermal buprenorphine in patients with inadequately controlled chronic pain related to cancer and other disorders: a multicenter, randomized, double-blind, placebo-controlled trial. *Clin Ther* 25(1): 150–168.

Skaer TL. 2014. Dosing considerations with transdermal formulations of fentanyl and buprenorphine for the treatment of cancer pain. *J Pain Res* 7: 495–503.

Smallwood GH, Meador ML, Lenihan JP, Shangold GA, Fisher AC, Creasy GW, ORTHO EVRA/EVRA 002 Study Group. 2001. Efficacy and safety of a transdermal contraceptive system. *Obstet Gynecol* 98: 799–805.

Smith EW, Maibach HI, eds. 2005. *Percutaneous Penetration Enhancers*, 2nd Edition. Boca Raton: Taylor & Francis.

Smith MT, Wyse BD, Edwards SR, El-Tamimy M, Gaetano G, Gavin P. 2015. Topical application of a novel oxycodone gel formulation (tocopherol phosphate mixture) in a rat model of peripheral inflammatory pain produces localized pail relief without significant systemic exposure. *J Pharm Sci* 104(7): 2388–2396.

Smith TR, Goldstein J, Singer R, Pugach N, Silberstein S, Pierce MW. 2012. Twelve-month tolerability and efficacy study of NP101, the sumatriptan iontophoretic transdermal system. *Headache* 52(4): 612–624.

Soler LI, Boix A, Lauroba J, Colom H, Domenech J. 2012. Transdermal delivery of alprazolam from a monolithic patch: formulation based on in vitro characterization. *Drug Dev Ind Pharm* 38(10): 1171–1178.

Sonneville-Aubrun O, Simonnet JT, L'Alloret F. 2004. Nanoemulsions: a new vehicle for skincare products. *Adv Colloid Interface Sci* 108–109: 145–149.

Sozio P, Cerasa LS, Marinelli L, Di Stefano A. 2012. Transdermal donepezil on the treatment of Alzheimer's disease. *Neuropsychiatr Dis Treat* 8: 361–368.

Srinivas NR, Hubbard JW, Korchinski ED, Midha KK. 1993. Enantioselective pharmacokinetics of dl-threo-methylphenidate in humans. *Pharm Res* 10(1): 14–21.

Staskin DR, Dmochowski RR, Sand PK, Macdiarmid SA, Caramelli KE, Thomas H, Hoel G. 2009. Efficacy and safety of oxybutynin chloride topical gel for overactive bladder: a randomized, double-blind, placebo controlled, multicenter study. *J Urol* 181(4): 1764–1772.

Staskin DR, Rosenberg MT, Dahl NV, Polishuk PV, Zinner NR. 2008. Effects of oxybutynin transdermal system on health-related quality of life and safety in men with overactive bladder and prostate conditions. *Int J Clin Pract* 62(1): 27–38.

Steiner DJ, Sitar S, Wen W, Sawyerr G, Munera C, Ripa SR, Landau C. 2011. Efficacy and safety of the seven-day buprenorphine transdermal system in opioid-naïve patients with moderate to severe chronic low back pain: an enriched, randomized, double-blind, placebo-controlled study. *J Pain Symptom Manage* 42(6): 903–917.

Stewart WF, Van Rooyen JB, Cundiff GW, Abrams P, Herzog AR, Corey R, Hunt TL, Wein AJ. 2003. Prevalence and burden of overactive bladder in the United States. *World J Urol* 20(6): 327–336.

Stiasny-Kolster K, Kohnen R, Schollmayer E, Möller JC, Oertel WH. 2004. Patch application of the dopamine agonist rotigotine to patients with moderate to advanced stages of restless legs syndrome: a double-blind, placebo-controlled pilot study. *Mov Disord* 19(12): 1432–1438.

Stinchcomb AL, Paliwal A, Dua R, Imoto H, Woodard RW, Flynn GL. 1996. Permeation of buprenorphine and its 3-alkyl-ester prodrugs through human skin. *Pharm Res* 13(10): 1519–1523.

Sun W, Araci Z, Inayathullah M, Manickam S, Zhang X, Bruce MA, Marinkovich MP, Lane AT, Milla C, Rajadas J, Butte MJ. 2013. Polyvinylpyrrolidone microneedles enable delivery of intact proteins for diagnostic and therapeutic applications. *Acta Biomater* 9(8): 7767–7774.

Swart PJ, De Zeeuw RA. 1992. Extensive gastrointestinal metabolic conversion limits the oral bioavailability of the dopamine D2 agonist N-0923 in freely moving rats. *Pharmazie* 47: 613–615.

Tamelier J, Chary S, Turner KL. 2013. Importance of loading and unloading procedures for gecko-inspired controllable adhesives. *Langmuir* 29(34): 10881–10890.

Tavano L, Gentile L, Oliviero Rossi C, Muzzalupo R. 2013. Novel gel-niosomes formulations as multicomponent systems for transdermal drug delivery. *Colloids Surf B Biointerfaces* 110: 281–288.

Tenreiro-Pinto J, Pereira FC, Loureiro MC, Gama R, Fernandes HL. 2018. Efficacy analysis of capsaicin 8% patch in neuropathic peripheral pain treatment. *Pharmacol* 101: 290–297.

Timmerman W, Westerink BH, De Vries JB, Tepper PG, Horn AS. 1989. Microdialysis and striatal dopamine release: stereoselective actions of the enantiomers of N-0437. *Eur J Pharmacol* 162(1): 143–210.

Trenkwalder C, Winkelmann J, Inoue Y, Paulus W. 2015. Restless leg syndrome – current therapies and management of augmentation. *Nat Rev Neurol* 11(8): 434–445.

Trottet L, Merly C, Mirza M, Hadgraft J, Davis AF. 2004. Effect of finite doses of propylene glycol on enhancement of in vitro percutaneous permeation of loperamide hydrochloride. *Int J Pharm* 274(1–2): 213–219.

Tse FL, Laplanche R. 1998. Absorption, metabolism, and disposition of [$^{14}$C]SDZ ENA 713, an acetylcholinesterase inhibitor, in minipigs following oral, intravenous, and dermal administration. *Pharm Res* 15(10): 1614–1620.

Vikelis M, Mitsikostas DD, Rapoport AM. 2014. Sumatriptan iontophoretic transdermal system for the acute treatment of migraine. *Pain Manag* 4(2): 123–128.

Vikelis M, Springos KC, Rapoport AM. 2015. The iontophoretic transdermal system of sumatriptan as a new option in the acute treatment of migraine: a perspective. *Ther Adv Neurol Disord* 8(4): 160–165.

Vučen SR, Vuleta G, Crean AM, Moore AC, Ignjatović N, Uskoković D. 2013. Improved percutaneous delivery of ketoprofen using combined application of nanocarriers and silicon microneedles. *J Pharm Pharmacol* 65(10): 1451–1462.

Walczak A, Siger M, Ciach A, Szczepanik M, Selmaj K. 2013. Transdermal application of myelin peptides in multiple sclerosis treatment. *JAMA Neurol* Jul 1: 1–6. doi:

Walsh L, Ryu J, Bock S, Koval M, Mauro T, Ross R, Desai T. 2015. Nanotopography facilitates in vivo transdermal delivery of high molecular weight therapeutics through an integrin-dependent mechanism. *Nano Lett* 15(4): 2434–2441.

Walters KA, ed. 2002. *Dermatological and Transdermal Formulations*. New York: Marcel Dekker.

Walters KA, Abdalghafor H, Lane ME. 2012. The human nail: barrier characterisation and permeation enhancement. *Int J Pharm* 435(1): 10–21.

Walters KA, Hadgraft J, eds. 1993. *Pharmaceutical Skin Penetration Enhancement*. New York: Marcel Dekker.

Wang Z, Mu HJ, Zhang XM, Ma PK, Lian SN, Zhang FP, Chu SY, Zhang WW, Wang AP, Wang WY, Sun KX. 2015. Lower irritation microemulsion-based rotigotine gel: formulation optimization and in vitro and in vivo studies. *Int J Nanomedicine* 10: 633–644.

Warshaw EM, Paller AS, Fowler JF, Zirwas MJ. 2008. Practical management of cutaneous reactions to the methylphenidate transdermal system: recommendations from a dermatology expert panel consensus meeting. *Clin Ther* 30(2): 326–337.

Warshaw EM, Squires L, Li Y, Civil R, Paller AS. 2010. Methylphenidate transdermal system: a multisite, open-label study of dermal reactions in pediatric patients diagnosed with ADHD. *Prim Care Comp J Clin Psychiatry* 12(6). pii: PCC.10m00996. doi: 10.4088/PCC.10m00996pur.

Watkinson AC. 2013. A commentary on transdermal drug delivery systems in clinical trials. *J Pharm Sci* 102(9): 3082–3088.

Watkinson AC, Bunge AL, Hadgraft J, Lane ME. 2013. Nanoparticles do not penetrate human skin – a theoretical perspective. *Pharm Res* 30: 1943–1946.

Watts RL, Jankovic J, Waters C, Rajput A, Boroojerdi B, Rao J. 2007. Randomized, blind, controlled trial of transdermal rotigotine in early Parkinson disease. *Neurology* 68(4): 272–276.

Wiedersberg S, Guy RH. 2014. Transdermal drug delivery: 30+ years of war and still fighting! *J Control Rel* 190: 150–156.

Wilens TE, Morrison NR, Prince J. 2011. An update on the pharmacotherapy of attention-deficit/hyperactivity disorder in adults. *Expert Rev Neurother* 11(10): 1443–1465.

Wilkinson M, Pfaffenrath V, Schoenen J, Diener HC, Steiner TJ. 1995. Migraine and cluster headache--their management with sumatriptan: a critical review of the current clinical experience. *Cephalalgia* 15(5): 337–357.

Williams AC, Walters KA. 2008. Chemical penetration enhancement: possibilities and problems. In Walters KA, Roberts MS. (eds) *Dermatologic, Cosmeceutic, and Cosmetic Development: Therapeutic and Novel Approaches*. New York: Informa Healthcare, pp. 497–504.

Wimbiscus M, Kostenko O, Malone D. 2010. MAO inhibitors: risks, benefits, and lore. *Cleveland Clin J Med* 77: 859–882.

Winblad B, Cummings J, Andreasen N, Grossberg G, Onofrj M, Sadowsky C, Zechner S, Nagel J, Lane R. 2007. A six-month double-blind, randomized, placebo-controlled study of a transdermal patch in Alzheimer's disease--rivastigmine patch versus capsule. *Int J Geriatr Psychiatry* 22(5): 456–467.

Woitalla D, Kassubek J, Timmermann L, Lauterbach T, Berkels R, Grieger F, Müller T. 2015. Reduction of gastrointestinal symptoms in Parkinson's disease after a switch from oral therapy to rotigotine transdermal patch: a non-interventional prospective multicenter trial. *Parkinsonism Relat Disord* 21(3): 199–204.

Wokovich AM, Shen M, Doub WH, Machado SG, Buhse LF. 2011. Evaluating elevated release liner adhesion of a transdermal drug delivery system (TDDS): a study of Daytrana™ methylphenidate transdermal system. *Drug Dev Ind Pharm* 37(10): 1217–1224.

Wong TW. 2014. Electrical, magnetic, photomechanical and cavitational waves to overcome skin barrier for transdermal drug delivery. *J Control Rel* 193: 257–269.

Woo FY, Basri M, Masoumi HRF, Ahmad MB, Ismail M. 2015. Formulation optimization of galantamine hydrobromide loaded gel drug reservoirs in transdermal patch for Alzheimer's disease. *Int J Nanomed* 10: 3879–3886.

Yang Q, Guy RH. 2015. Characterisation of skin barrier function using bioengineering and biophysical techniques. *Pharm Res* 32(2): 445–457.

Yu X, Jin Y, Du L, Sun M, Wang J, Li Q, Zhang X, Gao Z, Ding P. 2018. Transdermal cubic phases of metformin hydrochloride: in silico and in vitro studies of delivery mechanisms. *Mol Pharm* 15: 3121–3132.

Zhang YT, Han MQ, Shen LN, Zhao JH, Feng NP. 2015. Solid lipid nanoparticles formulated for transdermal aconitine administration and evaluation in vitro and in vivo. *J Biomed Nanotechnol* 11(2): 351–361.

Zhou W, He S, Yang Y, Jian D, Chen X, Ding J. 2015. Formulation characterization and clinical evaluation of propranolol hydrochloride gel for transdermal treatment of superficial infantile hemangioma. *Drug Dev Ind Pharm* 41(7): 1109–1119.

Zobrist RH, Schmid B, Feick A, Quan D, Sanders SW. 2001. Pharmacokinetics of the R- and S-enantiomers of oxybutynin and N-desethyloxybutynin following oral and transdermal administration of the racemate in healthy volunteers. *Pharm Res* 18(7): 1029–1034.

# 2 Preclinical and Clinical Safety Assessment of Transdermal and Topical Dermatological Products

*Lindsey C. Yeh and Howard I. Maibach*

## CONTENTS

## 2.1   INTRODUCTION

Since 1979, after the U.S. FDA approved the first transdermal patch, there has been successful marketing of numerous transdermal drug delivery systems. Transdermal patches have advantages over oral medications including reduction of first-pass drug-degradation effects, reduction in adverse effects and convenient painless medication administration. Efforts have been made to improve transdermal transport with chemical enhancers, use of electric fields (iontophoresis and electroporation) and ultrasound. However, many limitations exist in the development of transdermal delivery systems, which partly account for the limited number of products marketed over the last 30 years. The assessment of the safety of transdermal and topical dermatologic products is often a long and incompletely developed process, but on the basis of three decades of experience, manageable.

## 2.2   PREDICTING SKIN PERMEABILITY

Transdermal and topical transport of medications depends on permeation through the stratum corneum (SC). Permeation of drug molecules across the SC is primarily via passive diffusion and through a combination of intercellular lipid domains and transcellular and shunt routes (the appendages). Some barrier properties of the SC are imparted from the lipids in the cell membranes. Lipids are major constituents of the membrane and removal of lipids from the membrane may destroy barrier properties. Lipophilic substances, more than hydrophilics, penetrate the lipid-rich cell membrane with relative ease. Small, polar, water-soluble molecules may gain access through small pores between the protein subunits. Shunt diffusion describes diffusion through the pilosebaceous units and sweat glands, which are argued to only minimally effect absorption through the SC since the opening of the appendages only account for 1/10,000 of the total body surface area. The triviality of shunt diffusion is supported by observations that diffusion is not impaired in those with congenital absence of sweat glands (Brisson, 1974). However, shunt diffusion may play a more significant role during periods of high flux or in molecules with low permeability constants such as large molecules. In vitro studies comparing compounds show variability in the role of shunt pathways (Stahl et al., 2012). The intercellular route is the primary transport route of molecules that are insoluble in lipid membranes such as electrolytes. Other than transport of electrolytes, intercellular routes play a smaller role in absorption.

Passive diffusion is determined by the molecular and physical properties of the solute, the vehicle, the skin and their respective interactions. Numerous factors can alter transport. Hydration of the SC, thus water and humidity, can influence transport. An approximately five-fold increase in permeability is found after maximum hydration of the epidermis. Paradoxically, dehydration also enhances absorption due to physical damage to the barrier. Keratolytics (e.g., salicylic acid) are absorption enhancers because they damage the SC. Local hyperemia increases flux by rapid removal of diffusing molecules across the epidermis, creating a greater concentration gradient. Increased temperature also increases absorption through increases in molecular motion. Dermatoses exhibiting parakeratosis (namely psoriasis and eczema) impair barrier function and topical penetration may be greater. The solvent (vehicle) plays a critical role in diffusion as it plays a factor in the partition coefficient. The level of occlusion provided by the vehicle effects hydration and temperature and the more occlusive the vehicle, the greater the absorption.

Mathematical models have been proposed to predict skin permeability. These models were produced based on data compiled from various sources, laboratories and databases, which inevitably resulted in experimental variation. In an attempt to describe and account for the processes involved, many of the mathematical models are complex and cumbersome to use. The models are largely derived from in vitro studies. However, the majority of models derived from in vitro studies may underestimate in vivo data. The observed data is one to even 10,000 times greater than the predicted data from some of these models (Farahmand and Maibach, 2009).

A simple mathematical model of transepidermal diffusion can be expressed using Fick's law of diffusion. Fick's law postulates that the magnitude of diffusion of a molecule across a membrane is directly proportional to the concentration gradient moving from an area of high concentration to an area of low concentration and to the surface area of the membrane through which diffusion is taking place. Rate of diffusion is inversely related to membrane thickness. J is representative of diffusion flux through a set area for a set time interval (amount of substance per unit area per unit time, $mol/m^2 \cdot s$). Dm is the diffusion coefficient, a constant characteristic of the inherent mobility of a molecule. L is the length of the diffusion pathway, which is the thickness of the membrane in percutaneous absorbability testing. The partition coefficient (Km) is the velocity of drug passage through membrane in $\mu g/cm^2/h$ and must be considered when calculating flux for molecules other than water. The higher the Km for a solute, the easier it is for the molecule to diffuse and leave solvent. Cs is the concentration gradient ($C_{donor} - C_{receptor}$) between donor and receptor chambers.

$$\text{Rate of Diffusion} = \frac{\text{Partition Coefficient} \times \text{Diffusion Coefficient} \times \text{Concentration Gradient}}{\text{Membrane Thickness}}$$

$$\text{Or} \quad J = \frac{Km \times Dm \times \left( C_{donor} - C_{receptor} \right)}{L}$$

The most basic of the models that represent in vitro skin diffusion is applied when an infinite volume of well stirred vehicle is available and the solute penetrates the skin or other membrane to the receptor compartment that is a sink for the solute. Models vary if the volume of the vehicle is finite or if the receptor compartment can be saturated. Losses in vehicle or solute volume are due to evaporation, volatilization or adsorption to skin surface

Interactions between solute-vehicle, vehicle-skin and solute-skin interactions lead to complex variations in time and space dependent change in diffusivity.

## 2.3  IN VITRO METHODS FOR PERCUTANEOUS ABSORPTION MEASUREMENTS

Many experimental models exist for the study of percutaneous absorption, each with their own advantages. In vitro studies are possible because the permeability properties of the skin are maintained even after excision because the stratum corneum is non-viable. A commonly used model is a two-chamber diffusion cell, which measures the passage of substance from one chamber through a membrane. The diffusion cell consists of the donor compartment, a permeation membrane and a receptor compartment. The donor compartment varies depending on whether the drug dose delivered is an infinite or finite dose. A finite dosage of the donor solution is representative of the typical delivery profile of a topical dosage form. The penetration of solution in a finite dose system has an initial period of lag time prior to the onset of peak delivery. Topical dosage delivery is affected by evaporation of solvent that concentrates the drug, which in turn changes the composition of the enhancer mixture since more volatile components evaporate more quickly. Evaporation may also cause supersaturates and precipitates of the drug on the skin surface. Infinite dosage is common in transdermal delivery systems. If the donor compartment is covered to prevent evaporation or if the permeant dose is large, the dose is then finite. The third type of donor is a patch design. Transdermal patches provide both infinite and finite delivery and are represented in the donor compartment as such.

Ideally, human skin would be used as the permeation membrane, however, multiple factors prevent the wide spread use of human tissue in studies. The use of human skin is subject to ethical considerations and conditions. A pragmatic substitute is the use of in vitro animal skin in preclinical studies for drug development, which are currently widely used and studied. Permeability across animal skins varies from human skin due to variations in histology and permeability. Alternatives to human skin include primate, porcine, mouse, rat, guinea pig and snakeskin with varying degrees of comparability to human skin. There inter-individual and intra-individual variations among the species are relatively small among skin specimens from inbred animal strains (Takeuchi et al., 2011).

Animal skin of the pig or miniature pig and rhesus monkey have been proven to be a good animal model, however rodents (mice, rats and guinea pigs) are used more commonly for in vitro dermal toxicity studies (Bronaugh et al., 2005, Simon and Maibach, 1998, Simon and Maibach 2000). The advantages of using rodents are their small size, easy handling and affordability. Permeability of drugs varies between species and between drugs. It is not possible to establish a consistent relationship across various drugs between diffusion through animal skin and diffusion through human skin. This poses a limitation to the applicability of in vitro animal skin models.

Structural differences exist between human and animal skin such as the quality and quantity of hair follicles and in different animal species, thickness of the dermis and epidermis as well as the quality of the dermal-epidermal junction compared to human skin. The lipid content of skin acts as the major barrier and lipid content between species and anatomical sites are highly variable. Studies suggest that laboratory animal skin is often more permeable than human tissue, while pig and monkey are most similar to that of human tissue (Bronaugh and Stewart, 1985, Simon and Maibach, 1998, Simon and Maibach 2000). Skin permeability has been reported to increase in the following order: man, weanling pig, monkey, dog, cat, horse, rabbit, goat, guinea pig and mouse (McGreesh, 1965; Marzulli et al., 1969; Bartek et al., 1972).

Mouse skin is more permeable than human skin due to the thinner SC and is therefore an inferior in vivo model compared to other animal models (Marzulli et al., 1969; Bronaugh et al., 1982b; Scott et al., 1986; Simon and Maibach, 1998). The SC of humans is 16.8µm while the SC of the mouse is only 5.8µm. Although the hairless mouse also has a SC that is less than half the thickness of the human, the skin structure somewhat resembles human skin because of the sparse, thin hair growth. Studies have shown that the permeation characteristics of the hairless mouse are similar to human tissue for some compounds while very different for others (Simon and Maibach, 1998).

Rat skin is more permeable than human skin (Marzulli and Maibach, 1975, Bartek et al., 1972). Rat skin remains a suitable model for absorption in certain circumstances. Comparison of in vivo and in vitro absorption studies in rats has shown good correlation between human and rat skin (Bronaugh et al., 1982a). The use of guinea pig as a model in absorption studies has been limited. The appearance of guinea pig skin is similar to human skin, but tends to have greater permeability than human tissue, however there is limited data regarding correlation with human skin (Wester and Maibach, 1985, Andersen et al., 1980). Rabbit skin is much more permeable than human skin and is therefore a poor model for absorption studies, but the rapid absorptive qualities of rabbit skin may make it desirable for testing dermal toxicity (Bronaugh et al., 1982b). In vitro studies of pig or miniature pig skin correlate well with human skin in vivo despite the larger diameter of skin follicles found in pig skin. The density of hair follicles in pig skin is the lowest density found in any laboratory model. A less obvious, but acceptable, in vitro model is shed snakeskin. Snakeskin has many advantages supporting its use. Although it is not of mammalian origin, the lack of hair follicles and rate of compound penetration are similar with human skin (Rigg and Barry, 1990, Takahashi et al., 1993). The molted skin of snakes is what is used in the studies. Since this is a natural process, there is no harm inflicted on the animal and a single snake provides multiple specimens, which also eliminates inter-individual variability.

Human skin membrane may better correlate with in vivo human skin permeation. Split thickness skin (typically 200–400 µm thick) epidermal membranes prepared or full thickness skin with dermatome can be used, however full thickness skin should be no more than approximately 1mm and only used if required for testing of the chemical. Availability of good-quality human skin is limited. Human skin can be obtained from outdated skin graft tissue, cadaver skin or skin derived from cosmetic or other surgical procedures. There is variation in permeability in human skin tissue depending on the donor site and age and race of the donor from which the skin was obtained. Skin permeability can even vary from the same individual or among specimens procured from the same site. Therefore, the choice of anatomical site should be provided.

When selecting and preparing specimens, it is best to select from a consistent site of the body and document age, sex, race of donor and how the specimen was obtained. Storage and preservation of human skin poses another challenge for in vitro human skin studies. The proper maintenance and preservation of human skin creates a model more similar to an in vivo situation (Wester et al., 1998). Human cadaver skin is partially or wholly viable and is metabolically and enzymatically active for up to eight days after death when stored in Eagles Minimum Essential Media with Earle's Balanced Salt Solution with gentamicin and refrigerated at 4°C. Both freezing of the skin at −22°C or heat-treating the skin at 60°C, mimicking a procedure used for separation of the epidermis from the dermis, are detrimental to the viability of the skin (Wester et al., 1998). The OECD guideline specifies that the barrier function must be maintained for the testing of chemicals, but does not list specific requirements regarding optimal storage. It states that freshly excised skin should be used within 24 hours, but the acceptable storage period may vary depending on the enzyme system involved in metabolism and storage temperatures (OECD, 2004). Human skin samples stored at 80°C for three weeks prior to use in in vitro studies on percutaneous penetration leads to an overestimation of penetration rate and total penetration due to structural changes in the upper and deeper regions of the dermis (Nielsen et al., 2011). Current recommendations from the European Centre of the Validation of Alternative Methods (ECVAM) on methods for assessing percutaneous absorption state that skin samples can be stored at 20°C. The Environmental Health Criteria on dermal absorption issued by the International Programme of Chemical Safety states that human skin could be stored up to one year at 20°C, which is based on studies by Bronaugh et al. (1986). Regardless of storage conditions, evidence of the integrity of the barrier function of skin must be proven. This can be accomplished by conducting a preliminary permeability investigation using a model diffusing compound, such as tritiated water, and comparing the results obtained to expected permeability values for that membrane type (Bronaugh et al., 1982a). Simple bio-engineering equipment for measuring transfer (transepidermal water loss) is widely used (Levin and Maibach, 2005, Nangia, et al., 2005).

Synthetic membranes (including cellulose media and synthetic polymers) have also been studied as options to use as the permeation membrane in studies of percutaneous absorption. Synthetic membranes reduce use of experimental animals and are easily available, stable and uniform between batches which all allow better control of experimental conditions (Sato and Wan Kim, 1984). Cellulose media is made from plant fiber and consists of glucopyranose rings joined by $\beta$-1,4-linkages giving it a relatively rigid structure. Commercially available cellulose media typically have a cut off of 8,000–15,000 Daltons for molecular dialysis and contain softener, preservative and plasticizer additives, which may interfere with drug permeation. These substances are water-soluble and can be removed by soaking the membrane in water, or boiling the water as recommended by the manufacturer. Generally, cellulose membranes are reported to be more permeable than biological membranes or aporous synthetic media (Touitou and Abed, 1985). Silicone has been considered a useful synthetic membrane for use in diffusion cell systems for its inert and lipophilic nature, making it an ideal environment for the permeation of lipophilic drugs, while still rate limiting due to its aporosity (Haigh and Smith). Overall, the use of synthetic membranes is limited due to the poor adaptability to in vivo situations.

The receptor chamber is typically filled with a solution of physiologic saline or phosphate-buffered solution. The chemical of interest must be soluble in the receptor fluid so that absorption of the test substance is not hindered. The receptor fluid also serves an additional function of supporting skin viability. Eagle's minimal essential medium (MEM), Hepes-buffered Hanks' balanced salt solution (HHBSS) or Dulbecco modified phosphate-buffered saline (DMPBS) sustain viability and histpathologic integrity in rat skin for 24 hours (Collier et al., 1989) and are appropriate options for receptor fluid. The receptor fluid may further preserve the viability of the skin with the addition of antimicrobials. Use of phosphate-buffered saline (PBS) as the receptor fluid showed autolysis of the epidermis and dermis within 24 hours and a loss of anaerobic and aerobic metabolic activity (Collier et al., 1989). The concentration of the drug in the receptor fluid must be kept below saturation in order that steady-state flux can be maintained (Crutcher and Maibach, 1969). This can be accomplished by changing the receptor fluid frequently (flow through systems) – as popularized by Marzulli, Bronaugh and others.

In attempt to mimic human exposure, OECD recommends that application of the compound covers 1–5 $mg/cm^2$ of skin for a solid and up to ten $1/cm^2$ for liquids in finite dosing. Infinite dosing would require application of large volumes per unit area. Another aspect to take into consideration is maintaining the skin at a constant temperature close to normal skin temperature of $32°C \pm 1°C$ and humidity should be between 30–70%. Depending on the cell design, temperature is regulated by water baths or heated block temperatures.

Duration of exposure should also mimic human exposure. Shorter time intervals are usually most consistent with in vivo exposure. Exposure for 24 hours is often required to adequately characterize the absorption profile. However, skin integrity may deteriorate after 24 hours.

## 2.4  IN VIVO METHODS FOR PERCUTANEOUS ABSORPTION MEASUREMENTS

The quality of animal skin as a model for evaluation of properties of percutaneous absorption, irritation and toxicity of drugs has been widely studied (Bronaugh et al., 2005). Although animal skin is not identical, it poses as an acceptable alternative in preclinical testing of transdermal drug delivery systems (TDDS). While the in vitro animal models provide information regarding flux of the drugs, the in vivo animal testing provide information on skin and clinical toxicology prior to use in humans in vivo. In vivo studies use a system that is physiologically and metabolically intact rather than an isolated system used in in vitro studies, which allows analysis with the vascular system and viable enzymes.

In vivo studies are cumbersome in that they require the use of live animals, and often the need for radiolabeled material. Overall, the skin of rats and rabbits are more permeable than human skin. Guinea pigs (post auricular), pigs and monkey skin permeability are most similar to human skin in vivo. Percutaneous absorption from in vivo studies can be assessed through multiple methods. Measurement of the amount of chemical present in skin layers, urine, blood or exhaled air can all be used to assess percutaneous absorption.

### 2.4.1  RADIOACTIVITY IN EXCRETA

Radiolabeled compounds are applied topically to enhance the ability to detect the compound in the excreta. The concentration of radioactivity or biological markers of exposure can be measured to determine the amount absorbed. Typically, compounds are labeled with $^{14}C$ or tritium. The total amount of radioactivity measured in urine and/or feces is determined and compared to a reference exposure. The reference exposure is determined by measuring the amount of radioactivity excreted after intravenous administration or inhalation. This method fails to account for the metabolism of the compound by the skin. The percentage of compound absorbed through topical administration is calculated with the following equation:

$$\text{Absorption}\,(\%) = \frac{\text{Total radioactivity after topical administration}}{\text{Total radioactivity after parenteral administration}} \times 100$$

### 2.4.2  RADIOACTIVITY IN BLOOD

In using plasma to determine absorption of chemicals, the compound is also radiolabeled. The amount absorbed is assessed through the radioactivity in the plasma. Plasma radioactivity can be calculated by comparing the area under the plasma concentration-time profile (AUC) of the topical and intravenous administration.

$$\text{Absorbed dose} = \frac{\text{AUC}_{\text{dermal}}}{\text{AUC}_{\text{excretion}}} \times \text{Dose}_{\text{ref}}$$

### 2.4.3 SURFACE RECOVERY

Surface recovery determines percutaneous absorption through the loss of material from the surface of the skin as it is absorbed in the skin. The topical transdermal delivery device is removed and the residual amount of drug in skin is determined. Penetration is reported as a percentage absorbed. This method is not suited for drugs that are susceptible to evaporation or precipitation (Touitou et al., 1998). The accuracy of this method is questionable since it cannot be determined if the residual amount of drug was completely accounted for. Many factors must be controlled for to accurately assess with this method including timing of and surface area of exposure.

### 2.4.4 TAPE STRIPPING

The tape stripping method determines the concentration of a chemical in the layers of the SC. A pre-determined area of skin is exposed to a chemical for a set period of time (often 30 minutes). At the end of each exposure period, the SC is removed by sequential tape application and removal of one–three strips of tape. Tape strips are then assayed for chemical content. The advantages of this method are that radiolabeled chemicals are not required. A problem to this approach is that the amount of SC removed from each stripping is dependent on a variety of factors including the properties of the adhesive tape, the vehicle in which the chemical is applied, pressure applied during application and anatomical differences in the cohesiveness of the SC (Kezic, 2008). Timing of tape strip application is also crucial. Diffusion that occurs during stripping can account for up to 30% of measured absorption (Reddy et al., 2002). The amount of SC collected can be corrected for by quantifying the amount of SC recovered gravimetrically or by monitoring transepidermal water loss or spectrophotometrically which would measure protein content on the tape. Tape stripping is also a poor choice of technique for determining percutaneous absorption in volatile and rapidly penetrating chemicals. Tape stripping can be used to determine permeability coefficient and for evaluating bioavailability and/or bioequivalence. Tape stripping has become a salient technique for determination of dermal absorption in vivo (Wang and Maibach, 2011).

### 2.4.5 MICRODIALYSIS

Microdialysis measures dermal absorption through measurement of concentration of dermally applied chemical in extracellular fluid (ECF) beneath the skin. Microdialysis is unique in that it provides direct assessment of drug levels in the dermis. A microdialysis fiber (a semipermeable membrane in the shape of a hollow tube) is implanted in the dermis of the skin. The fiber resembles a blood vessel in function and allows molecules to pass through the fiber. The fiber is connected to a pump and sample vial. The pump perfuses the microdialysis fiber with physiologic solution (Ringer's solution) that equilibrates with ECF of the surrounding tissue. The dialysate is then collected at specified time intervals for analysis. Microdialysis is best suited for hydrophilic and a handful of moderately lipophilic drugs. Lipophilic substances are poorly recovered due to the low solubility of lipophilic substances in the hydrophilic perfusates used in microdialysis and the fiber is not permeable to proteins, which limits the use of microdialysis for lipophilic substances and highly protein bound drugs. Comparison of microdialysis and Franz-type diffusion cells has shown good quantitative and qualitative correlation. The correlation of microdialysis and measurement of plasma concentration are less consistent. Microdialysis is a minimally invasive technique, but invasive nonetheless. The implantation of the microdialysis fiber elicits increased blood flow, histamine release, which may influence absorption, however blood flow and histamine levels normalize after 30 minutes. Skin thickness also increases and later decreases, but does not normalize throughout the experiment (Kreilgaard, 2002). Studies show data that is promising for the use of microdialysis in the assessment of bioequivalence/bioavailability (Holmgaard et al., 2010).

### 2.4.6 BREATH ANALYSIS

Breath analysis is able to determine topical bioavailability of a substance virtually instantaneously. Following topical exposure, expired air is measured through a system that analyzes the exhaled air. Chemical components that are exhaled are detected following dermal exposure. Breath analysis can be used to detect expiration of volatile organic compounds up to every four seconds after dermal exposure. The Teledyne 3Dq Discovery ion-trip mass spectrometer equipped with an atmospheric sampling glow discharged ion source is a system that is available for this type of analysis (Poet et al., 2000).

### 2.4.7 SPECTROSCOPIC METHODS

The quantification of in vivo skin penetration has expanded to the use of spectroscopic methods. The advantages of these spectroscopic techniques are the noninvasive nature and the ability to produce real-time data on cutaneous penetration. Attenuated total reflectance Fourier transform infrared (ATR-FTIR) spectroscopy employs infrared (IR) spectroscopy that was improved by Fourier transform methods that increased sensitivity and accuracy (Touitou et al., 1998). It is currently commercially available and is the most commonly used spectroscopic technique for the study of penetration kinetics. The device emits an IR beam that passes thorough an IR-transparent crystal and makes contact with the skin sample. IR radiation penetrates into the skin and the radiated SC absorbed IR energy. IR energy is absorbed at energies that correspond with the normal absorption spectrum of the compound of interest. The IR beams also internally reflect through the crystal and all beams reflect back towards the spectrophotometer. Only the absorption spectrum of the most superficial layer of the skin is reflected in the measurements. When tape stripping is used with ATR-FTIR, multiple sequential layers of the SC can be measured. The use of ATR-FTIR has shown good correlation between the use of ATR-FTIR and other methods of determining SC concentration (Touitou et al., 1998). Other methods of spectroscopic analysis are less widely studied and used.

The OECD Guideline for the Testing of Chemicals recommends that laboratory animals of the similar size and of the same sex be used in in vivo studies.

Permeation may vary between genders of the animal within the same species for certain substances, particularly estrogen containing compounds. If data is available indicating differences in sensitivity to the substance of interest, the sex that shows greater toxic response should be used. Laboratory animals are typically given food and water ad libitum and stored in individual metabolism cages that are kept at 22°C ± 3°C. The duration and surface area of exposure should be chosen to mimic the human exposure period. Collection of urine, feces and trap fluids are collected and analyzed at specified periods. The exposed area of skin is examined for irritation. At the end of the exposure periods, blood is collected for analysis and animals are terminated. Skin and organs can be removed for analysis.

## 2.5 PRECLINICAL TESTING OF TRANSDERMAL DRUG TOXICITY

The skin serves as a protective barrier and under most circumstances is able to protect from chemicals and foreign materials entering the body and altering the internal milieu. At high enough doses, the absorption of chemicals into the skin is able to cause local and systemic toxicity. To determine potential toxicity of drugs delivered transdermally, the potential exposure is compared to toxicity tests. The majority of systemic toxicity is tested through oral and inhalation administration of drugs (Neely, 1994). It can be difficult to achieve toxic doses through percutaneous absorption. The information regarding skin toxicity is limited and may require the use of route-to-route extrapolation from oral or inhalational animal studies. Route-to-route extrapolations attempt to relate toxic doses achieved from internal doses to, in this case, skin exposure.

Irritant contact dermatitis and allergic contact dermatitis are common types of local toxicity. Acute dermal toxicity results from short-term exposure, which is tested by exposing adult rats, rabbits or guinea pigs at different dose levels including a lethal dose of 2 g/kg body weight are administered. Animals are observed for toxic reactions such as lesions, changes in weight, mortality, etc. All animals should be necropsied at the conclusion of the studies. The dermal $LD_{50}$ of many chemicals is reported as 2 g/kg based on the toxicity studies maximum required dosage. If cases of mortality are related to the compound, further testing may be required. In vitro studies using reconstructed epidermis can also be used in testing local irritation or toxicity, which decreases the need and use of laboratory animals.

During the development of topical and transdermal drugs, once a therapeutically efficacious drug level is obtained, toxicological studies in animals followed by the evaluation of skin sensitization in humans are required. A major obstacle to transdermal drug delivery (TDD) is the development of skin irritation, allergic contact dermatitis (ACD) and sensitization (Lynch et al., 1987). For example, varying degrees of skin irritation were reported in patients during long-term (five days) application of transdermal patches (Hurkmans et al., 1985). Delayed hypersensitization reactions have been reported for transdermal therapeutic systems (TTS) (Ale et al., 2009). Ale provides detail on local tolerance – including management of intolerance.

The retention of high concentrations of propranolol in the skin following topical application may account for the irritation of transdermal propranolol (Ademola et al., 1993). Individuals with chronic inflammatory disorders (e.g., atopic dermatitis), in which the barrier properties of the SC are often compromised, may promote drug absorption (Gattu and Maibach, 2011, Chiang et al., 2012). Also, such individuals may be more vulnerable to irritation. Those with "dry skin," a common disorder in those over 50 years of age, frequently have a structurally defective SC (Rawlings, 2017). These individuals may also be at greater risk for adverse cutaneous reactions to skin applications of TTS and topicals. The wide range of structural and functional capacity of the skin from one individual to another complicates the evaluation of the potential adverse effects of topical or transdermal formulations. The cellular and humoral components of the peripheral immune surveillance system present in the skin are responsible for the genesis of a hapten-specific, cell-mediated immune response following the penetration of skin by and complexation of skin components with sensitizing chemicals or drugs (i.e., haptens). Current knowledge in skin immunology implies epidermal Langerhans and other dendritic cells as one of the major antigen-presenting cells of the skin (Streilein, 1989). Contact dermatitis can be broadly divided into two major groups: irritation (the most common) and ACD. In contrast to irritation, immunological reactivity is involved in ACD. Host reactions, including inflammation, vasodilation, influx of leukocytes accompanied by cutaneous erythema, and itching are the hallmarks of both types. The various components of a TTS (e.g., permeation enhancers) may compromise the skin by inducing skin irritation. Irritant contact dermatitis increases the potential ACD. Irritant dermatitis results from direct toxic injury to cell membranes, cytoplasm or nuclei. Irritation can occur from the drug, its vehicle or the adhesive used to secure the TTS to the skin.

A significant population of individuals who have a history of frequent adverse reactions to topical drugs, cosmetics or toiletries may also be susceptible to additional complications and reactions from TTS.

Skin metabolism poses several potential obstacles for the transdermal delivery of beta-blockers. Skin metabolism of beta-blockers may be clinically significant if the metabolites(s) are active, toxic or irritating (Ademola et al., 1993). Active metabolites have been recovered in the skin during a program aimed at the development of a TTS for beta-blockers (Ademola et al., 1992). In addition to the difficulty to attain and maintain constant blood levels, the presence of active metabolites may pose major toxicity problems in patients with organ dysfunction (e.g., renal failure) (Ademola et al., 1992).

In contrast to the more frequently performed dosed-feed, gavage and dosed-water studies, fewer acute and chronic toxicity evaluations of transdermal systems are available. Toxicology and carcinogenicity studies are performed using animal models to provide information that can be used to evaluate the safety of drugs.

This chapter presents some important considerations for toxicological and skin sensitization evaluation in the transdermal delivery of drugs. It will be assumed that (1) local and systemic toxicity depends on a chemical penetrating the skin, and (2) application of a transdermal topical drug to the skin requires penetration through the epidermal layer before reaching the dermis and entering the systemic circulation.

## 2.6 EVALUATION OF SKIN IRRITATION AND SENSITIZATION

Acute irritation (in the rabbit and/or man) provides an early screen. Cumulative irritation may be evaluated in humans by either of two methods: a truncated (ten-day) irritation test or a full 21-day irritation test. In the first test, a small panel (ten subjects) is employed to test the components of a TTS and the drug that are applied daily five days a week for two weeks. The transdermal systems should be applied to the proposed site of application specified in the label instructions. A test article that results in no erythema or edema in any of the ten volunteers is unlikely to result in clinically significant irritation under end use conditions. Most likely, a TTS will be changed daily or every few days, and will not be worn in exactly the same site with each application. Components of a TTS that fail to induce erythema or edema after ten applications to the same site are extremely unlikely to induce significant contact irritation. When any component of a TTS produces mild to moderate irritation, it is difficult to determine if such components will produce a clinically significant irritant reaction. Finally, judgment of the irritation potential of a component can be made by increasing the number of subjects and the duration of application. A related comparative drug formulation provides a clinical frame of reference.

The 21-day test consists of 25 volunteers in which the components of the TTS are applied daily, five days a week, with the Friday application left in place until Monday morning, under an occlusive dressing for 21 days. Components of TTS that have a profile between the extremes should be closely scrutinized during the early developmental stages. Here too a related comparative drug with extensive clinical use provides a frame of reference (Phillips et al., 1972).

Additional methods for evaluating the irritant potential of TTS include laser Doppler measurements of cutaneous microcirculation (Ademola et al., 1996; Liu et al., 1997; Di Nardo et al., 1996; Henningsen, 1991). The power of these measurements lies in their objective assessment and noninvasiveness for assessing skin irritation. A combination of these noninvasive procedures often aids evaluation of the irritant potential of components of transdermal systems. Kubota et al. (1991) concluded that it would be difficult to give a sufficient amount of timolol to expect systemic effect(s) with no concurrent erythema, because erythema develops when the drug was applied topically to the skin. Transdermal delivery of mepindolol via an investigational patch was well tolerated and induced pharmacodynamic effects of stable, prolonged, beta blockade within one week following daily application; however, propranolol, in contrast, was not well tolerated, and it induced only mild indications of beta blockade.

ACD involves a host of immunological reactions to an antigen. The guinea pig maximization test, a widely accepted test for evaluating contact allergic reactions, can be easily adapted for testing the components of TTS. Note that components of TTS that show an allergenic potential in this assay may still be used by millions of patients with minimal adverse effects, and hasty decisions should be avoided. Some preliminary judgments can be made with expert symptoms. See "Updating the Skin Sensitization in vitro Data Assessment Paradigm in 2009—a chemistry and QSAR perspective" for a detailed current status (Roberts and Patlewicz, 2010).

Since yeast, bacteria and fungi will be promoted under a transdermal patch, their growth and development of superficial infection following the application of a TTS is a realistic possibility. In addition, the increased temperature, hydration and other changes, such as $CO_2$ pressure and pH changes, provide suitable environmental factors for microbial growth. Localized superficial infections from *Staphylococcus aureus* or *Candida albicans* can develop under occlusion. The potential of a TTS for promoting the growth of an organism can be evaluated by quantitative bacteriological cultures of skin sites before and after use of the transdermal system. Finally, prickly heat (miliaria rubra), when there is a stimulus for sweating, can develop under occlusive conditions of a TTS. This will be more prevalent if the TTS is to be applied over a prolonged period.

## 2.7 MECHANISMS OF DERMAL HYPERSENSITIVITY, ALLERGIC CONTACT DERMATITIS AND ATOPIC DERMATITIS

Toxicity studies utilizing routes of administration other than the skin are designed to examine systemic effects of the chemical and assume that some or most of the chemical enters the body. In contrast, many dermal studies use short-term designs to examine the toxic effects or determine the irritation potential of a chemical only at the application site. Studies designed to evaluate both the local and systemic toxic effects of TTS are less common. The species most commonly used in dermal toxicity studies are rats, mice, Syrian hamsters and, less often, rabbits and guinea pigs. Large databases have been complied for rats and mice; a knowledge of the behavior, anatomy, genetics, husbandry, nutrition, spontaneous diseases, spontaneous tumor incidence and susceptibility to tumor induction has been acquired that provides a more reliable basis to assess the results of toxicological studies with these species (Haseman et al., 1984). The best comparison is with control data collected under similar dermal toxicity study conditions. However, the number of transdermal toxicity studies conducted to date is relatively small, and a comparison of the results to an established database using other routes of exposure is necessary. Hamsters, guinea pigs and rabbits commonly used in dermal toxicity studies to determine irritation (N.I.H., 1985) can be used to evaluate the toxicity potential of transdermal systems. Factors, other than the species and strains that determine the nature and severity of a toxic skin response to transdermal drugs, include the site of application and the duration of exposure. The usual areas of chemical application are the ear and the lateral and dorsal areas of the body. Rabbit ear skin has been used to examine the potential for dermal irritation (OECD, 1981). The skin of the lateral surface of the body is the site commonly used in studies to determine irritation (OECD, 1981). Irritation and allergic response studies are usually short term, and the sites may be covered by a device, or the animal may be restrained to eliminate the possibility of external contact with the dose site. Percutaneous absorption and skin response to transdermal systems may vary at different application sites. In contrast to the application of other formulations where consistency in area and dose are problematic, the application of TTS for the delivery of beta-blockers to the skin does not offer such problems.

In order to maximize the potential to observe a toxic effect in dermal studies, a TTS with a large surface area can be applied to a larger area of the skin to increase the total absorption of the drug. Data from these studies may be used to determine local and systemic toxic effects, as well as to establish transdermal doses for long-term studies.

Dermal sensitization reactions of the skin either defend the host against pathologic agents or damage host tissue and cause diseases. The protective effects of inflammatory reactions are a desirable part of host "immunity," while the detrimental effects arise from immune-mediated lesions defined as "immunopathologic" disease (Sell, 1981). The terms *allergy* or *sensitivity* commonly denote harmful immune reactions that involve the pathophysiologic interaction of antigens (i.e., substances that induce an immune response) with specific antibodies (e.g., gamma globulin proteins) or with sensitized T lymphocytes. The terms *allergy* or *sensitization* usually signify delayed cellular immune reactivity. The preferred term for delayed dermal sensitization or contact allergies is "allergic contact dermatitis" (Slavin, 1985; Malten, 1981).

A brief review of the immunologic structure of the skin follows. The primary role of the immune system is defense of the host against disease. The two major arms of the immune system are humoral immunity and cell-mediated immunity. Cytokines primarily regulate the active immune response. When the delicate balance of immunocytes and regulatory cytokines operates in a healthy balance, then the host is immunocompetent and able to ward off infectious diseases or cancer and neutralize foreign antigens. Immune response can also produce immuno-pathologic disorders, such as autoimmunity or allergies. It is believed that inappropriate and harmful dermal allergic reactions to chemical substances are the evolutionary price we pay to enable our immune system to ward off complex parasites and cancer (Singh, 1981). Thus, the same immune mechanism that furnishes both resistance against infection and "immune-surveillance of neoplasia" can also produce immunopathologic diseases (e.g., a double-edged sword effect). Cell-mediated immunity becomes harmful during ACD reactions that cause tissue damage, autoimmune disorders and granulomas (Lakin and Strecker, 1985). Similarly, humoral immunity can also damage host tissues during immediate hypersensitivity reactions, such as anaphylaxis, immune-complex disease and cytotoxicity of host cells. There are five general classifications of hypersensitivity based on immunopathogenic mechanisms of tissue damage:

1. Anaphylaxis: reaction time is rapid.
2. Ig-dependent cytotoxicity: reaction time is variable; injury involves cell destruction.
3. Immune mechanism: reaction time is 6–18 hours; basement membrane is destroyed.
4. Cell mediated: onset of action is delayed (allergic contact dermatitis).
5. Involves bimolecular binding: reaction time is variable.

The clinical expression and incidence of ACD varies considerably among individuals; species; regions of the body; exposure conditions; and with differences in age, gender and physiological conditions (e.g., pregnancy, menstrual cycle, etc.) in humans (Fisher, 1984; Fisher, 1986).

ACD reactions are induced by specificity antigens and are elicited by either specific antibodies from sensitized B lymphocytes (e.g., antibody-secreting plasma cells) or by sensitized T lymphocytes and macrophages in the case of cell-mediated immunity. Most contact sensitizers induce their reaction through antigenic stimulation in the form of a "hapten," which is an incomplete antigen since it requires a suitable carrier molecule in order to become antigenic. If a drug is able to penetrate the skin and covalently bind with amino acids in the skin, dermal hypersensitivity is possible. If the hapten-protein conjugate is of a sufficiently large molecular size to be recognized as a foreign antigen, a specific antibody and/or specific cell-mediated immune response will ensue that sensitizes the skin immune system to the hapten molecule. Upon re-exposure of the skin to the sensitizing chemical, a dermal hypersensitivity reaction may be elicited. This inflammatory reaction is generally delayed-onset type IV hypersensitivity that stems from a cell-mediated immune response.

ACD may appear after single or repeated contact of allergenic haptens with the skin of sensitized individuals. The sensitization or induction phase is characterized by an activation (differentiation and proliferation) of allergen-specific T-effector lymphocytes, which requires presentation of the hapten in association with 2 MHC antigens on the surface of Langerhans cells. T cell activation is modulated by interleukins (Il-1, Il-2), gamma interferon (gamma IFN), Prostaglandin E (PGE) and other immunoregulatory cytokines (Henningsen, 1991).

Atopic dermatitis, a common eczematous dermatosis, is characterized by severe itching, onset in infancy, inheritance, associations with elevated IgE, multiple positive immediate-type skin tests, allergic rhinitis and bronchial asthma. Alterations in the ability of the immune system to control hypersensitivity can have a significant effect on the resulting degree of inflammation. The effects of immune dysfunction on dermal sensitivity include tolerance to contact sensitizers and depression of elicitation of dermal sensitization. Corticosteroids are well known for their potent immunosuppressive effects, including their ability to suppress both the induction and elicitation phases of ACD (Ashworth et al., 1991). A number of excipients and chemicals have been shown to alter delayed-type hypersensitivity in animal models (Exon and Koller, 1983); sunlight and its component ultraviolet (UVB) (295–320nm) radiation have been found to persistently suppress contact hypersensitivity to allergens applied subsequently to non-irradiated skin in mice, through the generation of suppressor T cells. Tolerance or hyporesponsiveness can be genetically or environmentally related. Enhanced hypersensitivity can also result from various genetic or environmental influences on the immune system. There are few examples of immune-mediated effects of potential transdermal candidates or their excipients.

## 2.8   IN VIVO METHODS TO EVALUATE DERMAL SENSITIZATION

The diagnosis of dermal sensitization requires a complete medical history and physical examination to eliminate other possible causes of reactions that are observed. The objective of the skin sensitization test is to either diagnose or predict potential dermal allergies.

### 2.8.1 IMMEDIATE HYPERSENSITIVITY TEST (FOR DIAGNOSIS OF CONTACT URTICARIA SYNDROME)

Contact urticaria syndrome has two mechanisms: non-immunologic (NICU) and immunologic (ICU) – it is the latter of dramatic clinical significance – as it manifests not only by local urticaria, but also by distant organ involvement (asthma, rhinitis, conjunctivitis and anaphylaxis). NICU can be predicted by simple animal and human assays (Lahti and Maibach, 1984); ICU has no predictive assay at present.

### 2.8.2 HUMAN TESTS

Human tests can be used for the diagnosis of type 1 hypersensitivity in the skin through the identification of specific allergens that elicit an IgE-mediated inflammatory reaction. Major tests include the skin prick test, the intradermal test, skin titration and provocative tests. Provocative tests can be used to decide whether the drug or the excipients in the patch system causes a skin disorder. The tests can be used to identify the causative agent in the entire patch system; this will enable the reformulation of the patch system.

### 2.8.3 ANIMAL TESTS

Animal tests are available to diagnose immediate hypersensitivity reactions (Patterson, 1985).

### 2.8.4 DELAYED-TYPE HYPERSENSITIVITY TESTS FOR DIAGNOSIS OF ALLERGIC CONTACT DERMATITIS

Patch testing can be used clinically to diagnose delayed hypersensitivity to topical or transdermal drugs in humans. The principle behind the test is to place a patch containing a suitable concentration of the drug and excipient that is neither irritating nor sensitizing on the skin, using suitable formulations and patch system. Lachapelle summarizes science of diagnostic and photopatch testing in man (Lachapelle and Maibach, 2012).

### 2.8.5 HUMAN PATCH TESTING

Patch testing of humans can be used as a predictive test for formulations when prior testing produced a negative result in the guinea pig sensitization test. The patch system can be tested in a repeated insult patch test in 200 subjects at different times. The vehicle is typically aqueous (i.e., ethanol or acetone) or petroleum or the final formulation, which is used in guinea pigs. The induction phase involves the application of a nonirritating concentration of material under an occlusive patch on the forearm or back thrice weekly for three weeks. Challenge testing is performed two weeks later by applying a nonirritating concentration of the test substance on both the original site of application and on a native site on the other arm, challenges are recommended within one or two weeks to aid in interpreting results. The provocative test may also be incorporated to better predict the sensitizing potential of the transdermal patch itself (Lauerma and Maibach, 1995).

Primary skin irritation and allergic contact sensitization potential of transdermal triprolidine was evaluated by Robinson et al. (1991). Concern over potential irritation and ACD skin reactions necessitates thorough skin toxicity testing before and during initial clinical development. Rabbit skin irritation and Buehler guinea pig skin sensitization testing indicate that this formulation produced both skin irritation and ACD potential. Of 26 subjects enrolled in a rising dose clinical pharmacokinetic study, one subject exposed twice to the primary formulation presented delayed skin reactions suggestive of ACD. Positive diagnostic patch test results for four out of five suggested that the formulation had a high ACD potential. Subsequent predictive clinical patch testing was conducted with a buffered aqueous drug formulation that provided in vitro skin penetration of the drug equivalent to the primary formulation. These clinical studies demonstrated that the drug itself had no significant irritation potential, but still induced ACD reactions in a high proportion of test subjects. The incidence of adverse skin reactions to the drug was considered to be too high relative to the degrees of improved therapeutic benefit of this delivery form. On this basis, all technology development effort was discontinued. In our laboratory, we routinely used similar approaches to evaluate the skin toxicity or ACD to transdermal drugs.

An invention directed towards the reduction or prevention of skin sensitization by inhibiting the immunological processing of a sensitizing drug as an antigen has been described by Ledger and Cormier (1994). Contact allergy has also been prevented by the coadministration of a corticosteroid with a sensitizing drug (Amkraut and Shane, 1994).

Green developed a method that allows for the measurement of chemical irritation in humans (Green and Bluth, 1995). The chemicals were applied on filter paper and then occluded and alternated at three-minute intervals with test vehicles. The results revealed large differences in the reactivity to the lactic acid, capsaicin and ethanol.

A two-phase study was conducted to determine the contact sensitization potential of a nicotine system. The study comprised two phases separated by a two-week rest period. The patches were evaluated for signs of irritation and subjective complaints, such as itching or burning. Of the 186 subjects, only three exhibited evidence of delayed contact sensitization manifested by erythema with or without infiltration and confined solely to the sites of the active transdermal nicotine system (Friedrickson et al., 1995). Sigman et al., (1994) developed a structure activity relationship (SAR) to solve the problems of skin sensitization using contact allergens in a data evaluation system. Several related expert systems have found wide application (Hostýnek and Maibach, 1998, Roberts and Patlewicz, 2010).

### 2.8.6 ANIMAL MODELS

Guinea pig skin offers a suitable model for human contact hypersensitivity; however, the model has several structural differences compared with human skin, for example, more numerous hair shafts, and a smoother dermal and epidermal junction. Specific procedures for delayed ACD include guinea pig predictive models (Elmets et al.,

1992), Buehler topical patch technique, the maximization test, mouse ear swelling test and in vitro screening methods.

Many factors influence the interpretation of results from dermal hypersensitivity tests; guinea pig allergy test results cannot stand alone. Results should be interpreted with available human patch and provocative tests. Although the dermal sensitizing potential of topical and transdermal products presents an extremely low risk of induction to clinical dermatoses, prospective dose-response studies of these products in humans with repeated insult may show an apparent threshold concentration of active drug and excipient, below which there will be no sensitization. An indication of the relative safety of the transdermal products may be presumed.

The skin possesses cellular structures and physiologic functions that qualify it as a secondary immune organ, both in terms of innate resistance to infections and acquired immunity to foreign antigens. The specialized set of tissues in the skin accounts for epidermotrophism of sensitized T lymphocytes, antigen presentation by Langerhans cells, and actions of other dermal cells that may contribute to skin immunity (e.g., mast cells, keratinocytes and possibly dendritic epidermal cells). The distribution of immune phenotypes of lymphocyte subpopulations in normal human skin is defined as the "skin immune system." The primary role of skin as an immune organ has been well reviewed (Henningsen, 1991).

## 2.9 IN VITRO METHODS FOR ASSESSING SKIN IRRITANCY OF TRANSDERMAL THERAPEUTIC SYSTEMS

The following processes are involved in skin irritation: percutaneous penetration, protein denaturation, epidermal cell lysis, cytotoxicity, enzyme leakage from cells, the production of epidermal antigens, the production of cytokines and inflammatory mediators (Corsini et al., 1996). In contrast with in vivo studies, which often use subjective measurements, such as erythema or edema, some of these events can be measured as endpoints in cell culture assays.

Different in vitro tests can be used to assess the cell toxicity of topical or transdermal drugs, including morphology, cell proliferation, cell adhesion, cell differentiation, cell membrane, cell metabolism, SC integrity, cell function impairment and the release of inflammatory mediators. The endpoints used to assess cell toxicity are as follows: (1) the measurement of cell viability reflecting irreversible damage caused by necrosis, and (2) the inflammatory process occurring concomitantly with skin irritancy (Balls and Clothier, 2010).

## 2.10 TOXICOLOGY AND SKIN IRRITATION

Toxicological and skin sensitization evaluations of TTS in human subjects present the possibility of treating two or more similar sites on the subject's body with patches containing different formulations. The number of sites depends on both the size of a patch and the subject. Several different types of toxic interactions are possible between the components of transdermal systems and the skin. These toxic interactions can be broadly classified as being corrosive, irritative or sensitive in nature. The pathology usually includes dermal inflammation and, depending on the severity, a variable amount of necrosis. In vivo test procedures used to assess the dermal toxicity of chemicals are easily adaptable to assess the toxicity of transdermal systems. The mechanism(s) by which the components of the patch system produce their effects may not be known; however, these in vivo tests recognize that the interactions between the components of the transdermal system and the skin will be complex, simultaneously involving various degrees of corrosion, irritation and sensitization.

Caution should be exercised in the use of traditional tests to evaluate the dermal toxicity potential of TTS. Although these traditional tests have been the standards used to evaluate such effects for many chemicals, these procedures have been increasingly challenged as to their validity for human extrapolation and as to their animal use requirements. Attention should be focused on in vitro alternative approaches to such testing that might be both more predictive of the human response and more conservative in reducing the number of animals required.

It is also possible to develop in vitro models to predict some of the dermatotoxic effects of transdermal products in vivo. The rationale for developing such in vitro models is: (1) to evaluate specific aspects of the irritation or sensitization of each component of the transdermal system, (2) to supplement in vivo evaluation by serving as a first tier screen test to minimize in vivo testing and as a decision point on chemical/product development, or (3) to replace an in vivo procedure. Different types of in vitro models for the evaluation of dermal irritation include structure activity, biochemical, cellular, tissue, lower vertebrate or invertebrate, and tissue models (Balls and Clothier, 2010).

## 2.11 TOXICOLOGICAL EVALUATION OF TRANSDERMAL AND TOPICAL PRODUCTS

Skin irritation is a major drawback for the successful development of transdermal drugs. Preliminary skin irritation studies indicated that neither metoprolol nor the components of the patch systems caused any appreciable skin irritation in hairless rats (Ghosh et al., 1995). Feldstein et al. (1996) observed that a hydrogel pressure sensitive adhesive (PSA) showed neither toxicity, skin irritation or sensitization in the course of preclinical study of transdermal propranolol. The unusually intensive irritation observed in various attempts to develop transdermal propranolol led to increased attention to the problems of skin irritation of this drug. However, in contrast to the generally observed skin irritation of propranolol, Corbo et al. (1990) showed that neither propranolol nor the adhesive used in the transdermal device caused any appreciable skin irritation. Little attention has been placed on preformulation techniques of evaluating the skin irritation potential of the various components of transdermal systems. We have found that in addition to the irritation potential of the drug itself, the adhesive, enhancers and solvent systems, for example, are potential skin irritants. Factorial designs, simplex-lattice designs (Cornell, 1990) and other methods have been used to achieve the desired release patterns and a balance of cohesive and adhesive properties of transdermal adrenergic agonist and blockers (Nagels et al., 1993). Similar attention should be focused on the toxic and skin irritation effects of the components of transdermal systems during preformulation and development stages.

## 2.12  FACTORS AFFECTING THE SKIN TOXICITY OF TOPICAL PRODUCTS

The major factors that affect the percutaneous penetration of drugs can broadly affect the skin toxicity of components of transdermal delivery systems (TDS). These factors can be classified into biological and physical factors.

### 2.12.1  BIOLOGICAL FACTORS

**Skin Age.** Aging human skin is an area of increasing concern for both medical and cosmetic reasons. The ability of the body to absorb a topically applied medication is determined by diffusion through the skin and the underlying blood vessel. Both of these processes may be altered as a consequence of the age of the skin. The elderly represents a growing fraction of the total population, and the consequences of skin aging have great impact on their lives. Cutaneous aging is of interest as a target for therapy; however, the aged skin poses a complicating factor for topical drug delivery because of the potential for irritation. The aged skin, particularly photodamaged skin, may present a less effective barrier. The skin of the elderly cuts and bruises more easily, heals more slowly and does not regenerate as efficiently as that of younger individuals. The loss of dermal papillae leads to a decreased number of anchoring sites between the dermis and the epidermis; thus, the epidermis may be more readily sheared from the dermis (Kligman and Balin, 1989). On the other extreme, the barrier of preterm infants is incompletely formed, resulting in a highly permeable skin. The full-term baby, on the other hand, has an SC that is as effective as that of the mature adult. The water-retention capability of "old" skin is less than that of young adults (Rosenthal et al., 1990). Aged skin was less permeable to relatively "polar" permeants compared to young skin; however, for lipophilic solutes, no age-related differences were found. Preclinical assessment of TTS in the target age groups may be critical to the successful development of TTS. Age and gender differences were observed in the absorption of topical acetaminophenol in vitro. Konda et al. (2012) provide recent overviews of the effect of age on percutaneous penetration.

**Skin Condition.** Percutaneous penetration through damaged or diseased skin is expected, and has been shown, to be different than that through intact tissue (e.g., with 8-methoxypsoralene, increased absorption in frozen and pretreated skin [Shah et al. 1996]). Multiple pieces of evidence show that damage to the SC results in enhanced permeability (Gattu and Maibach, 2011, Chiang et al., 2012).

**Anatomical Site.** The permeability coefficient ($Kp$) of a penetrant across the SC is inversely proportional to the diffusion path length. Hence, one might expect the $Kp$ to be smaller at anatomic sites where the SC is thickest (e.g., plantar surfaces). Experimental evidence, however, provides no such correlation, but instead suggests that SC lipid composition is a more reliable indicator of permeability. Rougier et al. (1983) showed that in vivo permeability was inversely related not to skin thickness, but to corneocyte size, a parameter that can significantly influence the absolute magnitude of the diffusion path length.

**Skin Metabolism.** The skin possesses the capability of metabolizing components of TTS. For example, Ademola and Maibach (1995) have shown that betamethasone, the metabolite of betamethasone-17-valerate, is rapidly transported through the human skin in vivo. The rate of transport of the drug through the skin affects its anti-inflammatory activity.

**Circulatory Effects.** In principle, changes in blood flow through the dermis can affect percutaneous absorption and skin irritation. In reality, the SC is the rate-limiting barrier; only if transport across the SC is very rapid can blood flow control the systemic appearance of the penetrant. In contrast to the increased uptake due to augmented blood flow, vasoconstriction or reduced blood flow can theoretically decrease the percutaneous absorption of components of TTS. Slowly penetrating molecules tend to accumulate in the skin, causing irritation (Ademola and Maibach, 1995).

### 2.12.2 PHYSICOCHEMICAL FACTORS

**Hydration.** When the skin is hydrated, the tissue softens, swells and wrinkles. Hydration of the SC promotes percutaneous absorption of many chemicals through the skin; however, the influence of this factor on irritation of the skin should be assessed prior to development of TTS (Zhai and Maibach, 2001).

**Drug Binding.** The binding of a diffusing molecule to various components of the skin can retard percutaneous absorption and enhance skin irritation. If a drug intended for TDD exhibits strong binding to the SC, uptake into the circulation will be hindered. This may necessitate the use of a higher applied dose, so that the level of mobile, freely diffusing drug is increased, increasing the possibility of skin toxicity.

**Temperature.** The temperature of the SC typically falls in the range of 30–37°C. Transient temperature changes (e.g., during the use of cooling lotions) have negligible effects on the transport properties of the skin. However, temperatures above 65°C for prolonged times (> 1 min), result in severe structural alterations. The potential effects on skin temperature should be assessed during the development of skin care products. Other factors, such as gender and race, that have a bearing on the extent of penetration may also affect skin irritation of TTS.

## 2.13   SYSTEMIC TOXICITY AND ADVERSE SKIN REACTIONS

The design or review of animal toxicity studies should not only take into account the lack of hepatic first-pass metabolism, but should also note skin metabolism by using the transdermal route. This may well affect the interpretation of chronic toxicity and reproduction studies performed by oral administration. Human adverse reaction data from long-term studies should be presented, including any evidence of the product's efficacy or development of tolerance (Alikhan and Maibach, 2011).

### 2.13.1 SKIN CANCER

Skin cancer is the most common neoplasm occurring in the human population. It is estimated that of all the new cancers diagnosed annually, almost one-third originate in the skin. Carcinogenesis research has demonstrated the tumorigenic activities of a large number of chemical substances in experimental animals. These chemicals include diverse chemical classes, organic and inorganic, and natural and synthetic products. Preclinical assessment of the potential of chemical agents to act as skin carcinogens is, therefore, prudent. Many chemicals have been identified as initiating agents for cutaneous carcinogenesis in animal test systems. The initiating agents for murine skin include polyaromatic hydrocarbons (PAHs), nitrosamines, aromatic amines and various alkylating agents. The promoting agents include a wide variety of compounds, plant products, tobacco products, surface-acting agents, anthrones, organic peroxides and hydroperoxides, long-chain fatty acids and their esters, and phenolic compounds. Since transdermal products contain a number of excipients, enhancers and the active drug, these agents might act in a cooperative manner with initiators to accelerate the response to the occurrence of skin carcinogenesis, and this cooperativity should be evaluated in transdermal systems. Each component of the TTS should be examined independently and in combination, and the potential roles they play in the events considered necessary for initiation-like exposure to carcinogenesis, its transportation to the target cell, metabolic activation to ultimate carcinogenic metabolite, and DNA damage leading to an inherited change with the appearance of a preneoplastic lesion.

Tumor development in initiated skin can be accomplished if a tumor promoter is present in a TTS that is locally applied. One common feature of tumor-promoting agents is that they induce skin inflammation and epidermal hyperplasia (Agarawal and Mukhtar, 1991). The TTS may be tested by repeated application over a period of several weeks to determine the potential of the TTS component to act as a tumor promoter.

### 2.13.2 PHOTOCARCINOGENESIS

Photocarcinogenesis refers to the process by which UV radiation produces cancer. Since the depth of penetration of this form of radiant energy extends no further than the dermis, essentially all forms of cancer produced by UV radiation involve the skin. Therefore, topically applied drugs, including transdermal products, may potentially be photocarcinogenic. The potential of a TTS to act as a photocarcinogen can be tested in animal models, where the animals are exposed to an artificial UV light source over a period of months. This protocol will produce primarily squamous cell carcinoma and fibrosarcomas. Basal cell carcinomas can be produced in rats by the application of TTS components and by the administration of ionizing radiation (Elmets et al., 1992).

## 2.14 CLINICAL PHARMACOLOGICAL CONSIDERATIONS OF SKIN PENETRATION ENHANCEMENT

Since the intended site(s) of action differ between a topically applied product intended for local or for systemic administration, an important difference between topical and transdermal drug products is the mass transfer rate of the drug within and across the skin. For topical drug products, formulations should promote drug uptake and retention by the skin at the site of application. In this setting, a high flux (i.e., the amount of drug transported through a unit area of skin per unit time) is not required; even through drug retained in the SC might eventually result in some systemic entry. For transdermal products, a high flux is desired so that drug can penetrate the SC in order to be available in sufficient amounts to the systemic circulation for therapeutic effect.

For physicochemical reasons, such as high molecular weight and polarity, most drugs are not suitable for transdermal administration. Thus, the enhancement of penetration of selected drugs might significantly expand the list of drugs that could be delivered transdermally.

The application of clinical pharmacological principles to the development of a transdermal product rests on the assumption that drug effect is related to the concentration of total or unbound drug in an accessible biological fluid, such as blood, plasma or urine. A transdermal product with or without penetration enhancement technology should be capable of producing therapeutically relevant plasma and tissue concentrations of a drug or its active metabolite(s). The development of a drug for transdermal delivery has generally followed its development and approval for other routes of administration. Although development of a new drug initially for administration by the transdermal route is by no means unlikely, the clinical pharmacological issues for most transdermal drug products relate to potential changes in drug pharmacokinetics and pharmacological effects when the route of administration and the delivery rate of a drug are changed. The conversion of a formulation delivered by another route of administration to a transdermal formulation also raises issues related to congruity in metabolic paths between the nontransdermal and the transdermal routes.

Changes in the time course of pharmacodynamic concentration-effect relation can occur with the development of a transdermal formulation. If changes occur in important metabolite or enantiomer patterns, the apparent concentration-effect relation may also change. Consequently, documentation of a relation between drug concentration in an accessible fluid, such as plasma or blood, and a pharmacological effect of interest will facilitate the development of a transdermal formulation. Similar concentrations arise with the conversion of immediate to controlled release oral formulations (Skelly et al., 1990). It is apparent that the development of a transdermal formulation may result in substantial change in the time course of the pharmacological effect of the drug. Clinical experience with transdermal nitroglycerin products suggests that continuous administration of a drug by the transdermal route also raises issues of clinical tolerance (Abshagen, 1996). Some of the differences observed between the metabolism of the drug in the skin and the liver may account for some of the observed pharmacological effects. Therefore, the addition of penetration enhancement methods to a transdermal product requires the reevaluation of the effect-time profile and the primary relations between pharmacological effect and plasma concentration. It is possible that the primary concentration-effect relationship may change in the presence of an enhancer. The choice of a chemical enhancer may have a significant influence on product design and development strategy. Agents that maximally interact with the SC and minimally with viable tissues are desirable. Smith summarizes percutaneous penetration enhancers (Smith and Maibach, 1995).

Iontophoresis and ultrasound techniques are physical methods used to enhance the percutaneous penetration of drugs. However, a major concern with the use of iontophoresis is that the device may cause painful destruction of the skin with high-current settings. High-quality electrodes with adequate skin adhesion, uniform current distribution and well-controlled ionic properties are essential to the safe use of the method.

### 2.14.1 REGULATORY CONSIDERATIONS

The application of permeation enhancers in a transdermal or topical formulation may change the time course of clinical effects. Specific recommendations for the pharmacokinetic and biopharmaceutical data relevant to a new drug or new dosage form have been defined by the U.S. Food and Drug Administration (FDA) guidelines for the format and content of the human pharmacokinetics and bioavailability section of a New Drug Application (NDA). Further information concerning NDA efficacy documentation for a new transdermal formulation with penetration enhancement technology may also be obtained from the applicable reviewing division in the Center for Drug Evaluation and Research (CDER) at the FDA. The use of unapproved permeation enhancers may also call for an additional need to document safety in an NDA. TDD systems are regarded as a "new drug" within the meaning of the Federal Food, Drug, and Cosmetic Act, Section 200.31, and thus require submission of scientific data to substantiate their clinical safety and efficacy. Furthermore, all such drugs or controlled-release dosage forms must demonstrate their controlled-release characteristics to support drug labeling in accordance with FDA requirements.

In addition, these delivery systems require demonstration of safety, both in terms of local irritations and systemic toxicity. The FDA may waive the demonstration of animal systemic toxicity, but it may require additional clinical testing for safety in human subjects if systemic toxicity is already defined in the scientific literature. Clinical testing to demonstrate safety and efficacy are required for TTS and may also be required to support new efficacy claims for drugs already marketed. Clinical efficacy data must be submitted to support a new medical claim or any claim of superior efficacy.

In certain instances, additional metabolism studies in humans may be required to define the cutaneous metabolism of the drug where significant alteration in metabolic pathways is suspected due to different hepatic-portal elimination or gastrointestinal (GIT) metabolism (Shah and Skelly, 1992). In the UK, TTS are regarded as medicinal products and require the same regulatory procedures and experience the same official scrutiny as more conventional preparations. Drug regulations in the UK are based on the Medicines Act of 1988. This act requires that the quality, safety and efficacy of a medicinal preparation be demonstrated to be satisfactory in the context of therapeutic indications and dosage schedule. Each new product, whether it is a new chemical entity or a new presentation of a known drug, is assessed on its own merits. Two main areas of regulation are encountered before a product is available for sale in the UK: the clinical trial certificate and product licenses.

Biopharmaceutical considerations are critical for dermal delivery systems because they determine specific kinds of clinical or toxicological studies that will need to be performed. General and specific FDA guidelines should be reviewed for current FDA specific regulatory insights.

The following International Conference on Harmonization (ICH) Guidances are considered key Nonclinical Documents for developing non-clinical programs:

- ICH M3(R2) – Nonclinical Safety Studies for the Conduct of Human Clinical Trials and Marketing Authorization for Pharmaceuticals (U.S. Food and Drug Administration, 2009).
- ICH S1 (A, B, C [R2]) – Carcinogenicity Studies (U.S. Food and Drug Administration, 1996/1998/2008).
- ICH S2 (R1) – Genotoxicity Testing and Data Interpretation for Pharmaceuticals Intended for Human Use (U.S. Food and Drug Administration, 2012).
- ICH S5A and B – Detection of Toxicity to Reproduction for Medicinal Products (U.S. Food and Drug Administration, 1995/1996).
- ICH S7A and B – Safety Pharmacology Studies for Human Pharmaceuticals (U.S. Food and Drug Administration, 2001/2005).
- ICH Q3A(R), Q3B(R2) & Q3C – Guidance for impurities, residual solvents & degradants (toxicological qualification) (U.S. Food and Drug Administration, 2006/2008).

In addition to the guidelines listed, specific recommendations for topical products may be contained in indication-specific U.S. FDA Center for Drug Evaluation and Research guidance documents (e.g., chronic ulcer, head lice infestation).

## 2.15   SUMMARY

Transdermal drug delivery systems provide many advantages in medication administration, however there are several barriers and limitations to the development of these transdermal drugs due to the difficulty of safety testing. International committees and the FDA have tried to simplify their view of the science and what is relevant in transdermal drug delivery systems for the industry. Those are included in the FDA and ICH guidelines. The FDA guidelines for safety testing can be referenced at www. fda.gov. Since bioequivalence usually relate to a generic, the basic preclinical work is usually in animals and is usually accomplished by the innovator. One of the first steps in the safety assessment of any transdermal and topical (dermatological) product formulation is assessing skin irritation and sensitization potential. There are in vitro and in vivo tests and mathematical models that are useful for predicting the relative degree of absorption, irritation or sensitization evoked by the formulation prior to human testing. However, these are limited by the use of animal models, which serve as acceptable surrogates and are useful in optimizing the safety of product formulations and selecting those worthy of clinical evaluations in man, however they are not necessarily accurate in the prediction of or the absence of skin irritation or sensitization in man. Ultimately, the safety of the transdermal or topical product must be evaluated in man under end-use conditions following single and multiple applications in normal volunteers, such as in phase I safety studies. Following the demonstration of an acceptable profile of acute skin tolerance (acceptable irritation profile and lack of sensitization), further studies of the product formulation should be carried out in the disease population in phase II and phase III studies. The potential for local adverse skin reactions to be evoked in response to the product should be evaluated in the target population, and variables such as age, gender, skin conditions and anatomical site should be considered and play a significant role in response. Finally, for new drugs or previously approved drug products that employ new excipients, the product formulation should be evaluated for systemic toxicity and subacute and chronic skin toxicity, such as skin cancer and photo-carcinogenesis. Generally, the regulatory requirements and safety data package for an OTC monograph product are minimal, greater for an abbreviated new drug application (ANDA) filing, and increase exponentially for an NDA product registration.

Integration of all pharmacology and toxicology elements is necessary for final safety assessment. Generally, in vivo toxicity is assessed in two species (rodent and non-rodent) and relevance of the test species for pharmacology and toxicology studies needs to be justified as per published guidances. In developing the nonclinical development program, indication is a key consideration to determine the nature of nonclinical studies (dose, route, duration and population). Clinical route of administration is the preferred route for nonclinical studies.

## GENERAL READING

Maibach, H.I. *Toxicology of Skin*. Philadelphia: Taylor & Francis, 2001.

Schwindt, D. and Maibach, H.I. *Cutaneous Biometrics*. New York: Kluwer/Plenum, 2001.

Shah, V.P. and Maibach, H.I. *Topical Drug Bioavailability, Bioequivalence, and Penetration*. New York: Plenum, 1993.

Wang, R.A., Knack, J.B. and Maibach, H.I. *Health Risk Assessment: Dermal and Inhalation Exposure of Toxicants*. Boca Raton, FL: CRC, 1993.

Wilhelm, K.P., Zhou, H. and Maibach, H.I. *Dermatoxicology*. 8th ed. New York: Informa, 2012.

## REFERENCES

Abshagen, U. (1996) Controlled Clinical Studies of Tolerance Development and Dosing Problems in Nitrate Therapy. *Herz* suppl. 1: 23–30.

Ademola, J. and Maibach, H.I. (1995) Cutaneous Metabolism and Penetration of 8-MOP, Betamethasone-17-Valerate, Retinoic Acid, Nitroglycerine, and Theophylline. In: *Exogenous Dermatol.*, Eds. C. Surber, P. Elsner, and A. Bircher. Marcel Dekker, Inc., New York, pp. 201–215.

Ademola, J., Wester, R.C., and Maibach, H.I. (1992) Transport and Metabolism of Theophylline in Human Skin In Vitro. *J. Invest. Dermatol.* 98: 310–314.

Ademola, J., Wester, R.C., and Maibach, H.I. (1993) Metabolism of Propranolol During Percutaneous Absorption in Human Skin. *J. Pharm. Sci.* 82: 767–770.

Ademola, J., Montenegro, L., Scrofani, N., Bonina, F., and Maibach, H.I. (1996) Evaluation of Skin Blanching of Topical Corticosteroid Using Stratum Corneum Measurements. *Int. J. Pharm.* 140: 51–60.

Agarawal, R. and Mukhtar, H. (1991) Cutaneous Chemical Carcinogenesis. In: *Pharmacology of the Skin,* Ed. J. Mukhtar. CRC Press, Boca Raton, FL, pp. 372–384.

Ale, I., Lachapelle, J., and Maibach, H.I. (2009) Skin Tolerability Associated with Transdermal Drug Delivery Systems: An Overview. *Advances in Therapy*. 26(10): 920–935.

Alikhan, F.S. and Maibach, H. (2011) Topical Absorption and Systemic Toxicity. *Cutan Ocul Toxicol.* 30(3):175–86.

Amkraut, A. and Shane, J. (1994) U.S. Patent 5,077,054.

Andersen, K.E., Maibach, H.I., and Anjo, M.D. (1980) The Guinea-Pig: An Animal Model for Human Skin Absorption of Hydrocortisone, Testosterone and Benzoic Acid? *Br J Dermatol.* 102(4):447–53.

Ashworth, J., Booker, J., and Breatthnach, S.M. (1991) Irritant Contact Dermatitis in Warehouse Employees. *Occup. Med.* 43: 32–34.

Balls, M. and Clothier, R. (2010) A FRAME response to the Draft Report on Alternative (Non-animal) Methods for Cosmetic Testing: Current Status and Future Prospects—2010. *Altern Lab Anim.* 38(5): 345–353.

Bartek, M.J., LaBudde, J.A., et al. (1972) Skin Permeability In Vivo: Comparison in Rat, Rabbit, Pig and Man. *J Invest Dermatol.* 58(3): 114–123.

Brisson, P. (1974) Percutaneous Absorption. *Can Med Assoc J.* 110(10): 1182–1185.

Bronaugh, R.L. and Stewart, R.F.F. (1985) Methods for Invitro Percutaneous Studies IV: The Flow-Through Diffusion Cell. *J Pharm Sci.* Jan; 74(1): 64–67.

Bronaugh, R.L., Stewart, R.F., et al. (1982a) Methods for In Vitro Percutaneous Absorption Studies. I. Comparison with In Vivo Results. *Toxicol Appl Pharmacol.* 62(3): 474–480.

Bronaugh, R.L., Stewart R.F., et al. (1982b) Methods for In Vitro Percutaneous Absorption Studies. II. Animal Models for Human Skin. *Toxicol Appl Pharmacol.* 62(3): 481–488.

Bronaugh, R.L., Steward, R.F., and Simon, M. (1986) Methods for In Vitro Percutaneous Absorption Studies. VII: Use of Excised Human Skin. *J Pharm Sci.* 75(11): 1094–1097.

Bronaugh, R.L., Dragicivec, N., and Maibach, H.I. (eds). (2005) *Percutaneous Absorption: Drugs, Cosmetics, Mechanisms, Methods.* 4th ed. CRC Press.

Chiang, A., Tudela, E., and Maibach, H.I. (2012) Percutaneous Absorption in Diseased Skin: An Overview. *J Appl Toxicol.* 32(8): 537–563.

Collier, S.W., Sheikh, N.M., Sakr, A., Lichtin, J.L., Stewart, R.F., and Bronaugh, R.L. (1989) Maintenance of Skin Viability During In Vitro Percutaneous Absorption/Metabolism Studies. *Toxicol. Appl. Pharmacol.* 99: 522–533.

Corbo, M., Liu, J., and Chien, Y. (1990) Bioavailability of Propranolol Following Oral and Transdermal Administration in Rabbits. *J. Pharm. Sci.* 79: 584–590.

Cornell, J.A. (1990) *Experiments with Mixtures, Designs, Models, and the Analysis of Mixture Data.* John Wiley, New York.

Corsini, E., Brucloleri, A., Marinunch, M., and Galli, C.L. (1996) Endogenous Interleukin-1 Alpha Associated with Skin Irritation Induced by Tributyltin. *Tox. and Appl. Pharmacol.* 138: 268–274.

Crutcher, W. and Maibach, H.I. (1969) The Effect of Perfusion Rate on In Vitro Percutaneous Penetration. *J Invest Dermatol.* 53(4): 264–269.

Di Nardo, A., Wertz, P., Ademola, J., and Maibach, H.I. (1996) The Role of Ceramides in Proclivity to Toluene and Xylene-Induced Skin Irritation in Man: Dermatosen. *Occup. Environ.* 43.

Elmets, E.A., Casarett, C., Doulls, C.D., Klassens, M.O., Amadur, A., and Doull, C. (1992) *Buehler Topical Patch Technique, Maximization Test, Mouse Ear Swelling Test and In Vitro Screening Methods,* Eds. Macmillian, New York, pp. 423–425.

Exon, J.H. and Koller, L.D. (1983) Effects of Chlorinated Phenols on Immunity in Rats. *Int. J. of Immunopharmacol.* 5: 131–136.

Farahmand, S. and Maibach, H.I. (2009) Estimating Skin Permeability from Physicochemical Characteristics of Drugs: A Comparison Between Conventional Models and an In Vivo-Based Approach. *Int J Pharm.* 375(1–2): 41–47.

Feldstein, M.M., Tohmakhchi, V.N., Malkhazov, L.B., Vasiliev, A.E., and Platé, N.A. (1996) Hydrophilic Polymeric Matrices for Enhanced Transdermal Drug Delivery. *International Journal of Pharmaceutics.* 131(2): 229–242.

Fisher, A.A. (1984) Dermatitis Due to Transdermal Therapeutic Systems. *Cutis.* 34: 526–530.

Fisher, A.A. (1986) Assessment of Contact Dermatitis. In: *Contact Dermatitis*, 3rd ed. Ed. A.A. Fisher, Lea and Febiger, Philadelphia.

Friedrickson, R.A., Hurt, R.D., Lee, G.M., Wingendes, L., Croghon, I.T., Lauger, G., Gomez-Dahl, L., Hahl, L., and Offord, K.P. (1995) High Dose Transdermal Nicotine Therapy for Heavy Smokers: Safety Tolerability and Measurement of Nicotine and Caffeine Levels. *Psychopharmacol.* 122: 215–222.

Gattu, S. and Maibach, H.I. (2011) Modest but Increased Penetration Through Damaged Skin: An Overview of the In Vivo Human Model. *Skin Pharmacol PHysiol.* 24: 2–9.

Ghosh, T.K., Adir, J., Xiang, S., and Onyilfur, S. (1995) Transdermal Delivery of Metoprolol II. In Vitro Skin Permeation and Bioavailability in Hairless Rats. *J. Pharm. Sci.* 84: 158–160.

Green, B. and Bluth, J. (1995) Measuring the Chemosensory Irritability of Human Skin. Journal of Toxicology: Cutaneous and Ocular Toxicology. 14(1): 23–48.

Haseman, J.K., Crawford, D.D., Huff, J.E., Boorman, G.A., and McConnel, E. (1984) Results from 56 Two-Year Carcinogenicity Studies Conducted by the Natl. Toxicology Program. *J. Tox./Envi. Health.* 14: 621–639.

Henningsen, G.M. (1991) Dermal Hypersensitivity: Immunologic Principles and Current Methods of Assessment. In: *Dermal and Ocular Toxicology: Fundamentals and Methods*, Ed. David W. Hobson. CRC Press, Boca Raton, FL, pp. 183–189.

Holmgaard, R., Nielsen, J.B., and Benfeldt, E. (2010) Microdialysis Sampling for Investigations of Bioavailability and Bioequivalence of Topically Administered Drugs: Current State and Future Perspectives. *Skin Pharmacol Physiol.* 23(5): 225–243.

Hostýnek, J.J. and Maibach, H.I. (1998) Scope and Limitation of Some Approaches to Predicting Contact Hypersensitivity. *Toxicol in Vitro.* 12(4): 445–453.

Hurkmans, J.F.G.M., Boddie, H.E., Van Driel, L.M.J., Van Doorne, H., and Junginger, H.E. (1985) Skin Irritation Caused by Transdermal Drug Delivery Systems During Long Term (5 days) Application. *Br. J. Dermatol.* 112: 461–467.

Kezic, S. (2008) Methods for Measuring In-Vivo Percutaneous Absorption in Humans. *Hum Exp Toxicol.* 27(4): 289–295.

Kligman, A.M. and Balin, A.K. (1989) An Overview of Aging and the Skin. In: *Aging and Skin*, Eds. A. Kligman and A.R. Balin, Raven Press, New York, pp. 1–10.

Konda, S., Meier-Davis, S.R., Cayme, B., Shudo, J., and Maibach, H.I. (2012) Age-related Percutaneous Penetration Part 2: Effect of Age on Dermatophrmacokinetics and Overview of Transdermal Products. *Skin Therapy Letter.* (17)6: 5–8

Kreilgaard, M. (2002) Assessment of Cutaneous Drug Delivery Using Microdialysis. *Adv Drug Deliv Rev.* 54 Suppl 1: S99–S121.

Kubota, K., Koyama, E., and Yasuda, K. (1991) Skin Irritation Induced by Topically Applied Timolol. *Br. J. Clin Pharm.* 31: 417–475.

Lachapelle, J.M. and Maibach, H.I. (2012) *Patch Testing and Prick Testing.* 3rd ed. Springer, New York, NY.

Lahti, A. and Maibach, H.I. (1984) An Animal Model for Nonimmunologic Contact Urticaria. *Toxicology & Applied Pharmacology.* 76(2): 219–224.

Lakin, J.D. and Strecker, R.A. (1985) In: *Allergic Diseases, Diagnosis and Management*, 3rd ed. Ed. R. Patterson. J.B. Lippincott, Philadelphia, p. 191. 76: 219–224.

Lauerma, A. and Maibach, H.I. (1995) Provocative Tests in Dermatology. In: *Provocative Testing in Clinical Practice*, Ed. S.C. Spector. Marcel Dekker, Inc., New York, pp. 749–760.

Ledger, P. and Cormier, M.J. (1994) Reduction or Prevention of Sensitization to Drugs. U.S. Patent 5,120,545.

Levin, J. and Maibach, H.I. (2005) The Correlation Between Transepidermal Water Loss and Percutaneous Absorption: An Overview. *J of Control Release*. 103: 291–299.

Liu, P., Ademola, J., and Maibach, H.I. (1997). Pharmacodynamic Measurements of 8-MOP in Human Skin. *Skin Pharmacology*. 10: 21–27.

Lynch, D.H., Robert, L.K., and Daynes, R.A. (1987) Skin Immunology: The Achilles Heel of Transdermal Drug Delivery. *J. Controlled Rel.* 6: 39–50.

Malten, K.E. (1981) Thoughts on Irritant Contact Dermatitis. *Contact Dermatitis*. 7: 238–247.

Marzulli, F. and Maibach, H.I. (1975) Relevance of Animal Models: The Hexachlorophene Story. In: *Animal Models in Dermatology*, Ed. H.I. Maibach. Churchill-Livingstone, New York, pp. 156–167.

Marzulli, F.N., Brown, D.W.C., and Maibach, H.I. (1969) Techniques for Studying Skin Penetration. *Toxicol. Appl. Pharmacol.* Supplement 3: 76–83.

McGreesh, A.H. (1965) Percutaneous Toxicity. *Toxicol. Appl. Pharmacol.* Supplement 2: 20–26.

Nagels, H., Klaus, K., Wolff Hans-Michael, Y., and Merkle, H. (1993). Optimization of HMPSA Formulation for Transdermal Bupranolol Delivery by Means of a [3,2] Simplex-Lattice Design. *Proceed. Inter. Symp. Contrl Rel. Bioac. Mater.* Abstract #1312, Drug Updates.

Nangia, A., Berner, B., and Maibach, H.I. (2005) Transepidermal Water Loss Measurements for Assessing Skin Barrier Functions During In Vitro Percutaneous Absorption Studies. In: *Percutaneous Absorption, Drugs-Cosmetics-Mechanisms- Methodology*. 4th ed., Eds., R.L. Bronaugh and H. I. Maibach. Taylor & Francis, Boca Raton, FL. Chp. 36, pp 489–495.

Neely, W.B. (1994) *Introduction to Chemical Exposure and Risk Assessment*. Lewis Publishers, Boca Raton, FL.

Nielsen, J.B., Plasencia, I., Sørensen, J.A., and Bagatolli, L.A. (2011) Storage Conditions of Skin Affect Tissue Structure and Subsequent In Vitro Percutaneous Penetration. *Skin Pharmacol Physiol*. 24(2): 93–102.

N.I.H. (1985) Guide for the Care and Use of Laboratory Animals. N.I.H. Publication No. 85-23. U.S. Dept. of Health and Human Services, Bethesda, MD.

OECD (1981) Acute Dermal Irritation/Corrosion. *OECD Guidelines for Testing of Chemicals* Section 4, no. 404. Organization for Economic Cooperation and Development, Paris.

OECD (2004) Skin Absorption: *in vitro* Method. *OECD Guidelines for Testing of Chemicals* Section 4, no. 428. Organization for Economic Cooperation and Development, Paris.

Patterson, R. (1985) Skin Allergies. In: *Allergic Diseases, Diagnosis and Management*, 3rd ed. Ed. R. Patterson. J.B. Lippincott, Philadelphia, pp. 666–670.

Phillips, L. 2nd, Steinberg M., Maibach H.I., and Akers, W.A. (1972) A Comparison of Rabbit and Human Skin Response to Certain Irritants. *Toxicol Appl Pharmacol*. 21(3): 369–382.

Poet, T.S., Corley, R.A., Thrall, K.D., Edwards, J.A., Tanojo, H., Weitz, K.K., Hui, X., Maibach, H.I., and Wester, R.C. (2000) Assessment of the Percutaneous Absorption of Trichloroethylene in Rats and Humans Using MS/MS Real-Time Breath Analysis and Physiologically Based Pharmacokinetic Modeling. *Toxico Sci*, 56: 61–72.

Rawlings, A.V. (2017) The Stratum Corneum and Aging. In: *Textbook of Aging Skin*. Eds., M. Farage, K. Miller, and H. Maibach. Springer, Berlin, Heidelberg, pp 67–90.

Reddy, M.B., Stinchcomb, A.L., et al. (2002) Determining Dermal Absorption Parameters In Vivo from Tape Strip Data. *Pharm Res*. 19(3): 292–298.

Rigg, P.E. and Barry, B.W. (1990) Shed Snake Skin and Hairless Mouse Skin as Model Membranes for Human Skin During Permeation Studies. *J Invest Dermatol.* 94: 235–240.

Roberts, D.W. and Patlewicz, G.Y. (2010) Updating the Skin Sensitization in vitro Data Assessment Paradigm in 2009—a chemistry and QSAR perspective. *J Appl Toxicol.* 30(3): 286–288.

Robinson, M.K., Parsell, K.W., Breneman, D.L., and Cruze, C.A. (1991) Evaluation of the Primary Skin Irritation and Allergic Contact Sensitization Potential of Transdermal Triprolidine. *Fund. and Appl. Toxicol.* 17: 103–119.

Rosenthal, D.S., Roop, D.R., Huff, C.A., Weiss, J.S., Ellis, C.N., Hamilton, T.A., Vorhees, J., and Yuspa, S.H. (1990) Changes in Photoaged Human Skin Following Topical Application of All-Trans RA. *J. Invest. Dermatol.* 95: 510–515.

Rougier, A., Dupuir, D., Lotte, C., and Roguet, R. (1983) In Vivo Correlation Between Stratum Corneum Reservoir Function and Percutaneous Absorption. *J. Invest. Dermatol.* 81: 275–278.

Sato, S. and Wan Kim, S. (1984) Macromolecular Diffusion Through Polymer Membranes. *Int. J. Pharm.* 22: 229–255.

Scott, R.E., Walker, M., and Dugard, P.H. (1986) In Vitro Percutaneous Absorption Experiments: A Technique for the Production of Intact Epidermal Membranes from Rat Skin. *J. Soc. Cosmet. Chern.* 37: 35–41.

Sell, S. (1981) *Immunologic Considerations in Toxicology*, vol. 1, Ed. R.P. Sharma. CRC Press, Boca Raton, FL, p. 123.

Shah, N., Ademola, J.J., and Maibach, H.I. (1996) Efforts of Freezing and Azido Treatment of In Vitro Human Skin on the Flux and Metabolism of 8-Methoxpswalen. *Skin Pharmacol.* 9: 270–280.

Shah, V.P. and Skelly, J.P. (1992) Regulatory Considerations in Transdermal Systems in the United States. In: *Transdermal Controlled Systemic Medicine Medications*, Ed. Y.W. Chien. Marcel Dekker, Inc., New York, pp. 399–420.

Sigman, C.C., Bagheri, D., and Maibach, H.I. (1994) Approaches to Structure and Activity Relationship in Skin Sensitization. In: *In Vitro Skin Toxicology*, Eds. A. Rougier, A. Goldberg, and H.I. Maibach. Mary Ann Liebert., Inc., New York, pp. 271–280.

Simon, G.A. and Maibach, H.I. (2000) The Pig as an Experimental Animal Model of Percutaneous Permeation in Man: Qualitative and Quantitative Observations- An Overview. *Skin Pharmacol Appl Skin Physiol*, 13: 229–234.

Simon, G.A., and Maibach, H.I. (1998) Relevance of Hairless Mouse as an Experimental Model of Percutaneous Penetration in Man. *Skin Pharmacol. Appl. Skin Physiol.* 11: 80–86.

Singh, B. (1981) Plant Cutaneous Sensitizers In: *Immunologic Considerations in Toxicology*, vol. 1, Ed. R.P. Sharma. CRC Press, Boca Raton, FL, pp. 123–130.

Skelly, J.P., Amidon, G.L., Barr, W.H., Benet, L.Z., Cater, J.E., Robinson, J.R., Shah, V.P., and Yacobi. (1990) In Vitro and In Vivo Testing and Correlation of Oral Controlled/ Modified Release Dosage Forms. *Pharm. Res.* 7: 975–982.

Slavin, R.G. (1985) In: *Allergic Diseases, Diagnosis and Management*, 3rd ed. Ed. R. Paterson. Lippincott, Philadelphia, p. 662.

Smith, E. and Maibach, H.I. (1995) *Percutaneous Penetration Enhancer.* 2nd ed. Informa Healthcare, New York, NY.

Stahl, J., Niedorf, F., Wholert, M., and Kietzmann, M. (2012). The In Vitro Use of the Hair Follicle Closure Technique to Study the Follicular and Percutaneous Permeation of Topically Applied Drugs. *Altern Lab Anim.* 40(1): 51–57.

Streilein, J.W. (1989) In: *Immune Mechanisms in Cutaneous Diseases*, Ed. D.A. Norris. Marcel Dekker, Inc., New York, pp. 73–96.

Takahashi, K, Tmagawa S., Katagi, T., Rytting, J.B., Nishihata, T., and Mizuno, N. (1993) Percutaneous Permeation of Basic Compounds through Shed Snake Skin as a Model Membrane. *J Pharm Pharmacol.* 45(10): 882–826.

Takeuchi, H., Mano, Y., et al. (2011) Usefulness of Rat Skin as a Substitute for Human Skin in the In Vitro Skin Permeation Study. *Exp Anim.* 60(4): 373–384.

Touitou, E., Meidan, V.M., et al. (1998) Methods for Quantitative Determination of Drug Localized in the Skin. *J Control Release.* 56(1–3): 7–21.

Touitou, E. and Abed, L. (1985) The Permeation Behaviour of Several Membranes with Potential Use in the Design of Transdermal Devices. *Acta Pharm. Helv.* 60: 193–198.

U.S. Food and Drug Administration/Center for Drug Evaluation and Research (1995) *Guideline, I., S3A: Toxicokinetics: The Assessment of Systemic Exposure in Toxicity Studies in International conference on harmonisation of technical requirements for registration of pharmaceuticals for human use.*

U.S. Food and Drug Administration/Center for Drug Evaluation and Research (1996) *Guideline, I. S1A: The Need for Long-term Rodent Carcinogenicity Studies of Pharmaceuticals in International conference on harmonisation of technical requirements for registration of pharmaceuticals for human use.*

U.S. Food and Drug Administration/Center for Drug Evaluation and Research (1998) *Guideline, I. S1B: Testing for Carcinogenicity of Pharmaceuticals in International conference on harmonisation of technical requirements for registration of pharmaceuticals for human use.*

U.S. Food and Drug Administration/Center for Drug Evaluation and Research (2001) *Guideline, I., S7A: Safety Pharmacology Studies for Human Pharmaceuticals, in International conference on harmonisation of technical requirements for registration of pharmaceuticals for human use.*

U.S. Food and Drug Administration/Center for Drug Evaluation and Research (2005) *Guideline, I., S7B: Nonclinical Evaluation of the Potential for Delayed Ventricular Repolarization (QT Interval Prolongation) Human Pharmaceuticals, in International conference on harmonisation of technical requirements for registration of pharmaceuticals for human use.*

U.S. Food and Drug Administration/Center for Drug Evaluation and Research (2006) *Guideline, I. S8: Immunotoxicity Studies for Human Pharmaceuticals in International conference on harmonisation of technical requirements for registration of pharmaceuticals for human use.*

U.S. Food and Drug Administration/Center for Drug Evaluation and Research (2008) *Guideline, I. S1C (R2): Dose Selection for Carcinogenicity Studies of Pharmaceuticals in International conference on harmonisation of technical requirements for registration of pharmaceuticals for human use.*

U.S. Food and Drug Administration/Center for Drug Evaluation and Research (2009) *Guideline, I. M3(R2): Guidance on nonclinical safety studies for the conduct of human clinical trials and marketing authorization for pharmaceuticals in International conference on harmonization of technical requirements for registration of pharmaceuticals for human use.*

U.S. Food and Drug Administration/Center for Drug Evaluation and Research (2012) *Guideline, I. S2 (R1): Genotoxicity Testing and Data Interpretation for Pharmaceuticals Intended for Human Use in International conference on harmonisation of technical requirements for registration of pharmaceuticals for human use.*

Wang, C.Y. and Maibach, H.I. (2011) Why Minimally Invasive Skin Sampling Techniques? *A Bright Scientific Future.* I. 30(1): 1–6

Wester, R.C., Christoffel, J., et al. (1998) Human Cadaver Skin Viability for In Vitro Percutaneous Absorption: Storage and Detrimental Effects of Heat-Separation and Freezing. *Pharm Res.* 15(1): 82–84.

Wester, R.C. and Maibach, H.I. (1985) Animal Models for Percutaneous Absorption. In: *Models in Dermatology.* Eds. H.I. Maibach and N.J. Lowe. Karger, Basel, pp. 159–169.

Zhai, H. and Maibach, H.I. (2001) Effects of Skin Occlusion on Percutaneous Absorption: An Overview. *Skin Pharmacol Appl Skin Physiol.* 14(1): 1–10)

# 3 Selection Considerations for Membranes and Models for In Vitro/Ex Vivo Permeation Studies

*Pei-Chin Tsai, Tannaz Ramezanli,
Dina W. Ameen, Sonia Trehan, Nathaly Martos,
Zheng Zhang and Bozena Michniak-Kohn*

## CONTENTS

## 3.1  INTRODUCTION TO HUMAN SKIN AND IN-VITRO PERMEATION OF ACTIVES

### 3.1.1  HUMAN SKIN

Skin, the largest organ in the body, functions as a protective barrier as well as maintains fluid homeostasis, provides thermoregulation of the human body, mediates sensory detection and is the major site for transdermal delivery of actives. Human skin consists of two major layers: (a) the epidermal layer, that is mainly composed of proliferating and differentiated keratinocytes and (b) an underlying dermal layer that is rich in fibroblasts, connective tissue and blood vessels.

The epidermis is a stratified squamous epithelium and is histologically divided into sub-layers: *stratum basale, stratum spinosum, stratum granulosum* and *stratum corneum*. The *stratum basale* is located right above the basement membrane that connects the epidermis and dermis. The basal layer is responsible for the constant renewal of the skin cells (the turnover takes approximately 40 to 56 days and is dependent on age), based on constant mitosis of the basal cells.[1] As the keratinocytes move outwards and upwards, they begin to generate daughter cells. The daughter cells then begin to differentiate, flatten their nuclei and produce lamellar bodies to form the *stratum spinosum*. As the journey of the cells continues, the *stratum granulosum*, a layer above the *stratum spinosum*, is formed. The granular layer contains anucleated keratinocytes that have only granular cytoplasm and the extracellular space between the cells is filled with the lamellar bodies that were released through exocytosis. In the final stage of keratinocyte differentiation, the cells reach the outermost layer, the *stratum corneum*. The cytoplasm of the cells in *stratum corneum* is rich in keratin and the cells are surrounded by intercellular lipids, forming "brick and mortar" structures. The *stratum corneum* contains about 40% protein, 40% water and 18–20% of lipids and forms the major barrier in skin for the transport of actives.[2]

Beneath the epidermis lies the dermis that is 3–5mm thick, supporting the overlying epidermis and consists of fibroblasts in an extracellular matrix (ECM) of woven fibrous proteins. It is divided into two layers: (1) papillary dermis which is superficial and contains blood vessels which provide nutrition for the epidermis above, and (2) the reticular dermis, which is thicker and contains sebaceous glands, sweat glands, hair follicles, blood vessels, lymph vessels and nerves. Overall, the dermis is a hydrophilic compartment of skin and may act as a diffusion barrier for highly hydrophobic drugs.

### 3.1.2 Skin Permeation

#### 3.1.2.1 Absorption Barrier and Skin Permeation

The human skin acts as an absorption barrier blocking the entrance of unwanted substances (e.g., pathogens and toxins) and limiting the penetration of a variety of small molecules and large hydrophilic molecules from the external environment. The rate-limiting step of the percutaneous absorption process is provided by the *stratum corneum*, although the more aqueous viable epidermis and dermis can in addition hinder the penetration of highly hydrophobic drugs.

The skin permeation of the substances is related to their molecular weight, lipophilicity, environmental pH and ionization status. In general, molecules with molecular weight smaller than 500 Daltons are able to permeate the *stratum corneum*.[3] Increasing the molecular weight over 500 Daltons causes a rapid decline in the absorption through the skin. Lipophilicity of the compounds is also a major factor that affects permeation. While hydrophilic substances have difficulty passing through the *stratum corneum*, highly hydrophobic compounds tend to be retained in the *stratum corneum*. Therefore, molecules with appropriate lipophilicity (Log P 1–3) are recommended for higher permeation across the skin. For weak acids or weak bases, the ionization status is affected by the environmental pH and therefore affects their permeability. Non-ionized forms of lidocaine[4], salicylic acid[5] and nicotine[6] were shown to penetrate through skin membranes significantly faster than their ionized forms as predicted by the pH-partition theory.

The overall skin permeation is a result of the passive diffusion of drugs through various routes (Figure 3.1). Permeation pathways for actives to transport across the skin barrier include (A) transcellular pathway (across cells), (B) paracelullar pathway (between the cells), (C) transappendageal pathway (along the shafts of hair follicles and sweat glands) and (D) micropores created by physical enhancement techniques (e.g., microneedles and thermal poration). It is generally thought that hydrophilic compounds permeate through the paracellular pathway whereas hydrophobic compounds tend to permeate through the transcellular pathway. Both small molecules and large proteins can be delivered through micropores created by physical enhancement techniques.

#### 3.1.2.2 Studying Percutaneous Absorption Using Franz Diffusion Cells

In vitro permeation utilizing Franz diffusion assays has been extensively used to compare delivery of drug into and through skins from different formulations and provided useful data for predicting in vivo percutaneous absorption. Franz

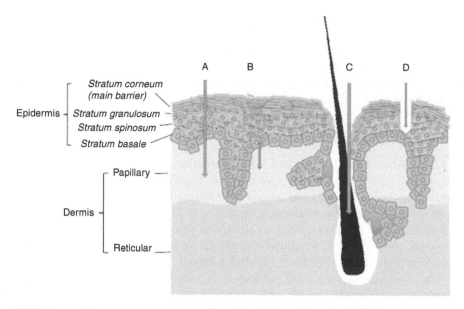

**FIGURE 3.1**  Schematic representation of skin structures and drug permeation pathways through human skin. (A) Transcellular pathway through cell membrane. (B) Paracellular pathway through tortuous route around the cells. (C) Drug transport through transappendageal pathway such as hair follicles and sweat glands. (D) Drug transport through micro-scale holes created by permeation enhancing techniques (e.g., microneedles, thermal poration).

diffusion assays generally use a vertical or a side-by-side diffusion apparatus that consists of two chambers (a donor and a receptor) separated by a membrane. The membrane can be excised human skin, animal skin, human skin equivalents (HSEs) or an artificial polymeric membrane. The advantages and disadvantages of various membranes will be discussed in detail later in the chapter. In the Franz diffusion test, the receptor compartment of the Franz diffusion cell is typically filled with phosphate buffer saline (PBS) or physiological solution that ensures sink conditions (drug concentration in the receptor fluid does not exceed 20% of the saturated solubility). The temperature of the membrane is maintained at physiological temperature (i.e., skin surface at 32°C). During the experiment, the active drug or formulation is applied to the epidermal side of the skin, and samples from the receptor compartment are taken at pre-determined intervals and replaced with equal volumes of receptor fluid. The amount of the drug permeated across the membrane and that remains in the tissue membrane at various time points can be analyzed using analytical methods (e.g., high-performance liquid chromatography [HPLC], liquid chromatography-mass spectrometry [LC-MS]) during or at the end of the experiment.

The passive transport of the drug through the membrane via a concentration gradient can be described by Fick's first law:

$$J = \frac{dM}{Sdt} = P(C1 - C2) = DK\left(\frac{C1 - C2}{h}\right)$$

where the flux $(J)$, is the amount of drug $(M)$, crossing through a unit area $(S)$ at an interval of time $(t)$; P is the permeation coefficient of drug; $C1$ and $C2$ are drug concentrations of donor and receptor compartment, respectively.

The permeation coefficient can be expressed with diffusion coefficient $(D)$, partition coefficient $(K)$ and thickness of membrane $(h)$:

$$P = \frac{DK}{h}$$

The flux at steady state can be obtained from the linear portion of the cumulative amount of drug permeated per area vs time. The flux, permeation coefficient, partition coefficient obtained from the in vitro Franz diffusion test may be useful to provide information about in vivo performance of transdermal drug products.

## 3.2 SELECTION OF MEMBRANE

For the in vitro permeation test, excised membrane such as human skin and animal skin are widely used. However, when biological membranes are not available, reconstructed HSEs and synthetic polymeric membranes can be used under certain conditions. The selection of membrane for the in vitro permeation test is governed by the availability, objective of the study and physicochemical properties of the tested drugs. Here in our chapter, a number of different biological and synthetic polymeric membranes are described in detail and the limitations and challenges are also addressed.

### 3.2.1 HUMAN SKIN

Human skin is regard as "gold standard" for in vitro/ex vivo percutaneous absorption studies by International Guideline OECD TG 428[7] and World Health Organization Environmental Health Criteria 235.[8] Several literature references have shown that the *stratum corneum* maintains its barrier function after the skin excision process.[9,10,11] The human skin used for percutaneous absorption studies can be obtained from cosmetic surgeries, biopsies and breast reductions or from cadavers. Viable skin is preferred if available, however frozen (non-viable) cadaver skin is usually easier to obtain. Moreover, depending on the objectives of the study and the physicochemical properties of the drug, different thickness of skin (full-thickness, split-thickness or *stratum corneum* alone) can be used.

### 3.2.1.1 Viable Human Skin

Fresh viable human skin can be obtained by surgical removal following cosmetic surgeries, biopsies or amputations. Abdominal or breast skin obtained from cosmetic surgical resection is a usual source of fresh viable skin. Tissues must be transferred as quickly as possible (while kept at a temperature of 4°C) to the laboratory facility where the ex vivo experimentation takes place. The skin has to be visually inspected to exclude any damage, and then the subcutaneous tissue is removed. The thickness of the excised skin tissue should not exceed 1mm; otherwise interference with the transport of lipophilic compounds across the membranes from dermal retention may occur.[12] In order to maintain skin viability, skin is preferably wrapped in gauze soaked with Eagle's Minimum Essential Media and Eagle's Balanced Salt Solution. In a study, Wester et al.[13] were able to maintain the viability of dermatomed skin (obtained immediately after death) for up to eight days. The skin was kept in Eagle's Minimum Essential Media and Eagle's Balanced Salt Solution at 4°C, and used the same solution as a receptor medium with 50 μg/mL gentamicin. The viability was sustained for eight days and was monitored by lactate produced due to anaerobic metabolism of glucose in the skin.

Viable skin has been shown to metabolize certain chemicals during percutaneous absorption. Kao et al.[14] showed that cutaneous metabolism has a significant effect on the penetration of benzo(alpha)pyrene based on its physicochemical properties. They found that the penetration of benzo(alpha)pyrene was greatly enhanced through viable skin preparations compared to non-viable skin. They speculated that when benzo(alpha)pyrene, a highly lipophilic compound, has undergone biotransformation in the skin, it is converted into metabolites with different solubility and partitioning properties causing them to permeate the skin at a different rate, or through another absorption route. In contrast, testosterone metabolites did not show such effects.

The use of viable skin allowed studying prodrug percutaneous absorption. Mavon et al.[15] compared the cutaneous permeation and metabolism of new vitamin E pro-drug, delta-tocopherol glucoside to that of vitamin E acetate using viable human skin. The skin used in this study was obtained from plastic surgery (abdominoplasty) and was maintained with a defined medium and remained viable for 72 hours. The viable skin was able to bioconvert delta-tocopherol glucoside to free tocopherol during the cutaneous permeation process whereas no metabolism was detected for vitamin E acetate. Therefore, the prodrug form of vitamin E was suggested to be an excellent antioxidant candidate for skin formulations.

### 3.2.1.2 Non-Viable Human Skin

Frozen, non-viable dermatomed human cadaver skin can be obtained from tissue banks. Such samples are used more frequently than fresh viable skin for in vitro permeation experiments due to ease of procurement and availability. Studies have shown the usefulness of non-viable cadaver skin in permeation investigations for many compounds.[16,17,18] The cadaver skin is usually dermatomed and stored at −20°C for later use (within 12 months or less). The barrier properties are maintained as long as the samples are stored correctly. Harrison et al.[18] showed that the skin maintained its water permeability characteristics when stored at −20°C for more than one year. Dennerlein et al. (2013)[19] reported that the permeation of 1,4-dioxane, anisole and cyclohexanone did not show any differences when either freshly excised or frozen skin was used (at −20°C for 30 days). However, storage conditions could potentially affect the barrier properties of skin. Neilson et al.[20] found that storing skin at −80 °C for three weeks increased caffeine permeability due to freezing-induced epidermal structural damage. It is considered that freezing may result in the formation of ice crystals that might damage the skin structure. Therefore, correct storage followed by testing the integrity of frozen non-viable skin is of crucial importance to confirm the reliability and accuracy of the in vitro data.

### 3.2.1.3 Full-Thickness and Partial Thickness Skin

Different thicknesses of skin can be used during in vitro permeation assays. Full-thickness skin (consisting of dermis, epidermis and *stratum corneum*), split-thickness (epidermis and *stratum corneum*) and heat/enzyme separated *stratum corneum* alone can be used. For a highly lipophilic compound, split-thickness and *stratum corneum* are more often used than full-thickness. This is because the dermis from the full-thickness skin may hinder the drug partitioning into the receptor medium, causing an underestimated permeation of the test compound in vitro.[7] Van de Sandt et al.[21] found that reduced skin thickness (from 0.9mm to 0.5mm) had a greater effect on the permeability of testosterone, a lipophilic drug, more than hydrophilic drugs, caffeine and benzoic acid. Higher amounts of testosterone permeated with thinner skin (average 0.5mm) than the thicker membranes. The same group studied the effect of skin thickness on the penetration of compounds of varying lipophilicity, caffeine ($logP = 0.01$), testosterone ($logP = 3.32$), propoxur ($logP = 1.52$) and butoxyethanol ($logP = 0.83$). Decreasing membrane thickness had no significant effect on caffeine penetration rate and the amount absorbed. However, it markedly increased the flux for more lipophilic drugs (i.e., butoxyethanol, propoxur, testosterone).[22] It is suggested that the dermal tissue, a hydrophilic membrane, acted as a barrier against the penetration of lipophilic compounds. Thus, using a full-thickness skin membrane is considered as adding resistance against lipophilic drug diffusion.[23] The resultant underestimated permeability is attributed to both increased diffusional path, and the compound reservoir formation in the dermis due to reduced partitioning into the receptor medium.[24]

### 3.2.1.4 Challenges of Using Human Skin

There are several major challenges associated with the use of human skin for in vitro percutaneous absorption studies. These include correct skin storage, compromised barrier integrity, inherent variability, inter and intra-subject variability and ethical concerns.

- *Correct skin storage*: Storage of skin at −20°C is needed to maintain the barrier properties of the skin samples. Multiple refreezing and thawing will often result in compromised barrier properties. Heat separated epidermal membranes can be stored at 4°C without significant changes to water permeability.
- *Compromised barrier integrity*: Skin barrier integrity may be impaired due to a disease, trauma, improper harvesting and/or handling, or inappropriate storage conditions. For these reasons, the OECD 428 guidelines stated

that cadaver skin integrity must be tested by appropriate methods, such as transepidermal water loss (TEWL), electrical resistance (ER) or tritiated water penetration.[7]

- *Inherent variability*: Skin is an inherently variable membrane, where differences in lipid content, number of hair follicles and degree of hydration may affect its permeability to test compounds. The variability associated with skin permeability poses as a major challenge for in vitro/ex vivo permeation studies. Differences in the skin permeability may be related to race,[25] and anatomic site.[16] However, less significant difference of variability was found with age and sex.[17]

- *Inter-, and intra-subject variability*: Southwell et al.[26] estimated inter-, and intra-subject to have a coefficient of variability of 66% and 43% respectively for a number of compounds of varying physicochemical properties permeating across human cadaver abdominal skin. Akomeah et al.[27] suggested that hydrophilic drug permeation might be more sensitive to inter- and intra-subject variability. This variability is related to skin structure differences affecting particularly the penetration routes of hydrophilic compounds. Another study was conducted by Meidan and Roper on a larger scale to determine the inter- and intra-donor tritiated water permeability. They found that intra-donor variability was higher than inter-donor, which is contradictory to the relevant previously published data.[28]

- *Ethical concerns*: The ethical issues associated with the use of living subjects for in vivo testing have necessitated justifiable use of human skin obtained from living or deceased donors. In both cases, written consent is obtained from the donor that the donated skin will be used for research purposes only.

### 3.2.2 ANIMAL SKIN

Animal models are important and practical models to study percutaneous absorption rate of chemicals and predict in vivo penetration behavior of the topical formulations. Animal skin is often used when human skin is not available. Even though excised animal skin is generally more permeable than human skin, it has several advantages for in vitro/ex vivo permeation screening. These advantages include easier access and less inter-subject variability. Moreover, the sex and age of the animals can be controlled and harvesting of skin from animals is less regulated.[11, 29] Various animal skin models from mammals, rodents and reptiles have been used for this purpose and overall monkey and pig skin were found to be a better model than rodent skin.[30] Table 3.1 depicts thickness of skin layers in several of these species and compared to human skin. In this section we briefly review common animal models for percutaneous penetration studies.

### 3.2.2.1 Pig Skin

Pig skin can be obtained easily and is an appropriate model for both in vitro and in vivo dermal/transdermal penetration studies. The animal is large enough for collection of many samples but not too large to make handling inconvenient. Human and porcine skins are similar in thickness of skin layers, follicular structure, a well-differentiated papillary body in dermis, number, size and distribution of dermal vessels, and large content of elastic tissue. There are some dissimilarities between human and pig skin, including poorer vascularization, smaller number of eccrine sweat glands and high fat content in pig skin. Due to high fat content of pig skin, lipid soluble compounds are more likely to remain in the fatty areas rather than getting exposed to systemic circulation.[31]

Barbero and Frasch[30] extensively reviewed variability in permeability and lag time between human and pig skin models for in vitro penetration studies. They investigated the suitability of pig, guinea pig and hairless guinea pig skin as surrogates for human skin and reported less variability with these models and a significant positive correlation between them and human skin. Another review in this area was performed by Maibach's group[29] and included permeability measurement of 77 compounds in 46 studies. They reported that the percutaneous permeability of the pig model for 86% of those chemicals fell within the range of ±1/2 log interval of human skin permeability.

Porcine ear skin is also a good model to investigate transfollicular delivery. Jacobi et al.[32] studied ear skin structure in German domestic pigs. They observed an average of 20 hairs per $cm^2$ of pig ear skin, which is very close to the follicular density reported for human vellus hairs in the literature (14–32 in per $cm^2$). Moreover, porcine ear skin was found to be a more suitable model than excised human skin for studying delivery and storage of topically applied chemicals in the hair follicles. This is mainly due to the contraction of human skin after excision. Whereas porcine ear skin connected to the cartilage does not contract.[33]

### 3.2.2.2 Primate Skin

Among all animals, monkeys are phylogenetically closest to humans; therefore, their skin is very similar to human skin. The regional variation in skin permeability that is observed with human skin also exists in monkeys. However, the use of primates is costly and limited due to ethical reasons.[29]

Wester et al.[34] tested percutaneous absorption of hydrocortisone, testosterone and benzoic acid in rhesus monkey and man, which resulted in similar total percentage absorption of compounds in both skin types. Bronaugh et al.[35] also examined percutaneous absorption of the fragrance diethyl maleate in rhesus monkey and human in vivo. In a 24-hour study, the absorption of the volatile fragrance was 54% of the applied dose in human skin compared with 69% penetration in the monkey skin.

### 3.2.2.3 Rodent Skin

Rodents are another popular model for transdermal screening and regulatory toxicity studies due to their availability, ease of handling, low costs and the reproducibility of the data.[36] However, rodent skin generally is more permeable and over-predicts percutaneous absorption of chemicals relative to human skin. Rodent skin has a thinner *stratum corneum*, higher hair follicle density and different intercellular lipid composition and organization in the *stratum corneum*.[11]

Jung and Maibach[29] reviewed percutaneous absorption of 110 compounds in 79 studies. They reported that rat skin was more permeable than human skin for the majority of these substances. Bond and Barry[37] studied suitability of hairless mouse skin as a surrogate for human skin under conditions of prolonged hydration. Their results showed that human skin retained its barrier properties over six–eight-days permeation study. In contrast, prolonged hydration of the rodent skin disrupted the *stratum corneum* and resulted in significant enhancement in skin permeability over a few days of hydration. Thus, it has been suggested that some rodent species can be useful for permeation screening if the exposure time is less than 12 hours.[11] Van Ravenzwaay and Leibold[38] compared the percutaneous absorption rate of a variety of the pesticides in human and rat epidermis. They observed higher permeability of rat skin for all the chemicals that were tested in vitro. They also reported that in vivo rat skin was less permeable than in vitro rat skin but more permeable than in vitro human skin in most of the cases.

In order to have a better estimation of the in vivo human penetration rate from transdermal screening on rat skin, several research groups suggested the Parallelogram method.[38,39,40] In this method the human dermal absorption is calculated using the combined in vitro and in vivo rat studies plus in vitro human studies:

$$Human_{in\ vivo} = \frac{(Rat_{in\ vivo}) \times (Human_{in\ vitro})}{(Rat_{in\ vitro})}$$

Ross et al.[41] utilized this method for several actives with different log P values and in most cases the estimated percutaneous absorption was ≤ 1.7-fold of the measured value in humans. The Parallelogram method can also be used for other animal models, such as the pig. This approach is valid when the ratio of in vivo to in vitro absorption for a given substance remains the same in both animal and human skin.[29]

### 3.2.2.4 Snake (Squamate) Skin
Shed squamate epidermis is another model that has been suggested as a surrogate for human epidermis. The epidermis of squamate reptiles consists of alpha and beta keratin and similarly to mammalian skin, both neutral and polar lipids are present in this membrane. The shedding process occurs every two–three months in the mature skin and therefore this membrane can be obtained without animal scarification. One animal can provide repeated sheds and inter-individual variability of the results are low. It is claimed that this membrane provides a permeability barrier similar to that of human skin and can be stored at room temperature without deterioration.[42] Therefore, this model can be used to predict transepidermal flux.

Rigg and Barry[43] investigated the effect of hydration and several chemical enhancers on membrane permeability for human skin, hairless mouse skin and shed skin from two species of snake: *Elaphe obsolete* and *Python molurus*. Their results showed that unlike hairless mouse skin, the permeability of human skin and snakeskin did not change significantly during prolonged hydration. Nevertheless, squamate membrane underestimated the effect of the penetration enhancers while the mouse model overestimated the changes.

**TABLE 3.1**
**Comparison of Various Animal Skin Thicknesses to Those of Human Skin**

| Species, and skin area | Stratum corneum ($\mu m$) | Epidermis ($\mu m$) | Whole skin (mm) | Reference |
|---|---|---|---|---|
| Human, abdomen | - | 79 | 1.33 | 49 |
| Human, forehead | - | 94 | 0.86 | 49 |
| Human, forearm | 17 | 36 | 1.5 | 50 |
| Human, thigh | 23 | 110 | 2.4 | - |
| Pig, back | 26 | 66 | 3.4 | 51 |
| Pig, ear | 10 | 50 | 1.3 | 51 |
| | 17–28 | 60–85 | 1.52–2.32 | 32 |
| Pig, outer ear | 9 | 62 | 1.18 | 48 |
| Mouse, back | 5 | 13 | 0.8 | 51 |
| Rat, back | 34.7 | 61.1 | 2.8 | 47 |
| Rat, abdomen | 13.8 | 30.4 | 1.66 | 47 |
| Rabbit, inner ear | 12 | 17 | 0.28 | 48 |

### 3.2.2.5 Rabbit Skin

Rabbit skin possesses rapid absorptive characteristics and is a good indicator of dermal toxicity.[44] Albino rabbit is known as a standard and valid model for assessing irritation of topically applied formulations.[45] However, rabbit skin is generally more permeable than human skin and can overestimate the percutaneous absorption.[46, 47]

Nicoli et al.[48] evaluated rabbit ear skin and reported comparable permeability for the tested compounds (lidocaine, triptorelin and thiocolchicoside) relative to pig ear skin. Rabbit ear stratum corneum has similar thickness to that of pig ear and human skin, but thinner epidermis and dermis layer (Table 3.1). Other variations include different lipid compositions of *stratum corneum* (higher lipophilicity) and higher hair follicle density. This membrane has shown lower permeability for hydrophilic agents such as caffeine and nicotine and higher absorption of the lipophilic chemicals.

### 3.2.2.6 Challenges of Using Animal Skin

A considerable amount of literature has been published on animal models for prediction of percutaneous absorption kinetics. Among all the alternative models for human skin, membranes from animal sources show higher resistivity to drug diffusion but lack stability and uniformity of the synthetic membranes. As we discussed in this chapter animal skin differs from human skin in features like thickness, hair density and biochemical composition. Elias et al.[52] have reported that lipid content of the animal skin is the major determinant for its barrier properties. As a result, the differences in diffusivity that exist among different species and sites of application are mainly due to variation in lipid composition. In general, the common laboratory animal skin is more permeable than human skin and the skin permeability increases in the following order: chimpanzee, man, pig, monkey, dog, cat, horse, rabbit, goat, guinea pig and mouse.[47]

### 3.2.3 Human Skin Equivalents (HSEs)

It would be ideal to conduct permeability tests using viable human skin samples that are of lower cost, are reproducible with little variability, easily available and have no issues with donor sourcing. In part, human skin equivalents (HSEs) have achieved some of these desired properties.[53] Test Guidance No. 28 issued by the Organisation for Economic Cooperation and Development (OECD) stated that reconstructed HSEs can be used for in vitro absorption if comparable results from the literature are obtained.[54] Reconstructed HSEs are viable three-dimensional (3D) tissue models that closely mimic normal human skin morphology and biochemical composition. Depending upon the structural composition and substrate used for model reconstruction, HSEs can be classified into two major types: (1) reconstructed human epidermis (RHEs) which consist of multiple layers of proliferated and differentiated keratinocytes on an inert filter membrane and (2) full-thickness HSEs that consist of keratinocytes on a fibroblast-populated collagen matrix. Based on the ability of HSEs to form organized and differentiated epidermal structures (especially the formation of *stratum corneum*), a number of studies have been conducted to evaluate them as penetration models and replacements for human and animal skins (Table 3.2).

#### 3.2.3.1 Reconstructed Human Epidermis (RHEs)

Reconstructed human epidermis (RHEs) consists of differentiated keratinocytes on acellular inert filter substrates. Although these models possess a differentiated *stratum corneum*, these epidermis-only skin equivalents have inferior barrier properties if compared with normal human skin.[55] Schmook et al.[56] compared the permeation profiles of drugs with different hydrophilicity using commercially available RHEs, SkinEthic™ (Episkin, France) to those using human, rat and porcine skin. The authors found that the flux from relatively hydrophilic compound (salicylic acid) was comparable to human skin. However, for more hydrophobic drugs such as clotrimazole and hydrocortisone, the flux was about 900- and 200-fold higher, respectively. In another study, a commercially available RHEs, EpiDerm™ (MatTek, Ashland, USA) revealed a five times higher flux compared to heat-separated human epidermis in a permeability study of flufenamic acid (lipophilic model drug).[57] In general, it is considered that RHEs exhibit higher permeability compared to that of human epidermis. Although the flux value is being overestimated, the RHEs could differentiate the relative ranking of the compounds. A validation study performed by ten laboratories demonstrated that the ranking of a wide spectrum of test substances (mannitol, benzoic acid, caffeine, nicotine, digoxin, flufenamic acid, testosterone, clotrimazole, ivermectin) permeating through three RHE models, Episkin (Episkin, France), EpiDerm and SkinEthic could reflect the permeation through human epidermis under both infinite and finite dose conditions.[55] In addition, the obtained permeation data had a tendency towards lower variability compared with human epidermis.

#### 3.2.3.2 Full-Thickness HSEs

The full-thickness HSE models contain keratinocytes grown on a dermal substrate populated with fibroblasts to form epidermal and dermal compartments.

**TABLE 3.2**
**Comparison of Drug Permeation on Commercial HSEs to Human Skin and Pig Skin**

| Commercial HSEs | Company | Model drug | Compared with human skin | Compared with pig skin | Ref. |
|---|---|---|---|---|---|
| *RHEs* | | | | | |
| EpiDerm | MatTek Corp (Ashland, USA) | Flufenamic acid | Flux is five times higher | | 57 |
| SkinEthic | Episkin (Lyon, France) | Terbinafine | ~ 24-fold higher in flux | ~37-fold higher in flux | 56 |
| | | Clotrimazole | ~ 900-fold higher in flux | ~ 900-fold higher in flux | |
| | | Hydrocortisone | ~ 200-fold higher in flux | ~ 500-fold higher in flux | |
| | | Salicylic acid | ~ 6-fold higher in flux | ~15-fold higher in flux | |
| Episkin | Episkin (Lyon, France) | Testosterone | ~100 times higher in permeation coefficient | | 67 |
| | | Caffeine | ~10 times higher in permeation coefficient | | |
| *Full-thickness* | | | | | |
| Graftskin™ LSE™ | Organogenesis (MA, USA) | Terbinafine | ~ 24-fold higher in flux | ~ 25-fold higher in flux | 56 |
| | | Clotrimazole | ~1000-fold higher in flux | ~ 1000-fold higher in flux | |
| | | Hydrocortisone | ~200-fold higher in flux | ~ 400-fold higher in flux | |
| | | Salicylic acid | ~ 2-fold higher in flux | ~ 3.5-fold higher in flux | |
| Phenion® FT | Henkel (Düsseldorf, Germany) | Testosterone | | ~20-fold higher in permeation coefficient | 58 |
| | | Caffeine | | ~200-fold higher in permeation coefficient | |

Commercially available models such as Graftskin™ LSE™ (Organogenesis, MA, USA), and Phenion FT® (Henkel Corp, Düsseldorf, Germany) have been evaluated for permeation testing. Schmook et al.[56] compared the permeation profile of terbinafine, clotrimazole, hydrocortisone and salicylic acid on Graftskin LSE and compared these with data from SkinEthic (Episkin, France), human, porcine and rat skin. When compared to human skin, the full-thickness Graftskin LSE demonstrated an adequate barrier for salicylic acid. However, the HSEs had at least 1,000- and

200-fold increase of flux for more hydrophobic drugs clotrimazole and hydrocortisone, respectively. In another study, Ackermann et al.[58] evaluated the use of Phenion FT® as a percutaneous absorption model by comparing permeation of testosterone, caffeine, benzoic acid and nicotine with that of pig skin and RHEs (i.e., EpiDerm, SkinEthic, Episkin). Overall, the Phenion FT® was more permeable than pig skin but was comparable with RHEs for lipophilic compounds such as nicotine and testosterone. The authors suggested that the retardant flux of lipophilic compounds was the result of additional uptake and a reservoir formed in the dermis as well as the presence of different lipid patterns in the epidermis. In spite of the fact that Phenion FT® exhibited inferior barrier properties compared with pig skin, the reproducibility of the permeation profiles was still good.

### 3.2.3.3   Challenges for HSEs as Permeation Models

Much effort has been made in the past to establish RHEs and full-thickness HSEs for permeation testing. Although the data suggests that HSEs could potentially reflect rank order of drug permeation and the reproducibility of HSEs is often better than that for human skin, the major hurdle of current HSE models lies in the overpredicted permeability parameters compared to those from human skin. This could be caused by different lipid composition and organization of the *stratum corneum* in current HSE models. Thakoersing et al.[59] analyzed their in-house HSEs and found an increased presence of monosaturated fatty acids and hexagonal lipid packing in their *stratum corneum*. This could be contributing to the lower barrier properties of HSEs. However, Batheja et al.[60] optimized HSE growth conditions with the addition of clofibrate, fatty acids and ascorbic acid, and showed that the ceramide profile and barrier properties of their in-house collagen-based full-thickness HSEs can be improved. Another major limitation of the HSEs is the lack of appendages such as hair follicles, pilosebaceous units and sweat glands. HSEs with appendages are yet to be developed. This is important as the use of nanoparticles has been intensively investigated for topically and transdermal treating several dermatological diseases[61] and studies have suggested that the delivery of drugs from nanoparticles occurs through the deposition in hair follicles.[62,63,64] Thus the incorporation of appendages in HSE models could further improve these models and add the follicular transport pathway to the HSEs.

Other limitations of current HSEs are short viability and shelf life, and handling issues due to a fragile supporting membrane. Improving these factors should allow the use of HSEs for in vitro permeation testing. However, continuous research in this field is undergoing, and advanced biomaterials (e.g., decellularized tissue) and advanced fabricating techniques (e.g., 3D printing) can provide functional HSEs for various drug screening purpose.[65,66] Therefore, we envision new technologies in the future to continuously improve pre-existing models and to achieve the application of specific models to meet the demand. Ultimately, HSEs with ideal barrier properties, less variation in permeability data and relevant in vitro/in vivo correlation will assist the development of topically applied drugs.

### 3.2.4   POLYMERIC MEMBRANES

In vitro/ex vivo permeation studies can be performed using samples of human skin, animal skin and HSEs. However, the use of biological skin specimens is limited by their availability, while HSEs are products containing viable tissues and have critical timeframes between sample arrival and use for permeation testing. For these specimens, batch-to-batch variation and its effect on drug permeation is also a concern. In contrast, polymeric membranes are readily available for permeation testing, usually do not require special storage conditions and do not require extensive treatment prior to use. Certain key properties of polymeric membranes are a feature of their chemistry or are acquired during the manufacturing process; therefore, the reproducibility of the drug permeability data from a polymeric membrane can be ensured. This feature provides additional control of the parameters in the permeation studies and allows the investigator to elucidate factors that affect permeation. However, these membranes do not have cells and express no enzymes or lipid/protein interactions as normal human skin would, so investigators need to realize the limitations when using these kinds of membranes in their permeability studies.

A wide spectrum of polymeric membranes is available on the market. These polymeric membranes can be categorized according to different criteria. For example, according to the composition, polymeric membranes can be grouped as "silicone based" (with the main component polydimethylsiloxane, PDMS),[68] "cellulose based" (e.g., regenerated cellulose, cellulose esters and cellulose nitrate),[69] and "synthetic polymeric" based (e.g., polyacrylonitrile, nylon, sulfone, polycarbonate and polypropylene membrane, and others). The polymeric membranes can also be characterized based on whether they are porous or non-porous: for example, silicone membranes are non-porous, while cellulose-based and synthetic polymeric membranes are often porous, having different thickness, pore size and molecular weight cut off (MWCO) values. Also, polymeric membranes can be grouped into high-flux and low-flux type, based on the value of flux.[70] Overall, polymeric membranes are widely used to study the drug release (which is different from drug permeability) from formulations that are applied in the Franz diffusion cell technique. In the following section, the studies on skin permeability using silicone membranes are further discussed since they are often employed to simulate the skin due to their skin-imitating lipophilicity and rate-limiting permeation properties.[71,72,73]

### 3.2.4.1 Silicone Membranes

Silicone membrane is based on silicone polymers whose backbone is composed of silicon-oxygen (Si-O) units. Among those silicone polymers, polydimethylsiloxane (PDMS) is the basic form, in which two methyl groups are linked to each silicon molecule. PDMS has unique properties such as high flexibility, low glass transition temperature and high gas permeability.[74] The properties of silicone polymers can be tuned by modifying the chemical structure of PDMS. For example, an important modification to PDMS is the incorporation of vinyl groups, which significantly increases the cross-linking efficiency with organic peroxide. Methyl-vinyl silicone is a widely used silicone rubber.

PDMS membrane has been used extensively to simulate and predict drug permeability to skin. One of the early foci was to investigate the effect of atomic charge on a compound's permeability. Chen et. al. reported an empirical model for drug permeation for aromatic compounds through PDMS using molecular modeling.[75] A total of 103 compounds in 15 ring classes, including benzene, quinoline, naphthalene, pyridine, naphthyridine, furan, benzofuran, imidazole, benzimidazole, indole, thiophene, pyrrole, pyrazole, pyridazine and pyrazine were studied. In this study flux was found to be significantly affected by atomic charge. Partial charge calculations combined with solubility and molecular weight provided a universal quantitative structure-transportability relationship (QSTR) model for the estimation of flux for all 15 classes of compounds. Later, the same research group refined the model and studied the maximum steady-state flux of 171 compounds through PDMS membranes.[76] The results further demonstrated that the simple QSTR equation is capable of accurately predicting the steady-state flux of a variety of compounds. Contribution of atomic charge to mass transport phenomena was further verified by the prediction of the apparent permeability calculated from the steady-state flux data.

Later, Geinoz et al.[77] investigated the relationship between hydrogen-bonding capacity and drug permeation across a silicone membrane, with the emphasis on the most distinctive structural parameters in a series of 16 permeants including substituted phenols and four drugs, i.e., diazepam, lidocaine, nicotine and orphenadrine. The substituted phenols were chosen as they vary significantly in H-bonding properties, while maintaining little change in other molecular parameters such as size and shape. This study demonstrated that the permeation of xenobiotics across PDMS membranes is controlled primarily by their hydrogen-bond donor capacity, in turn strongly influenced by intramolecular interactions. Lipophilicity also plays a role, which must be considered when heterogeneous drugs are included in the study.

The use of PDMS membranes in molecular simulations has contributed to the understanding of the effect of atomic charge, hydrogen-bonding capacity and lipophilicity. However, PDMS membranes are homogeneous, which differs from the heterogeneity of biological membranes. As an example, Frum et al. studied the permeation of five model penetrants (testosterone, oestradiol, corticosterone, aldosterone and adenosine) across PDMS membranes and they found that the permeability coefficients of all five drugs were distributed in a Gaussian-normal fashion, which was in distinct contrast with the non-Gaussian fashion that was obtained for mammalian skin.[78]

### 3.2.4.2 Challenges of Using Polymeric Membranes

The use of polymeric membrane in permeation testing allows the experimental conditions to be controlled more precisely since the biological variability is eliminated. The only variables are the inherent properties of the membrane and the physico-chemical properties of the drugs undergoing the testing. Polymeric membranes may be suitable for early formulation optimization and formulations comparisons and perhaps testing the effects of some excipients. The membranes offer longer shelf life, experimental convenience, are usually inexpensive and readily available. Compared to human and animal skin specimens, polymeric membranes have minimal concerns on safety and biohazard issues.

However, the use of polymeric membranes is associated with challenges such as undetermined in vitro/in vivo correlations (IVIVC), absences of metabolic activity, different barrier properties among materials and pore sizes, lack of cell components and fail to mimic transport pathways. The major drawback of polymeric membranes is the lack of biological structure and lipid composition, which highly limit the evaluation of interactions that occur when a drug is transported through lipoidal intercellular channels. In addition, polymeric membranes are not suitable to study excipient effect in formulation if the excipients are chemical penetration enhancers that are known to modify flux through interactions with the lipid organization of the *stratum corneum.*

## 3.3 OTHER ADVANCED IN VITRO MODELS

Evaluating the effect of potential drug candidates and many formulations using traditional skin samples from humans or animals can be a daunting task due to the low-throughput of the test. Advanced screening technology incorporating lipid infused synthetic polymeric membranes in a 96-well format may offer a potential solution for rapid drug screening. Moreover, the combinations of HSEs with microfluidic devices, also known as "skin-on-a-chip" models are in development. These models potentially mimic blood flow, skin physiology, skin metabolism and can be applied as screening tools to capture systemic pharmacokinetic and pharmacodynamics profiles of drugs. Some examples of these high-throughput models are discussed in the following sections.

### 3.3.1 SKIN-PAMPA MODEL

Parallel artificial membrane permeability assay (PAMPA) was first introduced by Kansy et al.[79] to assist the rapid determination of the passive membrane permeability of drugs. In the PAMPA model, a multi-well microtiter plate is used for the donor compartment and the receptor compartment is located on the top separated by a lipid-infused artificial membrane. To date, the PAMPA models have been correlated with drug permeation across a variety of barriers including gastrointestinal tract[80], blood brain barrier[81] and skin.[82] This method has drawn attention in the pharmaceutical industry for screening lead candidates during early-discovery phase based on the low cost and high-throughput. Ottaviani et al.[82] developed a skin-specific model, Skin-PAMPA, which incorporated different ratios of silicon oil and isopropyl myristate mixtures on polyvinylidene fluoride (PVDF) membranes. A correlation of permeability coefficients was reported between the Skin-PAMAPA model (70% silicon and 30% isopropyl myristate) and human skin for 19 compounds. In addition, the retention values of tested compounds on the Skin-PAMAPA model were correlated to the *stratum corneum*/water partition coefficient, which suggests that the model could reflect the affinity of compounds to the *stratum corneum* barrier.

### 3.3.2 STRAT-M™ MEMBRANES

Strat-M™ (EMD Millipore, Danvers, USA) membrane is a commercially available skin-mimic polymeric membrane that has shown in many cases to have good correlation of drug permeation to human skin. It is a synthetic polymeric membrane that consists of multiple layers of polyethersulfone (PES) (diffusion resistant) on top of a polyolefin (PO) layer (more diffusive) creating hydrophobic and hydrophilic domains similar to those of human skin. The porous structure in the membrane is impregnated with a blend of proprietary synthetic lipids, and the pore size decreases from top (PES layer) to bottom (PO layer). Uchida et al.[83] have demonstrated the correlation of Strat-M membrane to excised human and hairless rat skin specimens. In this study, permeation profiles and permeability coefficients (logP) of 13 chemicals exhibiting molecular weights of 152–289 and lipophilicities of −0.9 to 3.5 were obtained. Increased lipophilicities ($logK_{o/w}$) of the chemicals resulted in an increase in logP, and the logP relationships of Strat-M to human skin and hairless rat skin were almost 1:1 with a correlation of $r^2 = 0.929$ and $r^2 = 0.970$, respectively. In another study, Karadzovska and Riviere[84] cut Strat-M membranes to a diameter of 6mm and placed them into a 96-well filter plate. The permeation of six compounds (caffeine, cortisone, diclofenac sodium, mannitol, salicylic acid, testosterone) with molecular weights of 138–360 and $logK_{o/w}$ of −0.07–4.5 were compared with porcine skin placed in Franz diffusion cells. There was a good correlation ($r^2 = 0.73$) of the amount of drug remaining in the membrane between the 96-well format of Strat-M and porcine skin in Franz diffusion cells. In addition, the Strat-M could predict the vehicle ranking order for saturated concentrations of diclofenac sodium, mannitol and testosterone compared to the diffusion cells. However, little correlation of log absorption value was obtained between the 96-well Strat-M and the porcine skin in Franz diffusion cells.

### 3.3.3 PHOSPHOLIPID VESICLE-BASED PERMEATION (PVPA) MODEL

The phospholipid vesicle-based permeation (PVPA) model was essentially designed to mimic the human *stratum corneum*. This model is based on tightly fused liposomes on a polymeric membrane filter support (cellulose ester; 0.65μm pore size) in Transwell plates and is used to predict passive diffusion of drugs through a skin barrier. Engesland et al.[85] tested the permeation of model drugs, indomethacin, salicylic acid, ibuprofen, flufenamic acid, calcein and FITC-dextran across different PVPA models. They demonstrated, by modifying the lipid composition of the liposomes in the PVPA model to 50% egg phophatidylcholine/27.5% ceramides/12.5% cholesterol/2.5% cholesteryl sulfate/7.5% palmitic acid, a better mimic of the *stratum corneum* barrier was achieved. Moreover, they suggested that the liposomes could be viewed as simple models of cells that may mimic in vivo structures to a greater extent compared with the continuous lipophilic environment that is present in the PAMPA models. In addition, the prediction of partitioning between liposomes and the buffer may lead to better predictions of permeation as compared to those obtained from octanol and water experiments. However, a direct comparison of the permeation profile to human skin is still needed to establish the real correlations between the PVPA model and human skin.

### 3.3.4 SKIN-ON-A-CHIP

Recent innovations in microfluidics have provided novel ways to integrate three-dimensional (3D) tissue engineered models to create organ-on-a-chip platforms for drug screening applications. Microfluidic systems allow the precise manipulation of micro-liter volumes of liquid that can replicate blood circulation in membranes. Cultured multiple 3D organ substitutes in the microfluidic system, also known as "organ-on-a-chip" allows interconnecting the micro-chambers to mimic the entire process of ADME (Absorption, Distribution, Metabolism and Excretion) of drugs.[86] Atac el al.[87] have reported the successful culturing of commercially available full-thickness HSEs (EpiDermFT™; MatTek MA, USA), ex vivo human skin and single hair follicular units on a single microfluidic device. The dynamically perfused chip could overcome the short culturing period from conventional static tissue cultures. Moreover, the ability of the drug to pass through various tissue compartments has the potential to mimic systemic drug distribution. Abaci et al.[88] demonstrated the evaluation of skin toxicity effects of doxorubicin through their pumpless HSEs-on-a-chip model. The microchannels on the HSEs-on-a-chip can mimic the physiological residence time and blood flow in the tissue so that relevant drug concentrations can be measured following topical delivery of a drug. Transdermal transport and barrier properties of HSEs-on-a-chip were studied by topically applied fluorescein-tagged oligonucleotides on the epidermal surface of HSEs and the drug toxicity study was studied by adding clinically relevant doxorubicin plasma concentrations (i.e., 36µM) in the reservoirs of HSEs-on-a-chip. The authors stated that the HSEs were able to maintain intact barrier properties for three weeks and the toxicity effect of doxorubicin was confirmed through histology and immunostaining of biomarkers (i.e., Ki67 and loricrin). The development of ex vivo human skin or HSEs on microfluidic devices has the potential to allow the evaluation of ADME of drugs and also, for example, from nanoparticle containing drug delivery systems.[89]

### 3.3.5 CURRENT CHALLENGES FOR ADVANCED MODELS

More sophisticated, faster, efficient and physiological relevant screening tools for drug permeation are continuously being designed and tested. Although improvement has been observed in lipid/synthetic polymeric membranes such as the Skin-PAMPA and Strat-M models and fused liposomal system (PVPA), all of these systems still face the lack of active transport, cellular metabolism and skin appendages. Moreover, in order to establish higher screening efficiency from the 96-well format, the small amount of drug applied and low volume of the receptor phase often pose a problem for drug concentration quantification and require the tested drug to be radioactively labeled. Skin-on-a-chip, although promising for capturing the aspects of systemic drug transport and distribution, is still in early development. It faces challenges such as scalability issues, analytical detection limitations and the incorporation with other organs/tissues on a single chip as well as challenges with different requirements of media supplementation for each tissue.

## 3.4 CONCLUSIONS AND FUTURE DIRECTIONS

In order to develop efficient and safe transdermal drug products, in vitro/ex vivo skin permeation testing is required. This approach currently utilizes different skin membranes placed in Franz diffusion cells that these studies assist in the formulation optimization and provide useful information in the formulation selection process. Among the various membranes, human skin is still regarded as the gold standard by international regulatory agencies as providing the barrier function of

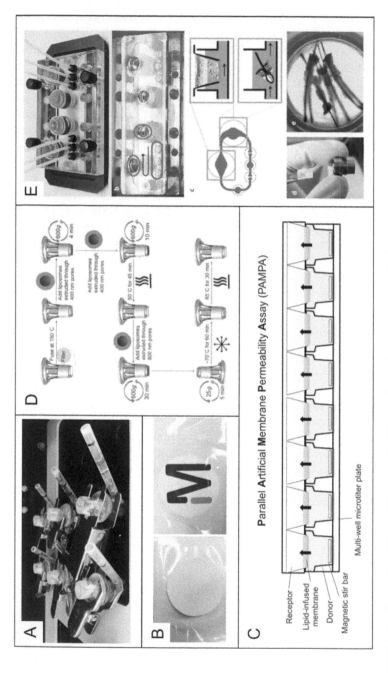

**FIGURE 3.2** Conventional Franz diffusion cells (A) and advanced permeation models: Strat-M membrane (B), Skin-Parallel Artificial Membrane Permeability Assay (Skin-PAMPA) (C), Phospholipid vesicle-based permeation (PVPA) model (D) and Skin-on-a-Chip model (E). (Figure 3.2D was adapted from Ref. [85] with permission of John Wiley and Sons; Figure 3.2E was adapted from Ref. [87] with permission of The Royal Society of Chemistry.)

*stratum corneum*, which is maintained after the skin excision process. When human skin is not available, animal skin can be a satisfactory surrogate especially if the same animal model is used for further in vivo studies of the formulation. Among animal skins, pig skin seems to be the best option due to its similarities to human skin in morphology and barrier properties. Moreover, pig skin has been shown to be a good model for transfollicular drug delivery. In terms of HSEs, the current models, although viable, over predict flux measurements for many drugs. Polymeric membranes such as silicone, although possessing low variability and the ability (in some cases) to provide quantitative structure-transportability relationships (QSTR), are homogeneous and non-viable which is significantly different to the heterogeneity of biological membranes.

Advanced models such as Skin-PAMPA, Strat-M, PVPA and skin-on-a-chip are under development to aim to provide more efficient, accurate and biorelevant assays for drug permeation prediction (Figure 3.2). Skin-PAMPA, Strat-M and PVPA improved polymeric-based membranes with incorporated lipid compositions that hope to mimic skin biology. The ability to incorporate these types of membranes into a high-throughput format is especially attractive. Moreover, microfluidic-based devices such as skin-on-a-chip provide a potential method to capture the processes of drug adsorption, metabolism, excretion and distribution.

Currently, no single model can predict and replicate the complex processes of skin drug permeation and even though very useful, all these models have limitations and have to be selected carefully and the data obtained have to be interpreted with caution.

## REFERENCES

1. Koster, M.I. Making an epidermis. *Ann N Y Acad Sci* **1170**, 7, 2009.
2. Kanerva, L., Elsner, P., Wahlberg, J.E., and Maibach, H.I. *Handbook of Occupational Dermatology.* New York: Springer-Verlag Berlin Heidelberg; 2013.
3. Bos, J.D., and Meinardi, M.M. The 500 Dalton rule for the skin penetration of chemical compounds and drugs. *Exp Dermatol* **9**, 165, 2000.
4. Menczel, E., and Goldberg, S. pH effect on the percutaneous penetration of lignocaine hydrochloride. *Dermatologica* **156**, 8, 1978.
5. Leveque, N., Makki, S., Hadgraft, J., and Humbert, P. Comparison of Franz cells and microdialysis for assessing salicylic acid penetration through human skin. *Int J Pharm* **269**, 323, 2004.
6. Hukkanen, J., Jacob, P., 3rd, and Benowitz, N.L. Metabolism and disposition kinetics of nicotine. *Pharmacol Rev* **57**, 79, 2005.
7. OECD. *Test No. 428: Skin Absorption: In Vitro Method.* In: Development O.f.E.C.-o.a., ed. 2004.
8. WHO. *Dermal Absorption (EHC 235).* In: World Health Organization I.P.o.C.S., ed. Germany 2006.
9. Marzulli, F.N., Brown, D.W.C., and Maiback, H.I. Techniques for studying skin penetration. *Toxicol Appl Pharmacol* **Supplement No.3**, 76, 1969.
10. Bronaugh, R.L., Stewart, R.F., Congdon, E.R., and Giles, A.L., Jr. Methods for in vitro percutaneous absorption studies. I. Comparison with in vivo results. *Toxicol Appl Pharmacol* **62**, 474, 1982.
11. Friend, D.R. In vitro skin permeation techniques. *J Control Release* **18**, 235, 1992.

12. Diembeck, W., Beck, H., Benech-Kieffer, F., Courtellemont, P., Dupuis, J., Lovell, W., Paye, M., Spengler, J., and Steiling, W. Test guidelines for in vitro assessment of dermal absorption and percutaneous penetration of cosmetic ingredients. European Cosmetic, Toiletry and Perfumery Association. *Food Chem Toxicol* **37**, 191, 1999.

13. Wester, R.C., Christoffel, J., Hartway, T., Poblete, N., Maibach, H.I., and Forsell, J. Human cadaver skin viability for in vitro percutaneous absorption: storage and detrimental effects of heat-separation and freezing. *Pharm Res* **15**, 82, 1998.

14. Kao, J., Patterson, F.K., and Hall, J. Skin penetration and metabolism of topically applied chemicals in six mammalian species, including man: an in vitro study with benzo[a]pyrene and testosterone. *Toxicol Appl Pharmacol* **81**, 502, 1985.

15. Mavon, A., Raufast, V., and Redoules, D. Skin absorption and metabolism of a new vitamin E prodrug, delta-tocopherol-glucoside: in vitro evaluation in human skin models. *J Control Release* **100**, 221, 2004.

16. Ritschel, W.A., Sabouni, A., and Hussain, A.S. Percutaneous absorption of coumarin, griseofulvin and propranolol across human scalp and abdominal skin. *Methods Find Exp Clin Pharmacol* **11**, 643, 1989.

17. Bronaugh, R.L., Stewart, R.F., and Simon, M. Methods for in vitro percutaneous absorption studies. VII: Use of excised human skin. *J Pharm Sci* **75**, 1094, 1986.

18. Harrison, S.M., Barry, B.W., and Dugard, P.H. Effects of freezing on human skin permeability. *J Pharm Pharmacol* **36**, 261, 1984.

19. Dennerlein, K., Schneider, D., Glen, T., Schaller, K.H., Drexler, H., and Korinth, G. Studies on percutaneous penetration of chemicals – impact of storage conditions for excised human skin. *Toxicology In Vitro* **27**(2), 708–713, 2013.

20. Nielsen, J.B., Plasencia, I., Sorensen, J.A., and Bagatolli, L.A. Storage conditions of skin affect tissue structure and subsequent in vitro percutaneous penetration. *Skin Pharmacol and Physiol* **24**, 93, 2011.

21. van de Sandt, J.J., van Burgsteden, J.A., Cage, S., Carmichael, P.L., Dick, I., Kenyon, S., Korinth, G., Larese, F., Limasset, J.C., Maas, W.J., Montomoli, L., Nielsen, J.B., Payan, J.P., Robinson, E., Sartorelli, P., Schaller, K.H., Wilkinson, S.C., and Williams, F.M. In vitro predictions of skin absorption of caffeine, testosterone, and benzoic acid: a multi-centre comparison study. *Regul Toxicol Pharmacol* **39**, 271, 2004.

22. Wilkinson, S.C., Maas, W.J., Nielsen, J.B., Greaves, L.C., van de Sandt, J.J., and Williams, F.M. Interactions of skin thickness and physicochemical properties of test compounds in percutaneous penetration studies. *Int Arch Occup Environ Health* **79**, 405, 2006.

23. USEPA. *Interim report dermal exposure assessment: Principles and applications exposure assessment group office of health and environmental assessment.* In: Agency U.S.E.P., ed. Washington, 1992. p. 1.

24. Bronaugh, R.L., and Stewart, R.F. Methods for in vitro percutaneous absorption studies. VI: Preparation of the barrier layer. *J Pharm Sci* **75**, 487, 1986.

25. Franken, A., Eloff, F.C., du Plessis, J., Badenhorst, C.J., and Du Plessis, J.L. In vitro permeation of platinum through African and Caucasian skin. *Toxicol Lett* **232**, 566, 2015.

26. Southwell, D., Barry, B.W., and Woodford, R. Variations in permeability of human skin within and between specimens. *Int J Pharm* **18**, 299, 1984.

27. Akomeah, F.K., Martin, G.P., and Brown, M.B. Variability in human skin permeability in vitro: comparing penetrants with different physicochemical properties. *J Pharm Sci* **96**, 824, 2007.

28. Meidan, V.M., and Roper, C.S. Inter- and intra-individual variability in human skin barrier function: a large scale retrospective study. *Toxicol In Vitro* **22**, 1062, 2008.

29. Jung, E.C., and Maibach, H.I. Animal models for percutaneous absorption. *J Appl Toxicol* **35**, 1, 2015.

30. Barbero, A.M., and Frasch, H.F. Pig and guinea pig skin as surrogates for human in vitro penetration studies: a quantitative review. *Toxicol In Vitro* **23**, 1, 2009.
31. Simon, G.A., and Maibach, H.I. The pig as an experimental animal model of percutaneous permeation in man: qualitative and quantitative observations—an overview. *Skin Pharmacol Appl Skin Physiol* **13**, 229, 2000.
32. Jacobi, U., Kaiser, M., Toll, R., Mangelsdorf, S., Audring, H., Otberg, N., Sterry, W., and Lademann, J. Porcine ear skin: an in vitro model for human skin. *Skin Res and Technol* **13**, 19, 2007.
33. Lademann, J., Patzelt, A., Richter, H., Antoniou, C., Sterry, W., and Knorr, F. Determination of the cuticula thickness of human and porcine hairs and their potential influence on the penetration of nanoparticles into the hair follicles. *J Biomed Opt* **14**, 021014, 2009.
34. Wester, R.C., and Maibach, H.I. Percutaneous absorption in the rhesus monkey compared to man. *Toxicol Appl Pharmacol* **32**, 394, 1975.
35. Bronaugh, R.L., Wester, R.C., Bucks, D., Maibach, H.I., and Sarason, R. In vivo percutaneous absorption of fragrance ingredients in rhesus monkeys and humans. *Food Chem Toxicol* **28**, 369, 1990.
36. Ghosh, B., Reddy, L.H., Kulkarni, R.V., and Khanam, J. Comparison of skin permeability of drugs in mice and human cadaver skin. *Indian J Exp Biol* **38**, 42, 2000.
37. Bond, J.R., and Barry, B.W. Limitations of hairless mouse skin as a model for in vitro permeation studies through human skin: hydration damage. *J Invest Dermatol* **90**, 486, 1988.
38. van Ravenzwaay, B., and Leibold, E. A comparison between in vitro rat and human and in vivo rat skin absorption studies. *Hum Exp Toxicol* **23**, 421, 2004.
39. van Ravenzwaay, B., and Leibold, E. The significance of in vitro rat skin absorption studies to human risk assessment. *Toxicol In Vitro* **18**, 219, 2004.
40. World Health Organization, *I.P.o.C.S. Dermal Absorption. Environmental Health Criteria 235*. Geneva: WHO Press; 2005.
41. Ross, J.H., Reifenrath, W.G., and Driver, J.H. Estimation of the percutaneous absorption of permethrin in humans using the parallelogram method. *J Toxicol Environ Health A* **74**, 351, 2011.
42. Roberts, J.B. Use of Squamate Epidermis in Percutaneous–Absorption Studies – A Review. *J Toxicol Cutan Ocul Toxicol* **5**, 319, 1986.
43. Rigg, P.C., and Barry, B.W. Shed snake skin and hairless mouse skin as model membranes for human skin during permeation studies. *J Invest Dermatol* **94**, 235, 1990.
44. Bronaugh, R.L., Stewart, R.F., and Congdon, E.R. Methods for in vitro percutaneous absorption studies. II. Animal models for human skin. *Toxicol Appl Pharmacol* **62**, 481, 1982.
45. Draize, J.H., Woodard, G., and Calvery, H.O. Methods for the study of irritation and toxicity of substances applied topically to the skin and mucous membranes. *J Pharmacol Exp Ther* **82**, 377, 1944.
46. Hui, X., Lamel, S., Qiao, P., and Maibach, H.I. Isolated human and animal stratum corneum as a partial model for the 15 steps of percutaneous absorption: emphasizing decontamination, part II. *J Appl Toxicol* **33**, 173, 2013.
47. Haigh, J.M., and Smith, E.W. The selection and use of natural and synthetic membranes for in vitro diffusion experiments. *Eur J Pharm Sci* **2**, 311, 1994.
48. Nicoli, S., Padula, C., Aversa, V., Vietti, B., Wertz, P.W., Millet, A., Falson, F., Govoni, P., and Santi, P. Characterization of rabbit ear skin as a skin model for in vitro transdermal permeation experiments: histology, lipid composition and permeability. *Skin Pharmacol and Physiol* **21**, 218, 2008.
49. Lee, Y., and Hwang, K. Skin thickness of Korean adults. *Surg Radiol Anat* **24**, 183, 2002.

50. Rougier, A., Dupuis, D., Lotte, C., Roguet, R., Wester, R.C., and Maibach, H.I. Regional variation in percutaneous-absorption in man – measurement by the stripping method. *Arch Dermatol Res* **278**, 465, 1986.

51. Boudry, I., Trescos, Y., Vallet, V., Cruz, C., and Lallement, G. Methods and models for percutaneous absorption studies of organophosphates. *Pathol Biol* **56**, 292, 2008.

52. Elias, P.M., Cooper, E.R., Korc, A., and Brown, B.E. Percutaneous transport in relation to stratum corneum structure and lipid composition. *J Invest Dermatol* **76**, 297, 1981.

53. Zhang, Z., and Michniak-Kohn, B.B. Tissue engineered human skin equivalents. *Pharmaceutics* **4**, 26, 2012.

54. OECD. *Guidance document for the conduct of skin absorption studies – Series on Testing and Assessment No.28*. In: *Development O.f.E.C.-o.a.*, ed. Paris 2004.

55. Schafer-Korting, M., Bock, U., Diembeck, W., Dusing, H.J., Gamer, A., Haltner-Ukomadu, E., Hoffmann, C., Kaca, M., Kamp, H., Kersen, S., Kietzmann, M., Korting, H.C., Krachter, H.U., Lehr, C.M., Liebsch, M., Mehling, A., Muller-Goymann, C., Netzlaff, F., Niedorf, F., Rubbelke, M.K., Schafer, U., Schmidt, E., Schreiber, S., Spielmann, H., Vuia, A., and Weimer, M. The use of reconstructed human epidermis for skin absorption testing: results of the validation study. *Altern Lab Anim* **36**, 161, 2008.

56. Schmook, F.P., Meingassner, J.G., and Billich, A. Comparison of human skin or epidermis models with human and animal skin in in-vitro percutaneous absorption. *Int J Pharm* **215**, 51, 2001.

57. Zghoul, N., Fuchs, R., Lehr, C.M., and Schaefer, U.F. Reconstructed skin equivalents for assessing percutaneous drug absorption from pharmaceutical formulations. *ALTEX* **18**, 103, 2001.

58. Ackermann, K., Borgia, S.L., Korting, H.C., Mewes, K.R., and Schafer-Korting, M. The Phenion full-thickness skin model for percutaneous absorption testing. *Skin Pharmacol and Physiol* **23**, 105, 2010.

59. Thakoersing, V.S., van Smeden, J., Mulder, A.A., Vreeken, R.J., El Ghalbzouri, A., and Bouwstra, J.A. Increased presence of monounsaturated fatty acids in the stratum corneum of human skin equivalents. *J Invest Dermatol* **133**, 59, 2013.

60. Batheja, P. *Polymeric nano spheres for skin penetration enhancement: In vitro and In vivo assessment in skin models*. PhD Thesis Rutgers–The State University of New Jersey, January 2010.

61. Zhang, Z., Tsai, P.C., Ramezanli, T., and Michniak-Kohn, B.B. Polymeric nanoparticles-based topical delivery systems for the treatment of dermatological diseases. *Wiley Interdiscip Rev Nanomed Nanobiotechnol* **5**, 205, 2013.

62. Shim, J., Seok Kang, H., Park, W.S., Han, S.H., Kim, J., and Chang, I.S. Transdermal delivery of mixnoxidil with block copolymer nanoparticles. *J Control Release* **97**, 477, 2004.

63. Lademann, J., Richter, H., Teichmann, A., Otberg, N., Blume-Peytavi, U., Luengo, J., Weiss, B., Schaefer, U.F., Lehr, C.M., Wepf, R., and Sterry, W. Nanoparticles--an efficient carrier for drug delivery into the hair follicles. *Eur J Pharm Biopharm* **66**, 159, 2007.

64. Otberg, N., Patzelt, A., Rasulev, U., Hagemeister, T., Linscheid, M., Sinkgraven, R., Sterry, W., and Lademann, J. The role of hair follicles in the percutaneous absorption of caffeine. *Br J Clin Pharmacol* **65**, 488, 2008.

65. Tsai, P.C., Zhang, Z., Michniak Kohn, B.B., and Florek, C. Constructing human skin equivalents on porcine acellular peritoneum extracellular matrix for in vitro irritation testing. *Tissue Eng Part A*, 2015.

66. Lee, W., Debasitis, J.C., Lee, V.K., Lee, J.H., Fischer, K., Edminster, K., Park, J.K., and Yoo, S.S. Multi-layered culture of human skin fibroblasts and keratinocytes through three-dimensional freeform fabrication. *Biomaterials* **30**, 1587, 2009.

67. Netzlaff, F., Kaca, M., Bock, U., Haltner-Ukomadu, E., Meiers, P., Lehr, C.M., and Schaefer, U.F. Permeability of the reconstructed human epidermis model Episkin in comparison to various human skin preparations. *Eur J Pharm Biopharm* **66**, 127, 2007.
68. Yamaguchi, Y., Usami, T., Natsume, H., Aoyagi, T., Nagase, Y., Sugibayashi, K., and Morimoto, Y. Evaluation of skin permeability of drugs by newly prepared polymer membranes. *Chem Pharm Bull* **45**, 537, 1997.
69. Jantharaprapap, R., and Stagni, G. Effects of penetration enhancers on in vitro permeability of meloxicam gels. *Int J Pharm* **343**, 26, 2007.
70. Ng, S.-F., Rouse, J., Sanderson, D., and Eccleston, G. A comparative study of transmembrane diffusion and permeation of Ibuprofen across synthetic membranes using Franz diffusion cells. *Pharmaceutics* **2**, 209, 2010.
71. Cronin, M.T., Dearden, J.C., Moss, G.P., and Murray-Dickson, G. Investigation of the mechanism of flux across human skin in vitro by quantitative structure-permeability relationships. *Eur J Pharm Sci* **7**, 325, 1999.
72. Garrett, E.R., and Chemburkar, P.B. Evaluation, control, and prediction of drug diffusion through polymeric membranes. I. Methods and reproducibility of steady-state diffusion studies. *J Pharm Sci* **57**, 944, 1968.
73. Du Plessis, J., Pugh, W.J., Judefeind, A., and Hadgraft, J. The effect of hydrogen bonding on diffusion across model membranes: consideration of the number of H-bonding groups. *Eur J Pharm Sci* **13**, 135, 2001.
74. Chorvath, I., Lee, M., Li, D., Nakanishi, K., Lee, Y., Oldinski, R.L., Romenesko, D.J., and Sage, J.P. *Thermoplastic silicone elastomers formed from nylon resins.* In: W.I.P.O., ed. Patent Cooperation Treaty 2001.
75. Chen, Y., Yang, W.-L., and Matheson, L.E. Prediction of flux through polydimethylsiloxane membranes using atomic charge calculations. *Int J Pharm* **94**, 81, 1993.
76. Chen, Y., Vayumhasuwan, P., and Matheson, L.E. Prediction of flux through polydimethylsiloxane membranes using atomic charge calculations: application to an extended data set. *Int J Pharm* **137**, 149, 1996.
77. Geinoz, S., Rey, S., Boss, G., Bunge, A.L., Guy, R.H., Carrupt, P.A., Reist, M., and Testa, B. Quantitative structure-permeation relationships for solute transport across silicone membranes. *Pharm Res* **19**, 1622, 2002.
78. Frum, Y., Eccleston, G.M., and Meidan, V.M. Evidence that drug flux across synthetic membranes is described by normally distributed permeability coefficients. *Eur J Pharm Biopharm* **67**, 434, 2007.
79. Kansy, M., Senner, F., and Gubernator, K. Physicochemical high throughput screening: parallel artificial membrane permeation assay in the description of passive absorption processes. *J Med Chem* **41**, 1007, 1998.
80. Bujard, A., Voirol, H., Carrupt, P.A., and Schappler, J. Modification of a PAMPA model to predict passive gastrointestinal absorption and plasma protein binding. *Eur J Pharm Sci* **77**, 273, 2015.
81. Campbell, S.D., Regina, K.J., and Kharasch, E.D. Significance of lipid composition in a blood-brain barrier-mimetic PAMPA assay. *J Biomol Screen* **19**, 437, 2014.
82. Ottaviani, G., Martel, S., and Carrupt, P.A. Parallel artificial membrane permeability assay: a new membrane for the fast prediction of passive human skin permeability. *J Med Chem* **49**, 3948, 2006.
83. Uchida, T., Kadhum, W.R., Kanai, S., Todo, H., Oshizaka, T., and Sugibayashi, K. Prediction of skin permeation by chemical compounds using the artificial membrane, Strat-M. *Eur J Pharm Sci* **67**, 113, 2015.
84. Karadzovska, D., and Riviere, J.E. Assessing vehicle effects on skin absorption using artificial membrane assays. *Eur J Pharm Sci* **50**, 569, 2013.

85. Engesland, A., Skar, M., Hansen, T., Skalko-Basnet, N., and Flaten, G.E. New applications of phospholipid vesicle-based permeation assay: permeation model mimicking skin barrier. *J Pharm Sci* **102**, 1588, 2013.
86. Lee, J.B., and Sung, J.H. Organ-on-a-chip technology and microfluidic whole-body models for pharmacokinetic drug toxicity screening. *Biotechnol J* **8**, 1258, 2013.
87. Atac, B., Wagner, I., Horland, R., Lauster, R., Marx, U., Tonevitsky, A.G., Azar, R.P., and Lindner, G. Skin and hair on-a-chip: in vitro skin models versus ex vivo tissue maintenance with dynamic perfusion. *Lab Chip* **13**, 3555, 2013.
88. Abaci, H.E., Gledhill, K., Guo, Z., Christiano, A.M., and Shuler, M.L. Pumpless microfluidic platform for drug testing on human skin equivalents. *Lab Chip* **15**, 882, 2015.
89. Bhise, N.S., Ribas, J., Manoharan, V., Zhang, Y.S., Polini, A., Massa, S., Dokmeci, M.R., and Khademhosseini, A. Organ-on-a-chip platforms for studying drug delivery systems. *J Control Release* **190**, 82, 2014.

# 4 Design, Development, Manufacturing, and Testing of Transdermal Drug Delivery Systems

*Timothy A. Peterson, Steven M. Wick and Chan Ko*

## CONTENTS

## 4.1 INTRODUCTION

Much of the scientific literature in the field of transdermal delivery pertains to skin permeation and methods of skin penetration enhancement, and rightly so, because these are fundamental questions that must be addressed for any transdermal drug candidate. However, in addition to the basic question of skin permeability, the development process must also address other questions related to the patch system such as: What is an appropriate patch design? What are appropriate materials for the patch construction? How will the patch be manufactured? How can quality be designed into the product and what parameters should be tested to prove the quality of the finished system? The goal of this chapter is to provide some practical insight into how these questions are currently being approached and provide some examples that are representative of the current state of the art.

There are many design issues which depend on the nature of the particular drug to be delivered. Therefore, several different design approaches for transdermal patches have been developed. While the design decisions must be grounded in good science, there may be multiple approaches to achieve the same end result. The potential design approaches and their advantages, disadvantages and applicability will be discussed, at length. Differences in drug properties often require the selection of different materials for patch components. Particular emphasis will be given to important factors in the selection of pressure sensitive adhesives for transdermal patches. Use of an adhesive is common to all transdermal patch designs and is vitally important to successful function. Adhesives and skin adhesion are complex topics that merit consideration in parallel with the drug delivery aspects of the patch design, rather than as afterthoughts. The manufacturing processes used to produce a finished transdermal patch are as varied as the system design and materials that go into the patch. The basic operations involved in the manufacture of each patch design will be described, along with important factors to consider in the scale-up from the laboratory to the manufacturing site. Finally, several tests have been found to be important in evaluating the quality characteristics of transdermal patches. Some of these are very similar to those used for other dosage forms, while others have been developed in other fields and applied to measure specific attributes of transdermal systems. In particular, appropriate tests to measure the adhesion characteristics of transdermal patches will be discussed.

## 4.2 TRANSDERMAL SYSTEM DESIGN ALTERNATIVES

Transdermal systems are designed with one primary objective: to deliver therapeutically effective and safe levels of a specific drug molecule into the systemic circulation (although there are a couple of exceptions in which the target is local delivery). While simple in concept, reducing this objective to practice involves the simultaneous optimization (and often trade off) of multiple product attributes.

Transdermal product development has matured greatly over the past 35 years. A variety of system designs have been utilized to deliver drugs across the skin as illustrated in Figure 4.1. However, a significant trend towards utilization of the matrix design has emerged, and most particularly, the drug-in-adhesive matrix design. Each

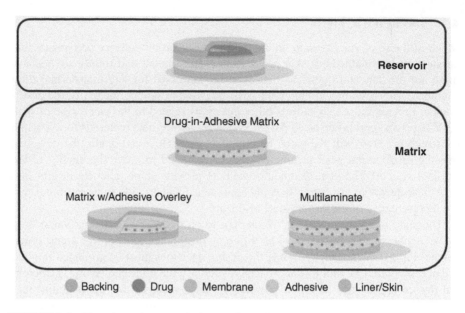

Reservoir

Drug-in-Adhesive Matrix

Matrix

Matrix w/Adhesive Overley

Multilaminate

Backing    Drug    Membrane    Adhesive    Liner/Skin

**FIGURE 4.1** Transdermal system design configurations.

of the new drugs introduced as a transdermal product since 1996 has utilized one of the matrix designs, with approximately 85% of those utilizing a drug-in-adhesive matrix design. While there are significant differences between each of the transdermal system designs, there are several aspects that are common to each of them. Each transdermal patch design incorporates four basic elements: a backing, an adhesive and a release liner, as well as the drug.

Although drug delivery is the primary objective of all transdermal dosage forms, the establishment and maintenance of skin adhesion is fundamental to all systems. Proper selection of the adhesive to assure sufficient skin adhesion throughout the wear period is required for the consistent and predictable delivery of drug to the systemic circulation. Most transdermal systems utilize adhesive polymers within one of the following general categories: polyisobutylene, polyacrylate or silicone (Tan and Pfister 1999, Grosh et.al. 1988). A listing of selected transdermal products marketed in the USA and the associated category of adhesive along with the type of patch design utilized within each of the respective systems is provided in Figure 4.2. A more thorough discussion of the significance of proper adhesive selection is offered later in this chapter.

The backing film and release liner serve to contain the formulation, and should be inert to other formulation components. These two layers function ideally when interaction with the drug delivery formulation is minimized. Factors to consider when selecting a backing film and a release liner are discussed later in this chapter.

The specific location of the drug within the system and the associated drug delivery formulation can be used to categorize a transdermal patch into one of the four design configurations.

| Transdermal System | Product Design Category | | | | | Adhesive Category | | |
| --- | --- | --- | --- | --- | --- | --- | --- | --- |
| | Reservoir | Matrix | | | | PIB | Acrylate | Silicone |
| | | w/ Adh Overlay | DIA | Multilaminate | | | | |
| Androderm$^R$ (testosterone) | ■ | | | | | | ■ | |
| BuTrans$^R$ (buprenorphine) | | ■ | | | | | ■ | |
| Catapres-TTS$^R$ (clonidine) | | | ■ | | | ■ | | |
| Climara$^R$ (estradiol) | | ■ | | | | | ■ | |
| Climara Pro$^R$ (estradiol / levonorgestrel) | | ■ | | | | | ■ | |
| Combipatch$^R$ (estradiol / norethindrone actetate) | | ■ | | | | | ■ | ■ |
| Daytrana$^R$ (methylphenidate) | | ■ | | | | | ■ | ■ |
| Duragesic$^R$ (fentanyl) | | ■ | | | | | ■ | |
| Emsam$^R$ (selegiline) | | ■ | | | | | ■ | |
| Exelon$^R$ (rivastigmine) | | | ■ | | | | ■ | ■ |
| Flector$^R$ (diclofenac epolamine) | | ■ | | | | | ■ | |
| Lidoderm$^R$ (lidocaine) | | ■ | | | | | ■ | |
| Minitran$^{TM}$ (nitroglycerin) | | ■ | | | | | ■ | |
| Neupro$^R$ (rotigotine) | | ■ | | | | | | ■ |
| Nicoderm CQ$^R$ (nicotine) | | | | ■ | | ■ | | |
| Ortho Evra$^R$ (ethinyl estradiol / norelgestromin) | | ■ | | | | ■ | | |
| Oxytrol$^R$ (oxybutynin) | | ■ | | | | | ■ | |
| NitroDur$^R$ (nitroglycerin) | | ■ | | | | | ■ | |
| Qutenza$^R$ (capsaicin) | | ■ | | | | | | ■ |
| Sancuso$^R$ (granisetron) | | ■ | | | | | ■ | |
| Transderm-Nitro$^R$ (nitroglycerin) | ■ | | | | | | | ■ |
| Transderm Scop$^R$ (scopolamine) | | | | ■ | | ■ | | |
| Vivelle Dot$^R$ (estradiol) | | ■ | | | | | ■ | ■ |

**FIGURE 4.2** Product design configuration and adhesives utilized within selected transdermal patches on the market in the USA.

## 4.2.1 RESERVOIR-TYPE PRODUCT DESIGN

The reservoir-type transdermal system design is characterized by the inclusion of a liquid reservoir compartment containing a drug solution or suspension, which is in turn separated from the release liner by a semi-permeable membrane and an adhesive. The adhesive component of the product responsible for skin adhesion can either be incorporated as a continuous layer between the membrane and the release liner (i.e., face adhesive) (Gale and Berggren 1986) or in a concentric configuration around the membrane (Chang et al. 1989).

The liquid reservoir formulation is relatively simple in design, providing a single liquid phase in which all the excipients and at least a portion of the drug reside. The drug is maintained within the formulation in a complete or partially solubilized state by means of a liquid excipient. The drug is preferentially permeable to the membrane and moves by means of passive diffusion through the membrane towards the skin. In the case of a suspension formulation, as drug is released from the solution phase, more of the suspended drug dissolves, thus replenishing the solution phase. The primary advantage of the reservoir-type configuration is the zero-order release kinetics of a properly designed system (Good 1986).

Correct selection of the membrane is critical for proper function of a reservoir-type patch design. The diffusion characteristics of the drug within the membrane determine the rate at which drug is released from the patch. The membrane must exhibit preferential permeability of the drug over the reservoir media. In certain cases, the membrane can be designed to allow passage of both the drug and one or more of the formulation excipients, which may be incorporated to function as penetration enhancers to modify the barrier functionality of the stratum corneum. Since the zero-order release characteristic of the reservoir-type product design relies on the maintenance of a constant drug concentration within the reservoir solution phase, drug delivery efficiency within these systems is highly dependent on the nature of the formulation and excipients used within each specific system. (The efficiency of drug delivery from a transdermal patch formulation is equal to the quantity of drug delivered within the application period divided by the total patch content.)

The membrane plays a critical role in drug release and drug delivery in the reservoir-type design. However, this patch configuration is particularly vulnerable to dose dumping. Rupture of the membrane layer or inadequate seals on the periphery of the reservoir could enable drug access to the skin and the possibility of uncontrolled absorption. Depending on the nature of the formulation and the barrier functionality of the stratum corneum, compromise of the membrane layer could lead to a significant increase in the rate of drug release from the reservoir and/or the rate of drug delivery to the systemic circulation. This type of failure has been a safety concern, particularly with fentanyl products (Edwards 2009), resulting in several product recalls and a further trend towards patch designs that avoid this potential defect.

### 4.2.2 MATRIX PRODUCT DESIGN

The matrix transdermal system design differs from reservoir-type transdermal system design by providing the drug in a solid polymeric formulation, instead of a liquid formulation sealed between polyer films. However, similar to the reservoir-type design, the drug can be maintained either within a solution or suspension phase.

Matrix transdermal system design is comprised of three related but distinct subcategories: drug-in-adhesive matrix, matrix with adhesive overlay and multilaminate matrix design.

### 4.2.2.1 Drug-In-Adhesive Product Design

The drug-in-adhesive (DIA) transdermal product design is characterized by the inclusion of the drug directly within the skin-contacting adhesive (Wick 1988, Subedi et al. 2010). In this transdermal system design, the adhesive fulfills the adhesion-to-skin function and serves as the formulation foundation, containing the drug and all excipients (Wilking et al. 1994, Nishida et al. 2010). The DIA system design is considered by many to be state-of-the-art in transdermal systems design with 11 of the last 13 new transdermal product introductions in the USA utilizing this design configuration.

The incorporation of the drug and all excipients directly within the adhesive requires that not only will the drug be released from the formulation in a reproducible manner, but also that the adhesion-to-skin characteristics of the formulation must be consistently maintained throughout the application period as the drug and/or the excipients are depleted from the DIA formulation. In order to adequately compensate for the inclusion of the drug and excipients within the adhesive, the adhesive polymer may be customized for each formulation. It is the simultaneous and often competing requirements for the DIA matrix to provide both adhesion and sufficient drug delivery that makes the DIA formulation among the most complex to formulate within the four basic transdermal patch designs. However, when properly formulated, the DIA patch design offers several physical advantages over the other patch designs.

Since the DIA patch design does not require an adhesive overlay or a concentric liquid reservoir seal, the DIA design offers maximum utilization of surface area for drug release to the skin. This design feature translates into a smaller overall patch surface for a given drug delivery rate.

In addition to the efficient utilization of surface area, DIA patch designs tend to be extremely conformable to the surface of the skin. A typical DIA patch design is very thin (i.e., Minitran™ (nitroglycerin), thickness = 165 micrometers; or NitroDur® (nitroglycerin), thickness = 200 micrometers). The proper selection of a backing film and a DIA formulation can combine to produce a thin, highly conformable and, ultimately, comfortable transdermal patch.

The major disadvantage associated with the DIA patch design relates to duration of drug delivery. The release of drug from a DIA formulation follows first order kinetics. That is, the release rate is proportional to the concentration of drug within the adhesive. As drug is delivered from the DIA formulation, the concentration will eventually begin to fall. If the formulation incorporates a reservoir of suspended drug particles or utilizes a multilaminate design concept, the concentration of drug-in-solution within the DIA formulation will be effected less rapidly. However, in either case, maintaining a relatively constant drug delivery profile from a DIA patch formulation is an issue which should be addressed within the clinical evaluation phase of development. It may be possible to partially compensate for the diminished duration of drug delivery by increasing the total drug content within the formulation. However, this approach will typically result in a product with a reduced efficiency of drug delivery.

#### 4.2.2.2   Matrix with Adhesive Overlay

In this type of patch design, the component of the product responsible for skin adhesion is incorporated in an "overlay" configuration and forms a concentric configuration around the polymeric drug matrix (Sanvordeker et al. 1982).

The matrix patch with adhesive overlay is among the simplest approaches to transdermal patch design. In its most basic form, the drug-containing polymeric matrix is held in contact with the skin by an adhesive tape overlay. Depending on the characteristics of the drug molecule and formulation excipients utilized within the polymeric matrix, it may be necessary to introduce an impermeable layer to minimize drug/excipient migration into the adhesive overlay. By utilizing a separate overlay material to provide skin adhesion, most of the formulation complexities associated with drug/adhesive or excipient/adhesive interactions are largely avoided. However, this simplicity generally comes at the cost of increased patch surface area, since the overlay must extend beyond the edges of the drug-containing polymer matrix.

The drug release characteristics of a matrix design are determined by the formulation of the drug-containing polymer matrix. There is no membrane layer that functions as a release-rate-moderating barrier. Release of drug from the polymer matrix exposes the drug directly to the surface of the skin where the rate of delivery is controlled by the stratum corneum. As with any other transdermal patch design, excipients may be added to the formulation to modify the barrier function of the stratum corneum, thereby modifying the rate of drug delivery. Since the excipients within a matrix with adhesive overlay design are not directly incorporated within the skin-contacting adhesive, the matrix with adhesive overlay design may offer an advantage in terms of excipient choice.

As in the reservoir-type design, the configuration of the matrix with adhesive overlay design implies specific physical characteristics. The most pronounced of these is the overall size. Separation of the adhesive from the drug-containing matrix necessitates that the overall patch surface area extends well beyond the matrix. The amount of this adhesive extension depends, to a degree, on the thickness of the drug-containing matrix. The thicker the matrix, the wider the concentric adhesive component must be in order to maintain adequate skin adhesion. Butrans$^R$, a more recent product introduction in this category, has a considerably thinner matrix, and consequently a more limited impact on overall patch surface area.

#### 4.2.2.3   MULTILAMINATE DRUG-IN-ADHESIVE PRODUCT DESIGN

A further subset of matrix patch design is the multilaminate DIA design. As depicted in Figure 4.1, the multilaminate DIA design encompasses either the addition of a membrane between two distinct DIA layers or the addition of multiple DIA layers under a single backing film (Peterson and Dreyer 1994). Catapres® (clonidine), Transderm-Scop® (scopolamine), Exelon® (rivastigmine) and Nicoderm® (nicotine) are specific examples of DIA patch constructions utilizing a multilaminate configuration. Multilaminate patch design may be useful for two primary reasons: to provide more control over the delivery rate (by virtue of having a membrane or a second DIA layer incorporated within the design) or to utilize a skin-contacting DIA layer that is relatively unaffected by the drug and excipient content within the patch and thereby maintains better skin adhesion. A recent example of this type of design is the Exelon$^R$ patch.

## 4.3  PATCH DESIGN SELECTION PROCESS

Selection of the most appropriate transdermal product design alternative should be based on an examination of the specific characteristics of the drug candidate and the desired product characteristics. First and foremost, the questions necessary to clearly define the desired final product must be answered:

1. What is the range of dose to be systematically delivered?
2. What is the target population for the final dosage form?
3. What is the maximum patch size that will be accepted by the target population?
4. What is the preferred site of application for the product?
5. What is the preferred application period (daily, biweekly, weekly)?
6. What is the cost/risk associated with residual drug remaining within the patch construction at the end of the application period?

The product definition is sometimes alternatively referred to as a design specification or a quality target product profile (QTPP) in the FDA's language of Quality by Design (QbD). An example QTPP for a generic transdermal product is shown in Table 4.1. Once the preferred product definition has been established, an evaluation of the drug candidate should begin. Figure 4.3 illustrates the major milestones and flow of work required to evaluate a typical compound for the transdermal route of administration (Wick et al. 1993).

The first step is to conduct a "paper" feasibility assessment in which the skin permeability and maximum attainable flux is evaluated based on an appropriate mathematical model or an existing database of permeability data. Certain aspects of a drug's physicochemical properties, some of which are listed in Table 4.2, can be used as parameters for modeling skin permeability (Potts and Guy 1992, Farahmand and Maibach 2009) and predicting the maximum attainable delivery via the transdermal route.

The results of the paper feasibility assessment should be compared with the proposed product definition, and assessed within the context of any pharmacokinetic information (i.e., clearance, half-life, vol. of dist. or effective blood level) which is available. If the results look favorable, the candidate compound is further evaluated by means of an in vitro feasibility assessment as illustrated in Figure 4.4.

The paper and laboratory feasibility assessments are combined to predict the probability of success in formulating a product within the scope of the original preferred product definition. A benefit of this systematic approach to evaluating candidate compounds is found in improved accuracy predicting formulation development costs to the first clinical evaluation, and the ANDA or NDA submissions. It is imperative that compounds be appropriately eliminated from the formulation development process with minimal cost, maximum information and minimal risk of error.

**TABLE 4.1**
**Example Quality Target Product Profile (QTPP) for a Generic Transdermal Product**

| QTPP Element | Target | Justification |
|---|---|---|
| **Dosage form** | Transdermal Patch | Pharmaceutical equivalence requirement; same dosage form as RLD |
| **Route of administration** | Transdermal | Pharmaceutical equivalence requirement; same dosage form as RLD |
| **Strength** | X, Y and Z mcg/h | Pharmaceutical equivalence requirement; same dosage form as RLD |
| **Pharmacokinetics** | 90% confidence interval for AUC and $C_{max}$ is within 80-125% of RLD | Bioequivalence requirement; adapted from FDA Guidances for ANDA applicants developing transdermal systems |
| **Clinical adhesion** | Cumulative patch adhesion is non-inferior to RLD during X day wear period | Bioequivalence requirement; adapted from FDA Guidances for ANDA applicants developing other types of generic transdermal systems |
| **Local tolerability** | Skin irritation and sensitization of a placebo is non-inferior to RLD | Bioequivalence requirement; adapted from FDA Guidances for ANDA applicants developing transdermal systems |
| **Stability** | At least 24-month shelf life stored at room temperature | Equivalent or better than the shelf life RLD |
| **Drug product quality attributes** | Physical attributes<br>Identification<br>API Content<br>API Content Uniformity<br>Drug Release<br>Impurities and Degradation products<br>Excipient content<br>Residual solvents<br>Microbial limits<br>Adhesion (e.g., peel force, tack, liner release.) | Meets appropriate quality standards, compendial limits, or requirements for pharmaceutical equivalence |
| **Container closure system** | Suitable container closure system to achieve the target shelf life and ensure integrity during shipping | Requirement to assure product quality over the shelf life of the drug product |
| **Administration/ concurrence with labeling** | Same as RLD | Information provided in the RLD labeling. |

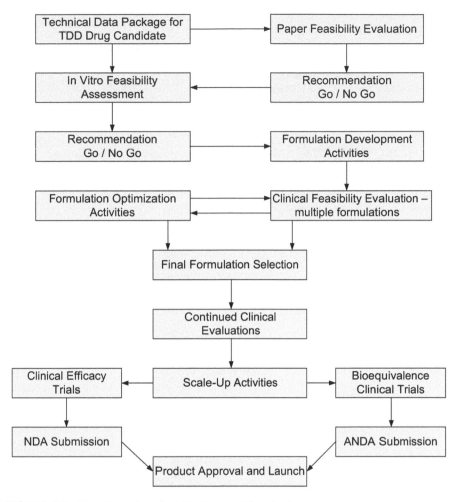

**FIGURE 4.3** Transdermal product development flowchart.

The ultimate decision regarding which of the four transdermal product design alternatives to pursue should be based on a thorough evaluation of the physicochemical characteristics of the specific drug candidate, the preferred product definition and consideration of the specific strengths and weaknesses of each design.

## 4.4 MATERIALS SELECTION FOR TRANSDERMAL DRUG DELIVERY SYSTEMS

Although the function and key properties of each individual patch component will be described separately, it is important to remember that a well-designed patch must incorporate materials that are compatible with one another. It is not enough to determine the best material for one aspect of the patch construction without considering how it will interact with the other materials in the patch. For example, the choice of

## TABLE 4.2
## Typical Data Requested on Compound During Feasibility Evaluation

**Technical Data Package Information**
- Chemical Structure & Molecular Weight
- Melting Point
- Boiling Point
- pKa(s)
- Known Decomposition Pathways
- Partition Coefficient
- Aqueous Solubility (as a function of pH)
- Additional Solubility Data
- Known Chemical Incompatibilities
- Toxicological Profile
- Solid State & Solution Stability
- UV Spectra
- Hygroscopicity
- Skin Penetration Data
- ADME Characteristics

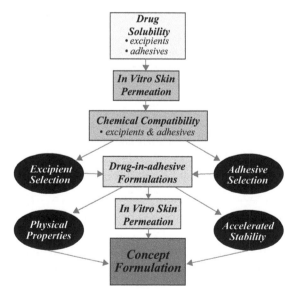

**FIGURE 4.4**  The in vitro feasibility scheme used in evaluating candidate compounds for transdermal delivery.

a particular penetration enhancer may lead to limitations in the choice of adhesive. There is tremendous interplay among the various material components in a transdermal patch; a decision on the use of any one material should consider its compatibility with other patch components, its effect on delivery, adhesion, and stability characteristics, its impact on the manufacturing process, its benefit to the patient or care giver, and its cost.

There are at least 23 different therapeutic agents currently available in transdermal patch form, and a total number of transdermal products that is substantially higher than that due to the prevalence of generic products. Yet each of these products incorporates a customized combination of construction and formulation that yields a viable transdermal drug delivery system. Table 4.3 summarizes the individual components utilized in a sampling of the transdermal products currently on the market.

## TABLE 4.3
## Components and Excipients in Transdermal Products Currently Marketed in the USA

| Drug | Product | Components | Excipients |
|---|---|---|---|
| Buprenorphine | BuTrans® (LTS/Purdue) | Outer Backing: Woven PET Overtape<br>Adhesive: Acrylate w & w/o aluminium cross-linker<br>Liner: Silicone-coated PET<br>Separating Layer:PET | Levulinic Acid, Oleyl Oleate, Povidone |
| Capsaicin | Qutenza® (LTS/ NeurogesX) | Backing: PET<br>Adhesive: Silicone<br>Liner: Release coated PET | Diethyleneglycol Monoethyl Ether, Dimethicone, Ethyl Cellulose |
| Clonidine | Catapres-TTS® (Alza/ Boehringer Ingelheim) | Backing: Pigmented Aluminized PET<br>Reservoir Matrix: PIB<br>Membrane: Microporous PP<br>Adhesive: PIB<br>Liner: Silicone-coated PET | Mineral Oil, Colloidal Silicon Dioxide |
| Diclofenac Epolamine | Flector® (Teikoku Seiyaku/ King) | Backing: Non-woven PET<br>Adhesive: Acrylate hydrogel<br>Liner: Silicone-coated PP | 1,3-Butylene Glycol, Dihydroxyaluminum Aminoacetate, Disodium Edetate, D-sorbitol, Fragrance (Dalin PH), Gelatin, Kaolin, Methylparaben, Polysorbate 80, Povidone, Propylene Glycol, Propylparaben, Sodium Carboxymethylcellulose, Sodium Polyacrylate, Tartaric Acid, Titanium Dioxide, and Purified Water |

*(continued)*

**TABLE 4.3**

**Components and Excipients in Transdermal Products Currently Marketed in the USA (Cont.)**

| Drug | Product | Components | Excipients |
|---|---|---|---|
| Estradiol | Climara® (3M/Bayer) | Backing: PE<br>Adhesive: Acrylate<br>Liner: Fluoropolymer-coated PET | Isopropyl Myristate, Glyceryl Monolaurate<br>Ethyl Oleate |
| Estradiol/ Levonorgestrel | Climara Pro® (3M/Bayer) | Backing: PE<br>Adhesive: Acrylate<br>Liner: Fluoropolymer-coated PET | Polyvinylpyrrolidone/Vinyl Acetate copolymer |
| Estradiol/ Norethindrone acetate | Combipatch® (Noven/ Novartis) | Backing: PET/EVA laminate<br>Adhesive: Silicone / Acrylate<br>Liner: Fluoropolymer-coated PET | Povidone, Oleyl Alcohol, Oleic Acid, Dipropylene Glycol |
| Ethinyl Estradiol/ Norelgestromin | Ortho Evra® (Janssen) | Backing: PE/PET laminate<br>Adhesive: PIB/Polybutene<br>Liner: Silicone-coated PET | Crospovidone, Lauryl Lactate, Non-woven PET fabric |
| Fentanyl | Duragesic® (Alza/Janssen) | Backing: PET/EVA laminate<br>Adhesive: Acrylate<br>Liner: Silicone-coated PET | None |
| Granisetron | Sancuso® (ProStrakan) | Backing: PET<br>Adhesive: Acrylate<br>Liner: Silicone-coated PET | None |
| Lidocaine | Lidoderm® (Teikoku Seiyaku/ Endo) | Backing: Non-woven PET<br>Adhesive: Acrylate hydrogel<br>Liner: Silicone-coated PET | Dihydroxyaluminum Aminoacetate, Disodium Edetate, Gelatin, Glycerin, Kaolin, Methylparaben, Polyacrylic Acid, Polyvinyl Alcohol, Propylene Glycol, Propylparaben, Sodium Carboxymethylcellulose, Sodium Polyacrylate, D-sorbitol, Tartaric Acid, and Urea. |
| Methylphenidate | Daytrana® (Noven) | Backing: PET/EVA laminate<br>Adhesive: Silicone / Acrylate<br>Liner: Fluoropolymer-coated PET | None |
| Nicotine | Nicoderm CQ® (Alza/Sanofi Aventis) | Backing: Pigmented PE/Alum/ PET/EVA laminate<br>Reservoir Matrix: EVA<br>Membrane: PE<br>Adhesive: PIB<br>Liner: Silicone-coated PET | None |
| Nitroglycerin | Minitran (3M/Medicis) | Backing: PE<br>Adhesive: Acrylate<br>Liner: Silicone-coated PET | Glyceryl Monolaurate, Ethyl Oleate |

**TABLE 4.3**

**Components and Excipients in Transdermal Products Currently Marketed in the USA (Cont.)**

| Drug | Product | Components | Excipients |
|---|---|---|---|
| | Nitro-Dur® (Merck) | Backing: PE laminate<br>Adhesive Acrylate w/resinous cross-linking agent<br>Liner: Silicone-coated PVC | None |
| Oxybutynin | Oxytrol® (Watson) | Backing: PET/EVA laminate<br>Adhesive: Acrylate<br>Liner: Silicone-coated PET | Triacetin |
| Rivastigmine | Exelon® (Novartis) | Backing: Flexible polymer film<br>Matrix Adhesive: Acrylate<br>Skin Adhesive: Silicone<br>Liner: Release coated polymer film | Silicone oil, Vitamin E |
| Rotigotine | Neupro® (UCB) | Backing: Pigmented Al coated PET film<br>Adhesive: Silicone<br>Liner: Fluoropolymer-coated PET film | Ascorbyl Palmitate, Povidone, Sodium Metabisulfite, and dl-alpha-Tocopherol |
| Scopolamine | Transderm-Scop® (PDR (Alza/Novartis) | Backing: Pigmented Aluminized PET<br>Reservoir Matrix: PIB<br>Membrane: Microporous PP<br>Adhesive: PIB<br>Liner: Silicone-coated PET | Mineral Oil |
| Selegiline | Emsam® (Somerset) | Backing: EVA/PE/PET film<br>Adhesive: Acrylate<br>Liner: Silicone-coated PET | None |
| Testosterone | Androderm® (Watson) | Backing: PET/EVA laminate<br>Membrane: Microporous PE<br>Adhesive: Acrylate<br>Liner: Silicone-coated PET | Ethanol, Carbomer 1342, Glycerin, Glycerol Monooleate, Methyl Laurate, Sodium Hydroxide, Water. |

*Acronyms:* PE = Polyethylene; PVC = Polyvinylchloride; PET = Polyethylene Terephthalate; PP = Polypropylene; EVA = Ethylene-Vinyl Acetate Copolymer; PIB = Polyisobutylene

### 4.4.1 PRESSURE SENSITIVE ADHESIVES FOR TDD SYSTEMS

#### 4.4.1.1 Three Different PSAs

Three types of pressure sensitive adhesives (PSAs) are commonly used in transdermal drug delivery (TDD) systems: polyisobutylenes, silicones and acrylics (Tan and Pfister 1999, Subedi, et al. 2010). These PSAs offer good drug solubility and diffusion properties, low skin irritation, good skin adhesion and the design flexibility required to obtain a TDD system with balanced properties.

Polyisobutylenes (PIBs) are paraffinic hydrocarbon polymers composed of long straight-chain molecules with only terminal unsaturation. Due to this structure, this material is relatively inert, odorless and nontoxic. Generally, PIB PSAs are composed of mixtures of high molecular weight PIBs that provide increased cohesive strength and low molecular weight PIBs that provide tack and good initial wet out for adhesion (BASF 2010). The PIB PSAs can be further modified by the addition of other resins and tackifiers.

Silicone PSAs are made of two major components: a resin and a polymer dissolved in solvent. The resin component is a three-dimensional structure having Si-O-Si siloxane bonds. Typically, Si resins and polymers have residual silanol (SiOH) functionality. A condensation reaction takes place between silanols on the resin and polymer to form the silicone PSA (Sobieski 1986, Ho and Dodou 2007). The molecular structure of silicone PSAs imparts unique properties such as low glass transition temperature ($T_g$) ($-120°C$) and a high degree of flexibility within the polysiloxane chains. Silicone PSAs are also known for their physiological inertness. Silicone PSAs may be modified by endcapping the reactive silanol groups to make them more compatible with amine-functional drugs (Pfister et al. 1992, Lin et al. 2007). Recently, "soft" silicone PSAs have been developed and incorporated in medical tapes (Grove et al. 2013) which result in very minimal skin trauma following removal (Figure 4.5) and may provide a useful adhesive option for TDD patches as well.

Acrylic PSAs are typically produced by copolymerizing acrylic esters with other co-monomers, either by a solution process or an emulsion process. By copolymerizing different co-monomers, acrylic PSAs with a wide range of adhesive properties and solubility characteristics can be prepared (Ulrich 1959). Acrylic PSAs prepared in this way are inherently tacky without requiring additional compounding. Single component adhesives have advantages over compounded PSAs in that they do not require a separate compounding step, and they inherently avoid concerns that a low

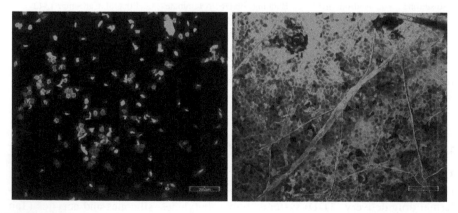

**FIGURE 4.5** Stained skin cells and hair on the surface of soft silicone adhesive tape (left) and acrylate adhesive tape (right).

molecular weight portion of a compounded PSA may migrate to the adhesive surface and negatively affect adhesion.

#### 4.4.1.2 PSA Selection

Transdermal drug delivery systems must provide good, reliable skin contact for a specified period of time in order to provide consistent drug delivery, then should be easy to remove when desired, without causing trauma to the skin. The PSA selection process should consider solubility characteristics (Grosh et al. 1988), adhesion properties and processing requirements (Gruhlke 1994).

#### 4.4.1.3 Surface Energy of Skin

When a PSA is brought into contact with the skin surface, the first requirement for adhesion is good wetting, which has both a thermodynamic and a kinetic component. The surface energy of human skin is difficult to measure because it is not smooth and each individual's skin surfaces can be quite different. Measurements of skin surface energy obtained by measuring contact angles with various liquids have been reported in the literature. The reported average critical surface tension ranges from approximately 27 to 37dyne/cm for clean human skin surface (Ginn et al. 1968, Venkatraman and Cogan-Farinas 1994). The effects of temperature and humidity on skin surface energies are also reported (Kenney et al. 1992). The relatively low value of skin surface energy obtained from these measurements indicates that, from a thermodynamic perspective, it is not easy to adhere to human skin. Adhesives used in transdermal systems are affected by the physicochemical properties of the drug and excipients to be released, and these in turn will influence both the surface and bulk viscoelastic properties.

#### 4.4.1.4 Characteristics of Excipient-Loaded PSAs

One of the challenges of TDD formulation development, particularly drug-in-adhesive matrix systems, is the impact of drug and excipients on the adhesive physical properties. The adhesive must be designed to accommodate these components both during storage and during the wear period as those materials are being delivered from the patch. The following sections describe the general impact that excipients can have on adhesive properties of various PSA materials.

#### 4.4.1.4.1 Plasticizing Effect

In regard to bulk viscoelastic properties, the effects of various excipients on the physical properties of selected acrylate, polyisobutylene and silicone pressure sensitive adhesives commonly utilized in transdermal systems have been evaluated (Wilking et al. 1994, Li et al. 2011). Typically, adding excipients to PSAs will plasticize the PSAs and lower their shear strength. The drug-in-adhesive patch design as well as reservoir designs in which the adhesive is allowed to equilibrate with the reservoir contents require a high level of performance from the pressure sensitive adhesive (Pfister and Hsieh 1990). The reduction in shear resistance may result in adhesive residue on the skin, edge lifting of the patch during wear or loss of adhesion. The maintenance of adequate adhesive physical properties is particularly important for three-day and seven-day wear patches.

#### 4.4.1.4.2 PSA Compliance

The bulk viscoelastic property of an adhesive can be characterized by measurement of adhesive compliance, sometimes also referred to as shear-creep compliance. Compliance is a measurement of the bulk adhesive viscoelastic flow under a given load and is useful for prediction of skin adhesion, cohesive strength of the adhesive, and for adhesive residue on the skin upon patch removal. The measurement of creep compliance consists of placing two samples of the PSA with a PET liner between plates of a shear creep compliance rheometer (Lucast and Taylor 1989). The plates, coupled to a strip chart recorder, are compressed and a 500 g load is applied. The creep compliance is calculated from the time-displacement curve using the following equation:

$$J = 2Ax/hf$$

where $A$ is the area of the adhesive sample in cm$^2$, $x$ is the displacement at time $t$ in cm, $h$ is the thickness of the adhesive sample in cm, $f$ is the applied stress in dynes and compliance, $J$, is reported in cm$^2$/dyne.

Compliance data is shown in Figure 4.6 for three PSAs with different levels of isopropyl myristate (IPM) loading. The compliance value of the silicone PSA without added excipient is $0.1 \times 10^{-5}$ cm$^2$/dyne, whereas for 1.5% and 2.5% IPM-added PSAs, the compliance values are $2.0 \times 10^{-5}$ and $4.5 \times 10^{-5}$ cm$^2$/dyne, respectively. Comparison of the compliance values for these excipient-loaded PSAs shows the plasticizing effect is greater for the silicone PSA than for PIB PSA which required 15% IPM to obtain the compliance value of $2.7 \times 10^{-5}$ cm$^2$/dyne, and 25% IPM to reach the compliance value of $5.0 \times 10^{-5}$ cm$^2$/dyne. The plasticizing effect is much less for the acrylic PSA which required 30% IPM to reach a compliance value of $2.6 \times 10^{-5}$ cm$^2$/dyne and 40% IPM to reach a compliance value of $5.0 \times 10^{-5}$ cm$^2$/dyne.

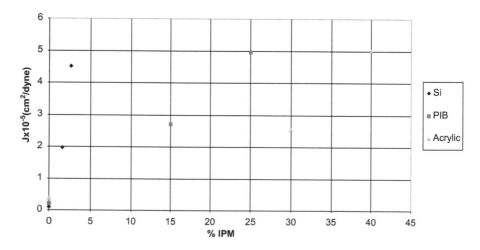

**FIGURE 4.6** Compliance vs % IPM.

This data shows that the acrylate PSA can incorporate higher levels of excipients, such as IPM, than the other PSAs commonly used in transdermal drug delivery systems.

### 4.4.1.4.3 180° Peel Adhesion to Stainless Steel

Testing the 180° peel adhesion from a stainless steel substrate is commonly performed to determine the adhesion of a transdermal patch. The 180° peel adhesion test is performed according to the instructions in USP General Chapter ‹3› (USP 36, 2012), in which a 25mm wide PSA on a 2mil thick PET backing is tested at 300mm per minute. The peel force is reported in N/25mm.

Test results for the three classes of adhesives are shown in Figure 4.7. The peel adhesion value for the silicone PSA without the added excipient is 7.25N/25mm, whereas for the 1.5% and 2.5% IPM-loaded PSAs, peel values are 6.8 and 6.2N/25mm, respectively. As higher levels of the model excipient are added to the PSAs, the values for 180° peel adhesion from the stainless steel substrate tend to be lower. This lowering of the peel values as increasing levels of excipients are added is similar in the case of the PIB and the acrylate PSAs. In the excipient-containing PSAs, in addition to the bulk plasticizing effect, there may also be a surface effect in which the excipient migrates to the PSA/stainless steel interface and may cause a substantial reduction in peel adhesion values.

### 4.4.1.4.4 PSA Cold Flow

Cold flow measures the shear flow properties of the adhesive under long-term storage. Cold flow can be evaluated by measuring the average displacement of a PSA with a microscope and suitable measuring device. This method involves placement of a weight over each PSA tape, and storage on a 45° incline. Samples are periodically removed for displacement measurements. Cold flow displacement is reported in microns of displacement per day (Leeper and Enscore 1982). Additional methods

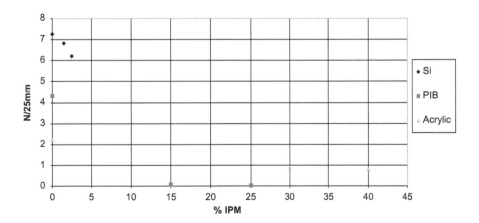

**FIGURE 4.7** 180° peel adhesion on stainless steel substrate vs % IPM.

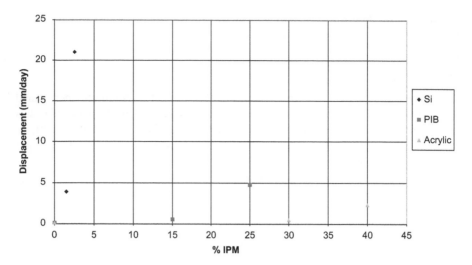

**FIGURE 4.8** Cold flow rate vs % IPM.

for measurement of cold flow may be adopted based on visual assessment, or gravimetric measurements of the packaging material and any residue left behind after patch contact during storage.

Since the presence of the drug and the enhancers significantly lower the shear resistance of the PSAs, it is important to measure long-time creep properties. The cold flow test can be used to assess the effect of loading enhancers into the PSAs. Cold flow data is shown in Figure 4.8 for the three different PSAs and for different levels of IPM. The cold flow data show that even though the compliance values were very similar for the three classes of PSAs, their cold flow behavior is substantially different. The cold flow rate was highest for the silicone PSA and lowest for the acrylate PSA. The key is minimizing cold flow properties without lowering skin adhesion. By minimizing cold flow, the adhesive will not migrate in the transdermal package during storage so the patch will not stick to its packaging materials.

Cold flow can also occur during the patch wear period, sometimes resulting in an undesirable ring of adhesive residue around the patch site which can accumulate lint and fibers from clothing.

*4.4.1.4.5 Skin Adhesion*

Adhesion to skin is evaluated in a skin wear panel utilizing a custom adhesion tester. The adhesive properties of the PSA tape or TDD patch are characterized by peeling it away from human skin and monitoring the peel force per unit width. Initial adhesion measures the quick stick characteristics of the adhesive and 24 hr dwell adhesion measures longer-term adhesive flow characteristics. After 24 hours of wear, or longer if desired, lift (i.e., an assessment of skin contact) is evaluated visually and assigned a score value. After the PSA tape or TDD patch has been removed, the amount of adhesive residue on the skin site is evaluated visually and also assigned a score value.

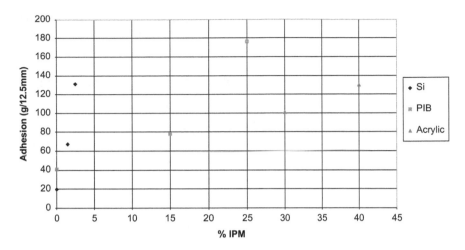

**FIGURE 4.9** Skin adhesion (Dwell time = 0) vs % IPM.

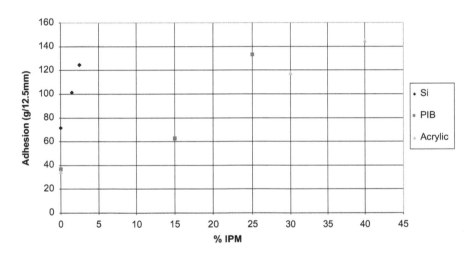

**FIGURE 4.10** Skin adhesion (Dwell time = 24 hours) vs % IPM.

In order to understand skin adhesion of pressure sensitive adhesives, many aspects of adhesion have been studied, such as tack, shear, adhesion to various substrates and viscoelastic properties (Urushizaki and Mizumachi 1991, Huie et al. 1985, Krug and Marecki 1983, Schiraldi 1990, Pierson 1990, Venkatraman and Gale 1998, Schulz et al. 2010). Many of these studies did not include excipients; however, several have been conducted using excipient-loaded PSAs for transdermal applications (Ko 1995). Figures 4.9 and 4.10 show skin peel adhesion data for initial (T=0) and dwelled (T=24 hours) samples from three classes of PSAs. The 0-hour adhesion value for the silicone PSA is 20.0 g/12.5 mm but with 1.5% IPM and 2.5% IPM, the skin adhesion values are 67.0 and 131.0 g/12.5 mm, respectively. The IPM plasticizes the PSA, allowing it to flow more easily and permitting more rapid wetting of the skin which increases the initial peel strength. The 24-hour peel adhesion values for the silicone PSA are 71.3, 101.1 and 124.5 g/12.5 mm for 0%, 1.5% and 2.5% IPM, respectively. For the 0% IPM PIB and acrylate PSAs, the 0-hour peel values were comparable (41.0 g/12.5 mm). After 24 hours of wear, the peel values of all IPM-loaded PSAs were comparable.

### 4.4.1.5 Failure Mode and Substrate Difference

The increase in skin adhesion values as IPM is added to all three classes of PSAs contrasts with the decrease in the peel values on stainless steel substrates. This may be due to the fact that the stainless steel substrate does not have the ability to take up IPM, which could lead to the formation of a weak boundary layer. In contrast, the surface of the skin is much rougher, thereby making displacement of the IPM from the contact surfaces easier. Also, excipients can be taken up by the skin, leaving less excipient accumulated at the interface to influence adhesion.

The failure mode in each case is also different. That is, when the tape is pulled away from the stainless steel surface, a clean interfacial failure occurs. In contrast, on skin, the failure mode is a mixture of skin interfacial failure and the cohesive failure of the stratum corneum. Figure 4.11 shows the stratum corneum removed from the skin after a peel test. Also, when the tape is being pulled from the skin, the skin substrate is deformed at the point of peel front. The diagram in Figure 4.12, which shows adhesive being removed from the stratum corneum layer, illustrates the cohesive failure of the stratum corneum layer plus the deformation of the skin at the point of peel. The skin peel adhesion's contribution can be expressed by the following equation: Skin peel adhesion = contribution from surface energies which can be expressed by work of adhesion ( $W_a$ ) + contribution from bulk viscoelastic property

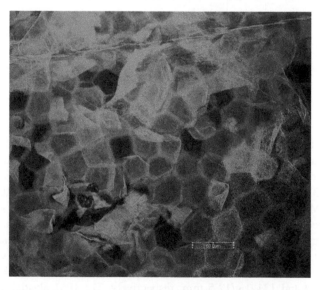

**FIGURE 4.11** Skin cells on surface of adhesive following removal from skin.

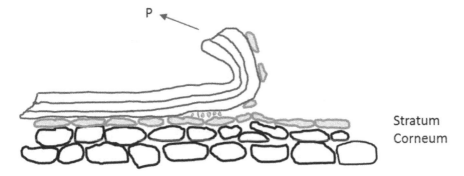

**FIGURE 4.12** Failure mode of a transdermal patch from the skin surface.

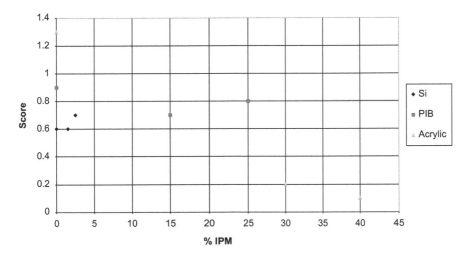

**FIGURE 4.13** Edge lift (dwell time = 24 hours) vs % IPM.

of tape + contribution from skin deformation + contribution from cohesive strength of stratum corneum. If the last two terms are removed, then the expression would be the same as that for the tape peel adhesion on any other substrate, such as stainless steel. The $W_a$ expression can be expressed by:

$$W_a = 2\left(\delta_s^d \delta_a^d\right)^{1/2} + \left(\delta_s^P \delta_a^P\right)^{1/2}$$

taking into account the polar and dispersive contribution of the surface energy ($\delta$); $s$ is for the substrate and $a$ is for the adhesive. The surface energy of PSAs and skin are discussed in the literature (Venkatraman and Cogan-Farinas 1994, Venkatraman and Gale 1998). However, for skin adhesion, the major adhesion contributing component is the bulk viscoelastic property of the PSA. As expected, in regard to the lift of the PSAs during wear (Figure 4.13), and residue of the adhesives on the skin surface

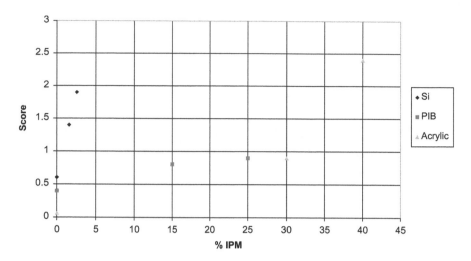

**FIGURE 4.14**   Residue on skin (dwell time = 24 hours) vs % IPM.

(Figure 4.14), as more IPM is loaded into the PSAs, the more residue remains due to the plasticizing effect of the excipients which reduces the cohesive strength of the adhesive. The lift of the acrylic PSA containing 40% IPM was low but the residue was high.

### 4.4.1.6   Prediction of Skin Adhesion

The correlation between physical properties of a PSA and actual skin adhesion appears strongest for the compliance property (Ko 1995). PSAs with compliance values in the same range had relatively similar skin adhesion values at $T=0$ for three different PSAs. This data suggests that, for the IPM loaded PSAs, and based on initial skin adhesion, the bulk viscoelastic property contribution plays a more important role than the surface properties.

### 4.4.1.7   Safety of TDD PSAs

The adhesives that are used for transdermal applications undergo safety and clinical evaluations to ensure they are suitable for pharmaceutical skin contact applications. They also have stringent limits on residual monomer and solvent levels. Limiting monomer and solvent levels is critical because residual monomers in the PSAs can irritate the skin or cause systemic toxicity. Also, residual monomers and catalysts can induce chemical interaction with the drug and negatively impact product stability or substantially change drug release profiles. The PSAs utilizing plasticizers, tackifiers and crosslinkers must be examined since they may induce dermatological responses. The typical preclinical safety evaluations for transdermal adhesives include: USP ‹86›/‹87› in vitro and in vivo biological reactivity testing (USP 36 2012), primary skin irritation, and repeat insult patch testing for sensitization potential. This preclinical testing helps assure that the adhesive can be safely incorporated into a transdermal system for human use.

### 4.4.2 PACKAGING COMPONENTS

The term packaging component is used here in its most general sense to include any component that is used to contain and protect the transdermal drug formulation but is not intended to contain any drug itself. Three types of packaging components will be described: release liners, backing films and pouch materials.

#### 4.4.2.1 Release Liners

Release liners are common to all types of transdermal patch designs and serve to protect the skin-contacting adhesive during storage. At the time of patch application, the liner is peeled away from the adhesive and discarded. Consideration is often given to the ease of the liner removal, particularly for drugs that target an elderly patient population. Examples include extending the liner around the periphery of the patch or slitting the liner in such a way that it can be easily grasped and removed.

In the most basic terms, release liners consist of a substrate that carries a very thin (500 Angstroms to several microns) release coating on at least one surface. The release coating provides a low energy surface that allows the liner to be easily peeled away from the adhesive. Common materials used as release liner substrates include papers, such as polycoated papers, or thermoplastic polymer films such as polyethylene terephthalate (PET), polypropylene, polystyrene, polyvinylchloride (PVC) or high density polyethylene. PET is generally preferred because of its resistance to drug uptake. Materials used as release coatings are usually polydimethylsiloxane (silicone) (Dean 1990, Sloboda 2011) or perfluoroether (Huie et al. 1985) polymers depending on choice of adhesives and ease of release desired. Perfluoroether polymers have the advantage of providing good release from silicone PSAs, which is one limitation of the silicone release coatings which tend to adhere aggressively to silicone PSAs.

There are several properties which are essential for any liner used in a transdermal patch system. Foremost among these is the ability to provide stable release from the adhesive throughout the shelf life of the product. It is also essential that the liner not interact with any other formulation components; there must not be any uptake, adsorption, reaction, etc. The overall stiffness of the substrate (i.e., choice of material and thickness) should be selected to facilitate handling of the patch and removal of the liner. Typical substrate thicknesses range from about 50 microns to 600 microns depending on the choice of substrate (PET liners are typically 50–125 microns). Finally, the liner materials should allow easy handling during all operations in the transdermal manufacturing process. For example, if the process calls for a solvent-containing adhesive to be coated onto the release liner and thermally dried, the substrate must be capable of enduring the drying process.

In some cases, a release liner may be used as an in-process material, as well as in the final product. For example, liners with release coating on both sides of the substrate are sometimes useful for adhesive processing without a subsequent lamination. This type of liner is known as a "differential" liner because the release coatings are designed such that adhesion to one side of the liner is greater than to the other.

#### 4.4.2.2 Backing Materials

The backing protects and contains the formulation throughout the shelf life and during the wear period. It forms the outermost (farthest removed from skin) layer in each of the four patch designs. The choice of backing material is critical because it influences the delivery profile, adhesion, wearability and appearance of the transdermal system. There are a great variety of polymeric materials in various configurations that may be suitable for use as transdermal backings, depending on the properties desired. Some of the most commonly used backings are actually laminates of several materials that provide the desired overall properties. For example, a backing might consist of an outer polyester layer to provide a vapor barrier, with an inner layer of ethylene-vinyl acetate copolymer to provide sealability. Other materials suitable for use as transdermal backings include: polyurethane, polyethylene or polyvinylydine chloride (PVDC) films, aluminum foil and various non-woven materials.

The key properties required in the backing material may vary depending on the patch design. For reservoir designs, the inner surface of the backing must be sealable to another film or membrane, in order to contain the liquid or semisolid contents of the drug reservoir. If the backing contacts the adhesive, such as in a monolithic drug-in-adhesive design, its surface properties must be such that the adhesive matrix has adequate adhesion to the backing. The adhesion between backing and adhesive should be significantly greater than the adhesion between the adhesive and skin. If not, residue results. If necessary, the surface properties may be altered through pretreatment, such as corona discharge or flame processing (Briggs 1982, Yializis et al. 1999) to improve adhesion.

Regardless of patch design, the backing must be compatible with the other formulation components and must be constructed of materials that avoid unwanted absorption of the drug or formulation excipients. Many drugs and excipients used in transdermal systems are quite hydrophobic and may have an affinity for hydrophobic polymers such as polyethylene. The conformability or flexibility of the backing is important in determining the wear characteristics of the patch. The ability to elastically deform and recover in response to the movement of the skin is important, both for the comfort of the patient and for ensuring adequate skin adhesion during the wear period. For example, if a patch is designed to be worn for extended periods or in an area of the body in which there is considerable skin movement, a highly flexible backing is imperative. For sites such as the upper torso or upper arm, flexibility may be less important. Finally, since most regulatory authorities require that patches be printed with at least the name of the active ingredient and the dosage, the backing must be capable of accepting print.

The backing is also the major contributor (but not the only contributor) to the overall occlusion provided by a transdermal patch (Casiraghi et al. 2002). Occlusion may be defined as the degree to which moisture vapor transmission is restricted at the patch site. A wide range of occlusive properties can be obtained in backing materials, ranging from non-wovens on the least occlusive or "breathable" end of the spectrum to polyester, aluminum foil and PVDC on the most occlusive end of the spectrum. The degree of occlusion will impact the skin adhesion time profile, drug delivery profile and skin irritation potential of the patch.

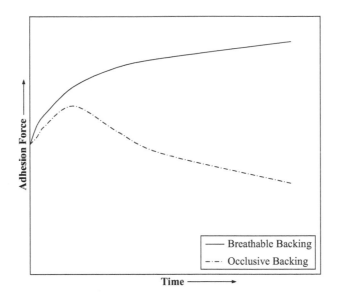

**FIGURE 4.15** Comparison of adhesion to skin for tapes containing the same adhesive and occlusive or breathable backings.

### 4.4.2.2.1 Skin Adhesion Time Profile

Figure 4.15 shows the skin adhesion profile of two medical tapes that use the same adhesive, however, their backings differ in occlusivity. The characteristic profile for an occlusive backing is an initial build in adhesion, followed by a gradual reduction in adhesion as the site beneath the patch becomes hydrated (Wilking et al. 1994) A "breathable" backing promotes an adhesion profile that continues to gradually build over the course of a normal wear period. As Figure 4.16 shows, there are three basic responses of adhesion vs time (Marecki 1987). In the ideal case (A), after the device is adhered to the skin, adhesion builds very quickly to an acceptable level and remains constant with time. In the second case (B), adhesion continues to build with time, such that skin may be traumatized on removal of the device. In the third case (C), after an initial increase, adhesion begins to decrease with time due to moisture buildup. Careful consideration must be given to match the backing and the adhesive such that adequate skin adhesion is maintained over the desired wear period.

### 4.4.2.2.2 Drug Delivery Profile

Skin hydration has long been recognized as a factor in skin penetration (McKenzie and Stoughton 1962) For many drugs, particularly hydrophobic drugs, as the skin becomes more hydrated, the drug permeation rate is enhanced (Bucks et al. 1989, Zhai et al. 2002) Therefore, it is possible for equivalent formulations that differ only in their backing material to provide very different drug delivery profiles.

### 4.4.2.2.3 Skin Irritation Potential

Long-term occlusion is a factor that may contribute to skin irritation (Hurkmanns et al. 1985, Zhai and Maibach 2001) Occlusion may also contribute to increased

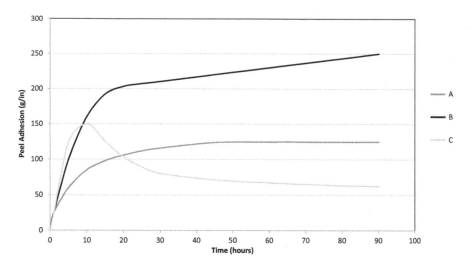

**FIGURE 4.16** Skin adhesion vs time. Ideal case (A). Unfavorable due to continued increase of adhesion (B). Unfavorable due to continued loss of adhesion (C).

growth of microorganisms on the skin surface (Kligman and Epstein 1975, Leow and Maibach 1997), which on rare occasions can lead to superficial infections and the development of pustules beneath the patch site. If there is a strong thermal stimulus for sweating, miliaria (prickly heat) may develop if the occlusion continues over a prolonged period (Leyden and Grove 1987). These effects are typically a rarity, and generally only occur after prolonged applications.

### 4.4.2.3 Pouch Materials

All currently marketed transdermal products are provided in single unit pouches. The function of the pouch is to protect and preserve the stability of the transdermal patch over the shelf life of the product. For some products, providing child resistance and/or easy access for the elderly is another pouch requirement. A pouch generally has a multilaminate construction and often utilizes a layer of aluminum foil for its barrier properties. Other pouch materials include various types of paper or polymer films such as polyethylene terephthalate, polyethylene, polypropylene or Barex$^R$. A common pouch construction is paper/foil/polyethylene (Bertrand 1983).

Above all else, the packaging film should not interact with the transdermal patch or any of the formulation ingredients through absorption, adsorption or chemical reaction. In addition, the packaging film should not permit the transmission of vapors, either into the pouch (e.g., water vapor) or out of the pouch in the form of vaporized formulation components. Another key property of the pouch material is its sealability. The packaging film is usually sealed to itself to form a pouch around each patch. Therefore, the inner surface of the pouch material must be sealable in some manner (i.e., thermal, ultrasonic, pressure, etc.). Finally, the outer surface of the pouch material must be capable of accepting print because the pouch must display the necessary product information and artwork.

Evaluation of the desired patch formulation with the proposed pouch materials should be done early in the development process in the form of controlled stability studies using ICH conditions.

### 4.4.3 MEMBRANES

Membranes are used primarily in reservoir or multilaminate patch designs to control the rate of drug release from the patch. In a lesser number of cases, the rate of drug release may be sufficiently rapid such that the membrane does not function to control the overall rate of delivery (i.e., the skin provides most of the rate control). In these instances, the primary function of the membrane in a reservoir patch design is to provide a means of containing the drug formulation, while in a multilaminate design, the principal membrane function is to provide a physical support.

Many different polymeric materials can be used to construct a membrane for use in a transdermal drug delivery patch. These materials can be grouped into two general categories: continuous films and porous films.

#### 4.4.3.1 Continuous Films

The mechanism of drug transport across these membranes can be described as a partitioning process from the upstream side of the membrane, followed by diffusion through the polymer film. Suitable materials for these membranes include: polyethylene, various polyurethanes, polydimethylsiloxane, polypropylene and ethylene-vinyl acetate copolymers. The latter have been used extensively and have proven useful for adjusting the rate of drug delivery through the membrane, since the permeability of many drugs depends on the composition of the copolymer (Higuchi and Hussain 1979, Mutalik and Udupa 2006). For many drugs, an increase in the percentage of vinyl acetate in the copolymer membrane will increase permeability (Peterson et al. 1990) primarily due to more favorable partitioning and the reduced crystallinity of the polymer as the vinyl acetate content rises.

#### 4.4.3.2 Porous Films

These membranes contain networks of interconnected pores as shown in Figure 4.17. They are made of materials such as polyethylene or polypropylene and are produced using a variety of processes, most of which involve some orientation or controlled stretching of the film to create or expand the porous structure. The drug transport mechanism in porous films involves diffusion through a vehicle used to fill the membrane pores, such as mineral oil, ethanol or other material that will wet the pores of the membrane.

Since the membrane material is often used to determine rate of drug release from a patch, it is essential that controls be placed on key membrane attributes such as composition, thickness, crystallinity, permeability, and pore size and distribution. These properties must be reproducible from batch to batch in order to obtain a consistent release rate. It is strongly recommended that some type of permeability measurement be included in the raw material acceptance specifications for any membranes that are used to control or influence the rate of drug delivery. An assessment of the stability of membrane permeability over time, both in the finished product as well as at the raw material stage, is also well-advised.

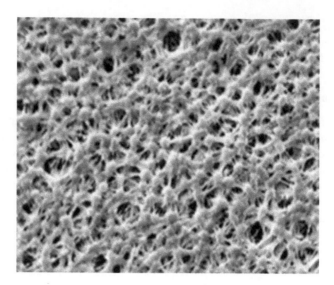

FIGURE 4.17   Electron micrograph (1500X) of microporous membrane surface.

A number of other factors also deserve consideration when selecting a membrane material. Reservoir patch designs require that the membrane be sealed to the backing to create a compartment for the drug formulation. Therefore, from a sealability standpoint, the membrane must be compatible with the backing. Depending on the patch design, one or both sides of the membrane will be in contact with an adhesive layer. Adhesion must be great enough to prevent delamination throughout the patch shelf life and wear period, as well as during removal. The membrane surface properties may be modified through means similar to those described in the section on backing films. The membrane must also be sufficiently robust in order to be handled during the patch manufacturing process without adversely affecting the membrane's permeability or other properties.

## 4.5   MANUFACTURING TECHNOLOGY IN TDD

The processes involved in the manufacture of transdermal patches are very different from those used in the manufacture of oral, topical or parenteral products and can also vary considerably depending on the type of transdermal system design. Many of the processes are more closely related to those found in the film and tape industries than to those used for other pharmaceutical dosage forms. This overview will briefly describe the major unit operations used to produce all different types of patch designs, give a more detailed overview of a typical drug-in-adhesive manufacturing process and address some of the issues involved in scale-up to a production site.

### 4.5.1   UNIT OPERATIONS

Typical process flow diagrams for the manufacture of each patch design are shown in Figure 4.18. Each major unit operation is shown as a separate step. The following are brief definitions of each unit operation, as they apply to transdermal manufacturing:

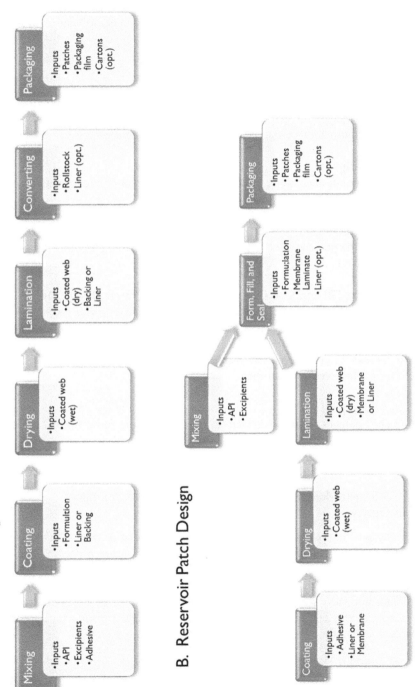

**FIGURE 4.18** Typical process flow diagrams for transdermal patches by design type.

#### 4.5.1.1 Mixing
In almost all transdermal patch designs, the active ingredient and any formulation excipients must be mixed into a carrier material (a polymer, solvent or matrix) at some point during the manufacturing process.

#### 4.5.1.2 Coating
Adhesives or drug-in-adhesive mixtures are coated onto a moving web, using a variety of methods. The adhesives are usually either a polymer melt or a polymer solution. The latter may be coated directly at room temperature, while hot melt coating requires an additional process to heat and/or mix the adhesive.

#### 4.5.1.3 Drying
If the coating solution contains volatile solvents, a thermal drying operation enables solvent removal.

#### 4.5.1.4 Converting
Converting is the process of obtaining patches of the desired size and configuration from a larger web.

#### 4.5.1.5 Form, Fill and Seal Converting (Reservoir Patch Design Only)
The form, fill and seal converting process is used to create reservoir patch designs in which a drug-containing gel or solution is metered onto the backing film; a laminated web consisting of a membrane, adhesive and release liner is brought in; and the backing is sealed to the membrane around the periphery of the metered gel or solution to form a reservoir compartment.

#### 4.5.1.6 Packaging
The finished patches from the converting operation or the form, fill and seal operation are placed in individual pouches, then placed in multiple-pouch packages for patient use.

### 4.5.2 A SAMPLE MANUFACTURING PROCESS FOR A DRUG-IN-ADHESIVE MATRIX DESIGN

The manufacturing technology used in the production of drug-in-adhesive matrix transdermal patches draws heavily upon tape manufacturing processes that have been developed over the past 80 years. The primary differences are the incorporation of a drug and other formulation excipients, and the much greater degree of precision and control required in order to ensure the quality of a drug product. The following provides a more detailed description of each unit operation and appropriate in-process testing for a monolithic drug-in-adhesive patch design:

#### 4.5.2.1 Mixing
A solution of adhesive polymer in a solvent is mixed with the active ingredient and any other formulation excipients to form a homogeneous solution or suspension. Typical equipment is a mixing vessel with some means for agitation (such as

a double planetary mixer), scaled appropriately for the desired batch size. Critical process parameters often include temperature, mix time and agitation speed (Van Buskirk et al. 2012). Key properties of the mixture are homogeneity, drug content on a weight-percent basis and particle size for suspension formulations.

#### 4.5.2.2 Coating

Following mixing, the solution is coated onto a web, usually the product release liner or the backing film. This is done in a continuous process in which the web is conveyed through a coating station where the solution is applied. There are a variety of coating techniques (refer to Figure 4.19 for some examples), which are known to those skilled in the art (Satas 1984; Satas and Tracton 2001) The choice of coating method is determined by the rheological properties of the coating solution, the desired coating weight (i.e., mass/area), the scale of the coating process (width and desired line speed) and the required uniformity. Typically, achieving the desired coating uniformity is the overriding concern for transdermal products. In order to consistently meet the USP requirements for content uniformity (no more than 6% relative standard deviation) it is advisable to select a coating method that is capable of routinely achieving uniformity of no greater than 2% RSD (Relative Standard Deviation). The methods most often used for drug-in-adhesive solutions are knife coating, Mayer bar coating and extrusion die coating. These are the typical choices because each is capable of coating viscous solutions (2,000–10,000cps) at the desired coating weight or thickness (usually 50 to 200 m), and most importantly, they are capable of achieving the necessary coating uniformity. For optimal coating uniformity and yield, it is possible to customize the coating die based on the rheological properties of the solution to be coated (Fenton 2013).

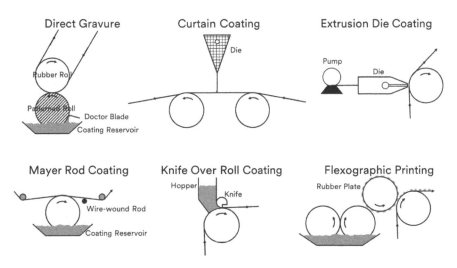

**FIGURE 4.19** Schematic diagrams of several coating methods useful in the production of transdermal drug delivery patches.

### 4.5.2.3 Drying

After the coating solution has been applied, the web typically proceeds into a drying oven(s) where the solvents are removed. The selection of oven conditions is generally a matter of balancing the following, sometimes conflicting, goals:

1. Achieving efficient removal of the solvent and any residual adhesive monomers, reducing their concentration to toxicologically acceptable levels.
2. Maintaining the smooth appearance of the coating.
3. Maintaining desired levels of any formulation components (such as drug or excipient) that may partially volatilize during the drying process.
4. Achieving web speeds that are sufficiently fast to keep manufacturing costs down.

The critical process parameters are oven temperatures, residence time (i.e., line speed), and for air impingement ovens, the velocity and amount of heated gas (usually air, but sometimes nitrogen) impinging on the web. Ovens of alternate design that utilize infrared radiation or heating by conduction may also be utilized. The drying process may be statistically modeled and optimized through the use of factorial experiments or response surface methodology (Gruhlke 1994, Lipp and Heimann 1996).

### 4.5.2.4 Lamination

After the web exits the oven, the release liner or backing is laminated to the exposed surface of the dried drug-in-adhesive matrix. This is done by bringing the two webs together between two rollers under moderate pressure. The laminate is then wound up in a roll and stored for further processing. Typical in-process tests at this stage might include: coating weight measurements, drug content, excipient content, and residual solvents and monomers testing.

### 4.5.2.5 Converting

This is the process of cutting patches, of the desired dimension, from the rollstock. In some cases, the rollstock from the coating, drying and lamination process must be slit to a narrower width prior to the converting operation. Converting equipment is typically built with the flexibility to perform several different operations in a single pass through the equipment. For example: an additional lamination, a liner slit or a cut to a different shape than the patch, printing of the patch or liner, and the actual patch die-cutting may all take place in a continuous process on the converter. In addition, the packaging operation (see the following section) may be integrated with converting.

### 4.5.2.6 Packaging

The patches from the converting process are placed onto a packaging film web at regular intervals, another packaging film web is brought in and the films are sealed together using heat, ultrasound, pressure or other means to form a pouch around the patch. The packaging film may be printed on-line, and the finished pouch is cut or sheeted from the web. Typically, there is also an operation in which the desired number of pouches are packaged in a carton, along with patient information, to form the ultimate container for sale to the patient. A full battery of finished product testing is performed at the completion of this step.

## 4.6 SCALE-UP FROM LABORATORY TO PRODUCTION

### 4.6.1 INFORMATION DATA PACKAGE

Scale-up from the laboratory to production-scale equipment can be an arduous task, especially if the transfer of information to the production site is incomplete or untimely. Typically, the transition to process-scale is accompanied by a transition in personnel who will be responsible for product manufacture and a change in physical location. An information data package can be a very useful mechanism for transferring important product information from the laboratory to the production site. For many of the personnel at the production site, this will be their first exposure to the new product. The information data package can serve as an aid in training employees and as a reference guide, as questions arise during the manufacture of the product. The contents of the information data package may vary slightly depending on the type of patch construction. The main elements that should be common to all transdermal patches are listed in Table 4.4.

There is no "proper" time to prepare the information data package; this varies, depending on the philosophy of each organization. The information to be included

---

**TABLE 4.4**
**Useful Items to Include in Laboratory Generated Information Data Packages**

1. Finished product specifications.
2. In-process specifications.
3. Raw material specifications and recommended (approved) vendors.
4. Material safety data sheets (MSDS) for all raw materials.
5. Test methods required for raw material, in-process, and finished product specs.
6. Test method validation reports.
7. Manufacturing process as it appears in all regulatory submissions.
8. Quantitative Composition for each dosage strength (patch size).
9. Example batch formula for each dosage strength (patch size).
10. Information on the packaging system.
11. Stability data and summary.
12. Pharmaceutical development report and rationale behind the chosen formulation.
13. Experimental results which show the impact of process parameters on the product.
14. Process conditions used in laboratory or pilot scale production.
15. Copies of lab and pilot scale manufacturing procedures.
16. Historically expected values for product, in-process, and raw material test results.
17. Summary of the clinical use of the product.
18. Regulatory status of the product, if not already approved.
19. Expected yield.
20. A historical account of challenges encountered at the lab scale, and how they can be solved or avoided.

also constantly evolves during the course of product development. However, since phase III clinical supplies must typically be produced on production equipment, the information data package should be completed in advance of phase III studies for developmental products. For generic products, information should be transferred prior to the production of bioequivalence supplies and the development of the process validation plan.

Effective communication between laboratory and production personnel is a critical ingredient in any successful product scale-up. The information data package can be a useful tool to aid in communication, but is not intended to replace the other, less formal and more frequent communications between lab and production personnel that are equally important.

### 4.6.2 Process Validation

Process validation is a requirement of the Current Good Manufacturing Practices described in CFR Title 21 Part 211, and is further elaborated in a guidance document (USFDA 2011). Similarly, the EMA has issued a draft process validation guideline (EMA 2012a). Both of these guidances attempt to bring the expectations for process validation into alignment with ICH Q8, Q9 and Q10. The FDA now defines process validation as the "collection and evaluation of data, from the process design stage through commercial production which establishes scientific evidence that a process is capable of consistently delivering quality product" (USFDA 2011). More than ever, a successful validation program entails more than simply testing three or more batches of product. The regulatory authorities are now embracing an approach which places more focus on the total life cycle of the manufacturing process, from the initial design of the process through the ongoing production of commercial batches.

From a regulatory standpoint, the development of a rational process validation plan and its successful implementation are the key activities in the scale-up process. Regulatory approval depends on the successful validation of the commercial manufacturing process. But beyond its importance in regulatory compliance, process validation is good business practice and good science. The validation process provides an opportunity to improve or optimize process efficiency while assuring only products of the highest quality will be produced.

A comprehensive validation plan goes far beyond the individual unit operations involved in the manufacturing process. It should also consider elements of the physical plant, such as the heating, air conditioning and ventilation systems; utilities; raw material and personnel flows; instrumentation and associated calibration systems; and cleaning and maintenance procedures (Hess 1988). The diversity of processes used in the manufacture of transdermal patches adds another layer of complexity and makes it difficult to formulate a "recipe" for the validation of all transdermal products. It also explains why little information specific to process validation for transdermal products is available in the literature. A full treatment of this topic goes considerably beyond the scope of this chapter. However, the basic preparations for process validation runs will be discussed.

**TABLE 4.5**
**Important Considerations in Process Validation**

1. What are the critical process variables?
2. What are the relationships between the critical process variables and critical quality attributes?
3. What is the magnitude and direction of each effect?
4. What are the optimum process conditions?
5. What are the stable operating windows around the optimum conditions, and what are appropriate control limits?

A good starting step is creating a flowchart for the overall manufacturing process in the greatest detail possible. Each operation with the potential to effect product quality, strength or purity should be included, even those steps that would not ordinarily be considered "processes," such as in-process testing or in-process packaging. Most importantly, each individual process should be well characterized, prior to the actual validation runs. There should be a strong understanding of the critical quality attributes, the critical process parameters and how they are related to one another. This will ensure that the time and expense invested in the validation lots will not be wasted and the runs repeated due to lack of process understanding. Table 4.5 lists a number of important considerations to address prior to the validation runs. Normally, these questions are best answered through a statistically based experimental approach, such as response surface methodology (Box and Draper 2007) If the questions have been addressed in advance, the "real" validation of the process will be complete and the formal process validation runs will be just that: a formality to confirm the validity of the process conditions obtained in the characterization experiments.

## 4.7　TESTING OF TRANSDERMAL DRUG DELIVERY SYSTEMS

The testing of transdermal drug delivery systems is both similar and unlike that of other pharmaceutical dosage forms. The content uniformity and release rate test methods are much like those used for oral dosage forms, while a number of physical tests related to adhesion are unique to transdermal systems. Both the USP General Chapters <3> and <725> (USP 36 2012) and the EMA Draft Guideline on Quality of Transdermal Products (EMA 2012b) provide guidance on the testing requirements for TDD patches. The following section describes a number of these tests that may be specified in transdermal product monographs; they are grouped into two categories: chemical and physical tests.

### 4.7.1　Chemical Tests

#### 4.7.1.1　Content
This assay is used to determine the average drug content of a composite sample containing multiple patches and is useful in monitoring the stability of transdermal patches.

#### 4.7.1.2 Content Uniformity

Transdermal patches must meet the pharmacopeial requirements for uniformity of dosage units. These requirements have been harmonized among the EP, JP and USP, and can be found in USP General Chapter <905> (USP 36 2012) This testing involves the individual assay of ten units with criteria for passing based on the mean assay value and the relative standard deviation. If this initial testing does not meet the criteria for passing, an additional 20 units may be tested with another set of criteria applied to the results obtained for all 30 units.

#### 4.7.1.3 Purity

The purity assay is typically a chromatographic method to assess any impurities that may have been introduced during the manufacture of the transdermal patch. Limits are typically set on the total impurities and on individual impurities, as appropriate. If the active drug has any optical isomers, an assay for chiral purity is also appropriate.

#### 4.7.1.4 Excipient Content

If the formulation contains excipients that are critical to the quality of the drug product, it is important to develop test methods for excipient content. For example, an excipient which acts as a permeation enhancer and is subject to partial volatilization during the drying process would be a good candidate for excipient content testing.

#### 4.7.1.5 Residuals

If the manufacturing process involves the use of processing solvents that are later removed, an assay for residual solvent is appropriate. Likewise, if the patch contains polymer materials that may contain residual monomers, such as an adhesive, it is appropriate to assay for their presence and set upper limits on their concentrations. Acceptable limits should be established for each residual based on its toxicological profile and the intended use of the product. Appropriate limits for various solvents based on a risk assessment classification scheme are discussed in USP General Chapter <467> "Residual Solvents" (USP 36 2012). The testing may be done as an in-process test or as a test on the final product.

#### 4.7.2 PHYSICAL TESTS

#### 4.7.2.1 Release Rate

Release rate testing for transdermal patches is described in the United States Pharmacopoeia General Chapter <725> (USP 36 2012) The test involves immersion of the patch in a receptor solution (typically aqueous) of specified volume, controlled temperature and consistent agitation with measurement of the drug in the receptor solution as a function of time. Specifications are generally adopted for at least three time points: an early time point to confirm the absence of dose dumping, an intermediate time point or two to characterize the release profile and a final time point to confirm that sufficient drug is released for the intended dose. USP Apparatus 5 ("Paddle over Disk"), Apparatus 6 ("Rotating Cylinder") and Apparatus 7 ("Reciprocating Holder") are described as appropriate for transdermal products.

The Paddle over Disk apparatus is probably the most popular and easiest to use with a variety of patch constructions and sizes.

### 4.7.2.2 Adhesive Properties

A number of important physical tests for measuring the adhesive properties of TDD patches were described earlier in Section 4.4.1.4 of this chapter. These include peel adhesion, tack and liner release (Wokovich et al. 2010) which are now typically required based on USP General Chapter 3. Other measurements such as compliance, shear, cold flow and in vivo measurement of peel force from skin may be useful tools during the development process.

### 4.7.2.3 Appearance

The final product specification should include testing which ensures the product conforms to a visual description including size, shape, color, patch configuration and labeling.

## 4.8 SUMMARY

The simple appearance of transdermal drug delivery patches does not fully reflect the complexity of the development process required to produce a therapeutically effective patch. Many choices and trade-offs must be made during the course of development regarding an appropriate patch design, materials, method of manufacture and appropriate product testing. It is not possible to follow a development "recipe" which applies to every TDD product. The physicochemical properties of each compound and the specific needs of the patients it is intended to treat require the TDD system developer to adapt the development process to suit the requirements of each compound. It is the authors' hope that this chapter has given newcomers a flavor for the complexity of the transdermal product development process, while also providing those working in the field with some additional insight and perspective.

## REFERENCES

BASF (2010) *Oppanol® PIB General Product Information*, BASF Corporation, Florham Park, NJ.

Bertrand (1983) Heat-Sealable Pouch Holds Coating-Sensitive Transdermal Medicine, *Packaging*, 28(13):68.

Box, G.E.P., and Draper, N.R. (2007) *Response Surfaces, Mixtures, and Ridge Analyses, Second Edition* [of Empirical Model-Building and Response Surfaces, 1987], John Wiley and Sons, New York, NY.

Briggs, D. (1982) *Surface Analysis and Pretreatment of Plastics and Metals* (D.M. Brewis, ed.), pp. 199–226, Macmillan, New York, NY.

Bucks, D.A.W., Guy, R.H., and Maibach, H.I. (1989) *Percutaneous Absorption, 2nd edition*, (R.L. Bronaugh and H.I. Maibach, eds.), pp. 77–93, Marcel Dekker, New York, NY.

Casiraghi, A., Minghetti, P., Cilurzo, F., Montanari, L., and Naik, A. (2002) Occlusive Properties of Monolayer Patches: In Vitro and In Vivo Evaluation, *Pharmaceutical Research*, 19(4):423–426.

Chang, Y., Patel, D.C., and Ebert, C.D. (1989) *Device for Administering an Active Agent to the Skin or Mucosa*, U.S. Patent 4,849,224.

Dean, J.W. (1990) *Handbook of Adhesives, 3rd edition* (I. Skeist, ed.), pp. 532–534, Van Nostrand Reinhold, New York, NY.

EMA (European Medicines Agency) (2012a) *Draft Guideline on Process Validation*, EMA/CHMP/CVMP/QWP/70278/2012-Rev1

EMA (European Medicines Agency) (2012b) *Draft Guideline on Quality of Transdermal Products*, EMA/CHMP/QWP/911254/2011

Edwards, J. (2009) *Watson's Fentanyl Patch Recall Is 6th So Far; Why Don't Patches Work?* CBSNews.com

Farahmand, S., and Maibach, H.I. (2009) Estimating Skin Permeability from Physicochemical Characteristics of Drugs: A Comparison Between Conventional Models and an In Vivo-Based Approach, *Int. Journal of Pharmaceutics*, 375(1–2):41–47.

Fenton, J. (2013). Transdermal Manufacturing – Maximizing Yield in Transdermal Manufacturing, *Drug Delivery Technology*, 13(2):68–72.

Gale, R.M., and Berggren, R.G. (1986) *Transdermal Delivery System for Delivery of Nitroglycerin and High Transdermal Fluxes*, U.S. Patent 4,615,699

Ginn, M.E., Noyes, C.M., and Jungermann E. (1968) The Contact Angle of Water on Viable Human Skin, *J. Coll. & Interface Sci.*, 146, 26.

Good, W.R. (1986) Transdermal Drug-Delivery Systems, *M.D.&D.I.*, 2:35–42.

Grosh S., Burton S., Ferber R., and Peterson T. (1988) Comparison of the Physical Properties of Three Adhesive Classes Commonly Used in Transdermal Drug Delivery Systems, *Proceed. Intern. Symp. Control Rel. Bioact. Mater.*, 15:215–216.

Grove G. L., Zerweck C.R., Houser T.P., Smith G.E., and Koski N.I. (2013) A Randomized and Controlled Comparison of Gentleness of 2 Medical Adhesive Tapes in Healthy Human Subjects, *Journal of Wound, Ostomy, and Continence Nursing*, 40(1):51–59.

Gruhlke, E. (1994) A Concept to Scale-up Drug-in-Adhesive Type Transdermal Drug Delivery Systems, *Proceed. Inter. Symp. Control. Release Bioact. Mat.*, 21:469–470.

Hess A. (1988) An Integrated Approach to Validation, *BioPharm*, 3:42–44.

Higuchi, T., and Hussain, A. (1979) *Device Consisting of Copolymer Having Acetoxy Groups for Delivering Drugs*, U.S. Patent 4,144,317.

Ho, K.Y. and Dodou, K. (2007) Rheological Studies on Pressure-Sensitive Silicone Adhesives and Drug-In-Adhesive Layers as a Means to Characterise Adhesive Performance, *Int. Journal of Pharmaceutics*, 333 (1–2):24–33.

Huie, S.A., Schmit, P.F., and J.S. Warren (1985) Testing Adhesive and Liner for Transdermal Drug Delivery, *Adhesives Age*, 28(6):30–35.

Hurkmanns, J.F.G.M., Bodde, H.E., and Van Driel, J.M.J. (1985) Skin Irritation Caused by Transdermal Drug Delivery Systems During Long-Term Application, *Br. J. Dermatol.*, 112:461–467.

Kenney, J.F., Haddock, T.H., Sun, R.L., and Parreira, H.C. (1992) Medical-grade Acrylic Adhesives for Skin Contact, *J. Appl. Poly. Sci.*, 355, 45.

Kligman, A.M., and Epstein, W. (1975) Updating the Maximization Test for Identifying Contact Allergens, *Contact Dermatitis*, 1:231.

Ko, C.U. (1995) *Pred. Percutaneous Penetration*, 4a, 6.

Krug, K., and Marecki, N.M. (1983) *Adhesives Age*, 11, 19.

Leeper, H.M., and Enscore, D. (1982) *Adhesives Age*, 2, 16.

Leow, Y.-H., and Maibach, H.I. (1997). Effect of Occlusion on Skin, *The Journal of Dermatological Treatment*, 8(2):139–142.

Leyden, J.J., and Grove G.L., (1987) *Transdermal Delivery of Drugs* (A.F. Kydonieus and B. Berner eds.), pp. 99–107, CRC Press, Boca Raton, FL.

Li C., Liu C., Liu J., and Fang L. (2011) Correlation Between Rheological Properties, In Vitro Release, and Percutaneous Permeation of Tetrahydropalmatine, *AAPS PharmSciTech*, 12(3):1002–1010.

Lin S.B., Durfee L.D., Ekeland R.A., McVie J., and Schalau G.K. (2007) Recent Advances in Silicone Pressure-Sensitive Adhesives, *Journal of Adhesion Science and Technology*, 21(7):605–623.

Lipp, R., and Heimann, G. (1996) Statistical Approach to Optimization of Drying Conditions for a Transdermal Delivery System, *Drug Development and Industrial Pharmacy*, 22(4):343–348.

Lucast, D.H., and Taylor, C.W. (1989) *Polym., Lami, & Coat. Conf.*, 721.

Marecki, N.M. (1987) *Pharm Tech Conf. Proc.*, 311.

McKenzie, A.W., and Stoughton, R.B. (1962) Method for Comparing Percutaneous Absorption of Steroids, *Arch. Dermatol.*, 86:88–90.

Mutalik, S., and Udupa, N. (2006) Pharmacological Evaluation of Membrane-Moderated Transdermal System of Glipizide, *Clinical and Experimental Pharmacology & Physiology*, 33(1–2):17–26.

Nishida, N., Taniyama, K., Sawabe, T., and Manome, Y. (2010) Development and Evaluation of a Monolithic Drug-In-Adhesive Patch for Valsartan, *Int. Journal of Pharmaceutics*, 402:103–109.

Peterson, T., Burton, S., Ferber, R., and Petersen, T. (1990) In-Vitro Permeability of Poly(Ethylene-Vinyl Acetate) and Microporous Polyethylene Membranes, Proceed. *Inter. Symp. Control. Release Bioact. Mat.*, 17:411–412.

Peterson, T.A., and Dreyer, S.J. (1994) Factors Influencing Delivery from Multilaminate Transdermal Patch Systems, Proceed. *Intern. Symp. Control. Rel. Bioact. Mater.*, 21:477–478.

Pfister, W.R., and Hsieh, D. (1990) *Pharm. Tech.*, 10, 54.

Pfister, W.R., Woodard, J.T., and Grigoras, S. (1992) Developing Drug-Compatible Adhesives for Transdermal Drug Delivery Devices, *Pharm. Tech.*, (1):42–58.

Pierson, D.G. (1990) *Tappi Journal*, 6, 101.

Potts, R.O., and Guy, R.H. (1992) Predicting Skin Permeability, *Pharmaceutical Research*, 9(5):663–669.

Sanvordeker, D.R., Cooney, J.G., and Wester, R.C. (1982) *Transdermal Nitroglycerin Pad*, U.S. Patent 4,336,243

Satas, D. (1984) *Web Processing and Converting Technology and Equipment*, Van Nostrand Reinhold Co., New York, NY, pp. 1–182.

Satas, D., and Tracton, A.A. (2001) *Coatings Technology Handbook*, Marcel Dekker, New York, NY, pp. 129–206.

Schiraldi, M.T. (1990) *Polym., Lami., & Coat. Conf.*, 63.

Schulz, M., Fussneggerb, B., and Bodmeiera, R. (2010) Drug Release and Adhesive Properties of Crospovidone-Containing Matrix Patches Based on Polyisobutene and Acrylic Adhesives, *European Journal of Pharmaceutical Sciences*, 41(5):675–684.

Sloboda, M. (2011) The Growing Importance of Release Liners in Pharmaceutical Manufacturing, *Pharm. Tech. Europe*, 23(2):40–44.

Sobieski, L. (1986) *PSTC Technical Seminar Proceedings*, Itasca, Il.

Subedi, R.K., Oh, S.Y., Chun, M.-K., and Choi, H.-K. (2010) Recent Advances in Transdermal Drug Delivery, *Archives of Pharmacal Research*, 33 (3):339–351.

Tan H.S., and Pfister W.R. (1999) Pressure-Sensitive Adhesives for Transdermal Drug Delivery Systems, *Pharm Sci Technolo Today*, 2(2):60–69.

Ulrich, E.W. (1959) *Pressure-Sensitive Adhesive Sheet Material*, U.S. Patent 2,884,126.

USFDA (United States Food and Drug Administration) (2011) *Guidance for Industry on Process Validation: General Principles and Practices*, USFDA, Rockville, Maryland.

Urushizaki, F., and Mizumachi, H. (1991) *Chem. Pharm. Bull.*, 39(1), 159.

USP 36 (2012) *The United States Pharmacopeia*, The United States Pharmacopeial Convention, Rockville, MD.

Van Buskirk, G.A., et.al. (2012). Passive Transdermal Systems Whitepaper Incorporating Current Chemistry, Manufacturing and Controls (CMC) Development Principles, *AAPS PharmSciTech*, 13(1):218–230.

Venkatraman, S.S., and Cogan-Farinas, K. (1994) Proceed. *ACS, PMSE*, 128, 70.

Venkatraman, S.S., and Gale R. (1998) Skin Adhesives and Skin Adhesion, *Biomaterials*, 19(13):1119–1136.

Wick, S.M. (1988) *Transdermal Nitroglycerin Delivery System*, U.S. Patent 4,751,087.

Wick, S.M., Hart, J.R., and Wirtanen, D.J. (1993) *Demonstrated In Vitro Feasibility Utilizing a Multitude of Drug-in-Adhesive Formulations*, U.S.-Japan Conference on Transdermal Drug Delivery, Maui, Hawaii.

Wilking, S.L., Husberg, M.L., Ko, C.U., and Wick, S.M. (1994) The Effect of Excipients on the Physical Properties of Selected Acrylate, Polyisobutylene, and Silicone Pressure-Sensitive Adhesives Commonly Utilized in Transdermal Drug Delivery Systems, *Pharm. Res.*, 11: S-226.

Wokovich, A. M., Shen, M., Doub, W.H., Machado, S.G., and Buhse, L.F. (2010) Release Liner Removal Method for Transdermal Drug Delivery Systems, *Journal of Pharmaceutical Sciences*, 99(7), 3177–3187.

Yializis, A., et.al. (1999) *Surface Functionalization of Polymer Films*, Proc. Annual Technical Conference – Society of Vacuum Coaters, 469–474.

Zhai, H., Ebel, J.P., Chatterjee, R., Stone, K.J., Gartstein, V., Juhlin, K.D., Pelosi, A., and Maibach, H.I. (2002) Hydration vs. Skin Permeability to Nicotinates in Man, *Skin Research and Technology*, 8(1):13–18.

Zhai, H., and Maibach, H.I. (2001) Skin Occlusion and Irritant and Allergic Contact Dermatitis: An Overview, *Contact Dermatitis*, 44(4):201–206.

# 5 Quality by Design (QbD) Principles in the Development of Transdermal Drug Delivery Products

*Muralikrishnan Angamuthu, H.N. Shivakumar and S. Narasimha Murthy*

## CONTENTS

## 5.1 INTRODUCTION

Drug shortage due to product recalls have been a severe burden not just to patients but also to medical care givers, national and international regulatory authorities. According to USFDA Enforcement Reports, a total of 519 pharmaceutical recalls have been realized till the end of third quarter in 2013, out of which 52 and 361 recalls have been classified as class I and II, respectively[1].

163

Several reasons may contribute to product recalls but the majority of high profile recalls (almost 46%) in the recent past had been due to lack of quality in drug products[2]. Pharmaceutical product quality is instrumental in ensuring patient safety and thus it has been realized of late that the quality should be built in the product rather than being finally tested[3]. In order to encourage continuous improvement in the pharmaceutical quality control systems, the International Conference on Harmonization (ICH) developed guidelines to globally harmonize technical requirements for the manufacture and use of pharmaceutical ingredients and drug products. The ICH guidelines have helped to transform conventional, univariate, trial and error-based product development approach into multivariate, science-based and risk-based practices governed by the principles of Quality by Design (QbD). In 2004, QbD framework was implemented in chemistry, manufacturing and controls (CMC) review process in *Pharmaceutical Current Good Manufacturing Practices (cGMPs) for the 21st Century* initiative to achieve a desired state in quality pharmaceutical manufacturing[2]. The concepts of QbD are well described in several regulatory guidelines including *PAT (Process Analytical Technology) – A Framework for Innovative Pharmaceutical Manufacturing and Quality Assurance*, ICH Q8 (R2) entitled *Pharmaceutical Development*, ICH Q9 entitled *Quality Risk Management* and ICH Q10 entitled *Pharmaceutical Quality System*[4,5,6,7]. The ICH Q8 guidelines are applicable to product design, process design, scale-up and tech transfer while ICH Q10 guidelines are relevant from process design through commercial manufacturing. On the other hand, the ICH Q 9 guidelines are known to regulate all the stages of the product development life cycle, as represented in Figure 5.1.

The ICH Q6A guidelines relate product quality to patient safety, wherein the product quality is defined as, "The suitability of either drug substance or drug product for its intended use." As per the guidelines, product quality includes attributes such as identity, strength and purity. Further, ICH Q9 guidelines relate process parameters to product quality, wherein the product quality is defined as, "The degree to which a set of inherent properties of a product, system or process fulfills the requirements." Thus, traditional product development in the past involved the use of a simplistic approach that linked "process and product quality" and consequently "product quality and patient safety." In contrast, QbD framework (over simplified in Figure 5.2) facilitates systematic approach for product development that begins with predefined objectives (drug product performance, patient safety & efficacy). Through sound science and quality risk management, QbD mediated development lay emphasis on thorough product, process understanding and enhanced process control[5]. QbD in its core can be defined as a scientific-based, risk-based, proactive, holistic approach towards pharmaceutical development with desired outcomes being "A maximally efficient, agile, flexible pharmaceutical manufacturing process that reliably produces high-quality drug products without extensive regulatory oversight," as identified by Janet Woodcock, Director of Center for Drug Evaluation and Research (CDER)[8]. Some of the differences between the traditional approach and the QbD approach are portrayed in Table 5.1 and Figure 5.3.

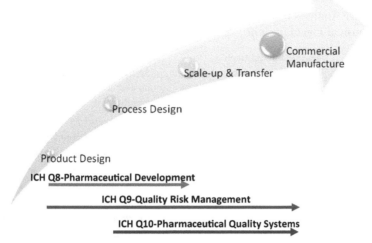

**FIGURE 5.1** Role of ICH guidelines in product development life cycle of transdermal patch systems. (Modified and adopted from reference no. 14.)

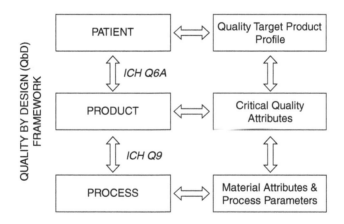

**FIGURE 5.2** Quality by design (QbD) approach that effectively links process to product quality and to patient safety and efficacy.

QbD aims to identify variables (both product and process related) that are critical to product quality (safety and efficacy) and facilitates a control strategy to consistently produce drug products with desired quality characteristics[3]. In order to accomplish this, drug product quality attributes are effectively linked to formulation variables (drug substance and excipient attributes) and manufacturing process variables to identify sources of variability at an early stage (and potential risks minimized). This relationship is vital to implement a flexible and robust manufacturing process that can consistently produce a quality drug product.

**TABLE 5.1**

**Comparative Analysis of the Traditional Approach and QbD Approach in Pharmaceutical Development**

| | Traditional Approach | QbD Approach |
|---|---|---|
| **Development principle** | Empirical, trial and error-based development involving univariate experiment design | Systematic, risk-based approach towards product development, multivariate experiment design feasible |
| | *Quality related decisions not based on science and risk evaluation* | *Quality related decisions based on process understanding and risk management (Design space concept)* |
| **Manufacturing process** | Fixed, validation on three batches, emphasis on quality reproducibility | Flexible within the design space, emphasis on control strategies for achieving product quality |
| | *Discourages quality improvement and innovation* | *Quality improvement feasible and changes made within company's quality system* |
| **Process Control strategy** | In-process tests, offline/end product testing, process validation | Continuous quality verification, PAT for real-time monitoring enabled with feed forward or feedback controls |
| | *Quality not efficiently controlled but only tested in the products, i.e., Quality by Testing (QbT)* | *Quality is ensured through product and process understanding and risk-based control strategy* |
| **Product specification** | Primary means of quality control, based on the batch data | Part of overall quality control strategy, based on overall product performance |
| **Control strategy** | Relies on intermediate and end product testing | Risk-based, control shifted up-stream, relies on real-time testing |
| **Regulatory filing and life cycle management** | Reactive (problem solving, corrective action) | Proactive approach with facilitated continual quality improvement |
| | *Post-approval changes require regulatory scrutiny* | *Continuous quality improvement possible within design space* |

Important steps in QbD-based product development would be to:

- Define quality target product profile (QTPP).
- Identify critical quality attributes (CQA), critical process parameters (CPP) including sources of variability.
- Control the manufacturing process to produce a consistent product.

Desired outcomes of a successful QbD program are as follows:

- Robust product and manufacturing process design.
- Systematic, risk-based and science-based product development.

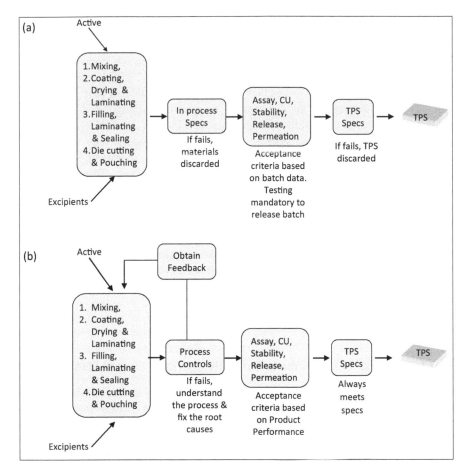

**FIGURE 5.3** Diagram depicting the manufacture of TPS using a traditional approach involving quality by testing (QbT) principles (a); Diagram depicting the manufacture of TPS using quality by design (QbD) approach (b). (Modified and adopted from reference no. 3.)

- Built-in product quality (for efficacy and safety).
- Render huge cost benefits.
- Establish operating design space and edge of failure.
- Enhance manufacturing process understanding and control strategy.
- Enhance process capability and robustness.
- Facilitate post-approval regulatory oversight.

Plethora of case studies has been documented in literature for inception of QbD in development of several drug products. However, a detailed review pertaining to application of QbD-based development in the transdermal drug products segment is scarce. In this context, the present chapter is an attempt to summarize essential elements involved in the development and manufacturing of transdermal patch products utilizing the QbD approach.

## 5.2 TRANSDERMAL PATCH SYSTEMS (TPS) – OVERVIEW OF QUALITY ISSUES AND REGULATORY PERSPECTIVES

TPS are self contained discrete drug delivery systems which are known to deliver drug into systemic circulation when applied to intact skin. TPS possess obvious advantages that other delivery routes lack, namely (1) avoidance of first-pass metabolism, (2) steady delivery of the therapeutics to systemic circulation, (3) enhanced patient compliance, (4) possible dose intervention and (5) avoidance of frequent dosing. Despite these attractive benefits, TPS constitute a niche area with only a handful of commercial products approved by U.S. FDA therapeutic areas like smoking cessation, hormone replacement therapy, cardiovascular disorders, contraception, pain and neurological disorders[9] (Table 5.2).

Though, first TPS were approved three decades ago, progressive research activities leading to broader adoption by pharmaceutical industries and governing regulations still remain primitive. Despite continuous bridging needs for TPS in mainstream clinical therapy, lack of control over drug product quality (like drug recrystallization, reservoir leakage and adhesive issues) still remain a major concern[10]. A snapshot of common quality issues associated with TPS in a chronological sequence is

**TABLE 5.2**
**List of Transdermal Patch Products Currently Approved by U.S. FDA**

| Brand Name | Active Ingredient | Dosage Form | Therapeutic Indication |
|---|---|---|---|
| Catapres TTS® | Clonidine | Transdermal Patch | Hypertension |
| Alora® | Estradiol | Transdermal Patch | Hormone Replacement |
| Climara® | | | |
| Estraderm® | | | |
| Estradiol® | | | |
| Menostar® | | | |
| Vivelle/Vivelle Dot® | | | |
| ClimaraPro™ | Estradiol/Levonorgesterol | Transdermal Patch | Hormone Replacement |
| Combipatch® | Estradiol/norethindrone acetate | Transdermal Patch | Hormone Replacement |
| Ortho Evra® | Ethinyl estradiol/ norelgestromin | Transdermal Patch | Birth Control |
| Duragesic® | Fentanyl | Transdermal Patch | Chronic pain |
| Sancuso® | Granisetron | Transdermal Patch | Anti-emetic |
| Daytrana® | Methylphenindate | Transdermal Patch | Attention Disorder |
| Nitro Dur® | Nitroglycerine | Transdermal Patch | Angina Pectoris |
| Minitran™ | | | |
| Oxytrol® | Oxybutynin | Transdermal Patch | Bladder Control |
| Exelon® | Rivastigmine | Transdermal Patch | Dementia |
| TransdermScop® | Scopolamine | Transdermal Patch | Motion Sickness |
| Emsam® | Selegiline | Transdermal Patch | Parkinson's Disorder |
| Androderm® | Testosterone | Transdermal Patch | Hypogonadism |

**TABLE 5.3**
**List of Transdermal Patch Products Currently Approved by U.S. FDA and Common Quality Issues Associated with Product Recalls**

| Year | Product | Company | Reason for recall | Recall volume |
|------|---------|---------|-------------------|---------------|
| 2004 | Duragesic® | Ortho-McNeil-Janssen Pharmaceutical Inc. | Defective Patches | About 1 million Patches |
| 2007 | Daytrana® | Noven Therapeutic LLC. | Defective Patches | Several lots |
| 2008 | Duragesic® | Ortho-McNeil-Janssen Pharmaceutical Inc. | Defective Patches | About 32 million patches |
| 2008 | Fentanyl Transdermal system | Actavis Pharmaceuticals Inc. | Defective Patches | Millions of defective patches |
| 2008 | Duragesic® | Ortho-McNeil-Janssen Pharmaceutical Inc. | Defective Patches | Unknown |
| 2008 | Neupro® | UCB (Pharma) Ireland Ltd. | Drug Recrystallization | Unknown |
| 2009 | Fentanyl Transdermal system | Watson Pharmaceuticals Inc. | Defective Patches | Unknown |
| 2010 | Nicotine Transdermal system | Aveva Pharmaceuticals Inc. | Chemical Impurities | Unknown |
| 2010 | Fentanyl Transdermal system | Watson Pharmaceuticals Inc. | Defective Patches | Unknown |
| 2011 | Fentanyl Transdermal system | Watson Pharmaceuticals Inc. | Defective Patches | One lot |
| 2012 | Duragesic® | Ortho-McNeil-Janssen Pharmaceutical Inc. | Drug Recrystallization | Unknown |
| 2013 | Daytrana® | Noven Therapeutic LLC. | Defective Patches | 335,910 patches |

depicted in Table 5.3. Quality problems in TPS have affected both safety and efficacy of drug products leading to several product recalls and/or market withdrawals. Of late, many transdermal products were recalled from the market owing to one or the other associated quality issues. For instance, a major issue associated with a reservoir transdermal patch is the leakage from the liquid reservoir as a result of aberration in the manufacturing process leading to faulty or defective patches. Reservoir TPS are basically composed of a central reservoir containing the active surrounded by a rate controlling membrane. Dose dumping leading to over dosing as a consequence of uncontrolled drug release from the faulty system is one of the common problems associated with reservoir TPS[9]. Manufacturing defects causing leakage of TPS lead to product recall in 2004 and 2008 as it was likely to expose patients to a potentially fatal overdose of fentanyl. The other concern associated with TPS is the potential for changes in the drug solid state causing crystallization that in turn could affect the stability. Crystallization is a specific problem that could arise from supersaturated TPSs which may be thermodynamically unstable where the drug has the tendency to crystallize during storage. Formation of crystals in transdermal patches in TPS was found to have a substantial effect on the product performance. Solid state instability of TPS induced by drug crystallization continues to be one of the reasons for the product recalls[11]. The formation of "snowflake" crystals in the rotigotine TPS led to product recall considering the severe impact crystallization could have on the product performance[9]. In retrospect, product recalls lead to severe drug shortage as well as significant financial damage to the manufacturer.

Current manufacturing practices involved in the development of transdermal products are highly specialized and require critical supervision. The mainstay of quality issues in TPS is related to a lack of rational selection of raw materials including adhesives. Staggered assessment of raw materials, intermediate products (ex. drug laminate, reservoirs) and final drug product may provide insights into effectively delineating potential quality issues during various stages of drug product development. In particular, detailed testing of adhesive materials can provide early assessment and help to minimize quality issues which critically affect functional performance (patch adhesion to skin) and product performance[12]. Raw material testing may generally include, but not be confined to, material authentication (using infrared spectroscopic analysis) and physicochemical characterization (molecular weight distribution, polydispersity index, intrinsic or complex viscosity). Intermediate product testing would necessarily include, but not be restricted to, evaluation of peel, tack, shear and adhesion. Finished product testing may include, but not be limited to, peel, shear, adhesion, tack, in vitro release testing (IVRT) and in vitro permeation testing[12].

U.S. FDA had issued a special guidance for industries, to inculcate QbD developmental approaches in design and development of TPS. Special emphasis was placed on initiatives to effectively control/limit drug residuals post usage period and consequently minimize associated risks. From a safety standpoint, primary quality concerns with TPS development may include lack of appropriate strategies to minimize residual drugs in TPS. Although, generic TPS may not be qualitatively (Q1) and quantitatively (Q2) similar to reference listed drugs (RLDs), it is critical for generic TPS to demonstrate bioequivalence (BE) and deliver the drug at the same rate as that of an RLD. In this context, generic TPS may essentially contain a surplus active pharmaceutical ingredient (API) in order to meet BE requirements by the way of maintaining adequate drug permeation/flux rate throughout its intended use period. From publicly available label information, typical residual drug levels in a TPS can potentially range from 10 to 95% of its initial drug loading which largely depends on product design. Looking back, drug residual in TPS had raised potential safety issues and resulted in occasional death of children who were inadvertently exposed to the discarded TPS[13].

Risk of skin irritation and sensitization is yet another critical quality issue which currently prevails in TPS. Manufacturers are required to adopt robust product development practices (QbD initiatives) to elucidate irritation and sensitization potential of excipients, adhesives and permeation enhancers used in TPS[12]. Last but not the least, proper sealing of multilaminate layers in each individual reservoir patch needs to be perfected which otherwise could lead to dose dumping and potential exposure to high levels of drug dose from TPS.

## 5.3 ROADMAP FOR QbD IMPLEMENTATION IN TPS DEVELOPMENT

In 1997, three pivotal scientific organizations, American Association of Pharmaceutical Sciences (AAPS), United States Food and Drug Administration (FDA) and United States Pharmacopeia (USP) jointly organized a workshop to revisit the regulatory principles governing transdermal drug product development[14] (guidance Industry). Owing to the renewed interest among the scientific community, a top line review is presented here featuring structured approaches for QbD implementation in transdermal drug product development detailing industrial, academic and regulatory aspects (Figure 5.4).

### 5.3.1 Identifying a Quality Target Product Profile (QTPP)

QTPP can be defined as "prospective summary of the quality characteristics of a drug product that ideally needs be achieved to ensure the desired quality, taking into account safety and efficacy of the drug product"[5]. Generally, desired labeling information is used to arrive at a Quality Target Product Profile (QTPP) which describes strength, indication, contraindication, dosage form, dose, frequency and pharmacokinetics[8]. In extension, QTPP for a drug product may include elements vital in clinical settings like the dosage form, route of administration, residual drug, safety advice and containers and closure systems for the intended market.

Certain critical quality attributes of a typical TPS like identification, strength, assay, uniformity, residual solvent levels, crystalline form, purity, stability, microbial burden, in vitro release and in vitro permeation could be labeled as QTPP. The QTPP should be established right after the identification of the lead drug candidate and is generally regarded as instrumental for setting a strategic foundation for product development. Predefined product quality profile/specifications would lead to a highly objective and efficient product/process design. Typical QTPPs for a transdermal

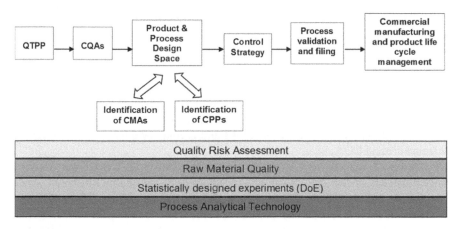

**FIGURE 5.4** Roadmap for QbD implementation in TPS development.

**TABLE 5.4**
**Quality Target Product Profile (QTPP) for Model Transdermal Patch Systems (TPS)**

| QTPP | TARGET ELEMENTS |
|---|---|
| Dosage form | *Transdermal patch* |
| Route of administration | *Transdermal* |
| Strength | *Permeation/flux rate* |
| Pharmacokinetics | *Bioavailability requirement* |
| Shelf life | *At least 24 months when stored at room temperature* |
| Product quality attributes | *Physical properties (appearance, size, shape, thickness)* |
| | *Patch performance* |
| | *(adhesion, ease of removal)* |
| | *Identification* |
| | *Assay* |
| | *Degradation products* |
| | *Residual drug/solvents* |
| | *Content uniformity* |
| | *Drug depletion/release rate* |
| Container closure system | *To achieve target shelf life and maintain patch integrity* |

patch system are listed in Table 5.4. For generic patch development, QTPP can be readily obtained from the reference listed drug (RLD).

## 5.3.2 IDENTIFYING CRITICAL QUALITY ATTRIBUTES (CQA)

The second goal after establishing QTPP is to identify CQA for the transdermal patch product. A CQA is defined in ICH Q8 as "a physical, chemical, biological or microbiological property or characteristic that should be within an appropriate limit, range, or distribution to ensure the desired product quality"[5]. Generally, three different types of tests are used to evaluate finished TPS that include product quality tests, in vitro drug product performance tests and in vivo drug product performance tests[9]. The product quality attributes for TPS may include, but are not limited to, visual description, identification, assay, impurities, content uniformity, residual solvent levels, polymorphism and microbial limits. A selection of CQA from a set of quality attributes is determined by its potential impact on patient safety and efficacy. Desired critical quality attributes must be ensured in every single product unit during manufacturing phase. Product specifications and regulatory guidance would help to determine critical CQA.

A risk-based analysis tool is highly useful in identifying CQA from a set of quality attributes of the TPS. Notably, the criticality of the quality attributes would be dependent on their potential impact on patient safety and efficacy. In addition to those listed in Table 5.5, additional product-specific CQA such as adhesion, cohesion, leakage, cold flow property, compatibility and patch size/shape may be considered on a case-by-case basis (Table 5.5). The relationship between typical CQA and the QTPP,

**TABLE 5.5**
**Typical CQA of a Transdermal Patch System**

Critical Quality Attributes (CQA)
Assay
Content uniformity
Impurities
In vitro drug release
Drug polymorph
Particle size
Cold flow
Assay of drugs in cold flow
Microbial test
Residual solvents
Residual monomer
Enhancers content
Adhesion test
Cohesion test
Patch tackiness

for a transdermal patch product, has been pictorially represented in Table 5.6. A risk assessment tool should be able to evaluate and rank some or all of various CQA.

### 5.3.3 IDENTIFYING PRODUCT AND PROCESS DESIGN SPACE

#### 5.3.3.1 Considerations for Product Design

Once the QTPP and CQA for TPS are identified, product design is undertaken utilizing a statistically designed experimental design to arrive at an optimum formulation design. Choice of formulation components would eventually determine drug delivery rate and minimize residual drug levels. The design of experiments (DoE) model is highly efficient in investigating the combined effects of critical material attributes (raw material) on product performance. Investigation of key variables governing formulation performance and formulation robustness followed by formulation optimization is the key goal during the formulation development phase. Identification of sources of variability would be an integral part of the developmental studies involving DoE.

The concept of design space is defined in ICH Q8 as "the multidimensional combination and interaction of input variables (e.g., material attributes) and process parameters that have been demonstrated to provide assurance of quality." Working within the design space is not considered as process deviation, whereas movement out of the design space is considered critical deviation and would eventually warrant post-approval changes in regulatory approval.

Design space is proposed by the applicant and is subjected to regulatory assessment and approval[5]. A model design space and control space for development of a typical transdermal patch system is represented in Figure 5.5.

**TABLE 5.6**

**Quality Target Product Profile (QTPP) Derived from the Product Requirement is Used to Identify the Critical Quality Attributes (CQA)**

| Product Requirement | Quality Target Product Profile QTPP | Critical Quality Attributes | | | | | | | |
|---|---|---|---|---|---|---|---|---|---|
| | | Assay | Impurities | Content Uniformity | Stability | Crystalline form | In vitro release | In vitro Permeation |
| | Transdermal patch | | | | | | | |
| | Strength | √ | | √ | √ | | | |
| | Dosing frequency | √ | | | | | √ | √ |
| | Shelf life at least 2 years at 25°C/60%RH | | | | √ | √ | | |
| | Container closure system | √ | | | √ | √ | | |
| | Safety | | √ | | √ | | | |
| | Pharmacokinetics | | | | | | √ | √ |
| | Residual drug | | | | | | √ | √ |
| | Meet the pharmacopeial requirements | | | | | | | √ |

(Modified and adopted from reference no. 12.)

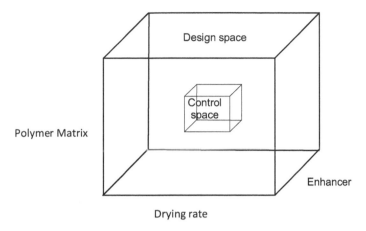

Design space

Control space

Polymer Matrix

Enhancer

Drying rate

**FIGURE 5.5** A schematic representation of a design space and control space in the product design of typical TPS.

An initial risk assessment must be performed to screen critical material attributes followed by execution of multivariate DoEs to systematically link quantitative effects of critical material attributes to critical quality attributes of the final product. The results are evaluated to establish the quality/grades of raw material and acceptable limits of raw material to be used in the formulation. This collectively results in the thematic representation of an effective design space (ideally products manufactured within the design space would possess QTPP built-in inherently). The established product design space illustrates the range for acceptable variability in product CQA and is furnished in the regulatory filing as in-process and product specifications. Drug delivery performance of TPS is largely governed by judicious choice of polymers, adhesives, penetration enhancers and other excipients. The effects of critical material attributes (including API) on typical critical quality attributes of TPS are summarized in Table 5.7.

### 5.3.3.2 Considerations for Process Design

Once the formula is optimized, the next step is to develop and optimize the manufacturing process. A layout of a commercial manufacturing process is outlined with due diligence paid to the intended scale of manufacturing. The selection of a manufacturing process greatly depends on both product design, scale of manufacture and equipments used. A general process flow diagram involved in the development of TPS is depicted in Figure 5.6. A typical unit operation involved in TPS manufacturing involves a set of critical process parameters (CPPs) that may potentially influence the CQA of the finished product when varied within the operating range. For instance, liquid mixing is an important step in the manufacture of "drug-in-adhesive" TPS that would determine drug content uniformity (quality attribute) of the finished product. Various process parameters and Process Analytical Technology (PAT) involved in the liquid mixing stage are pictorially represented in Figure 5.7.

**TABLE 5.7**
**Typical Material Properties that Affect CQA of TPS**

| Critical Material Attributes | Critical Quality Attributes of TPS |
|---|---|
| **Active Pharmaceutical Ingredient** | Drug delivery rate |
| Particle size/area | Drug crystallization |
| Polymorph | Presence of impurities |
| Impurities | |
| Solubility in formulation matrix | |
| **Pressure Sensitive Adhesive** | Delivery rate |
| Adhesive type | Patch Adhesion |
| Viscosity | Cohesion (cold flow) |
| Type/Ratio | Irritation/sensitization |
| Molecular weight | Residual drug |
| Residual monomers | Assay/impurities |
| **Excipients** | Delivery rate |
| Permeation enhancer | Crystallization |
| Crystallization inhibitor | Assay/impurities |
| Rate controlling membrane | |
| Solvent | |
| **Backing Membrane** | Patch integrity |
| **Release liner** | Flexibility |

In addition, detailed process parameters involved in the entire manufacturing process of "drug-in-adhesive" TPS and effective control strategies based on PAT tools are depicted in Table 5.8.

A control strategy includes a set of controls derived from current product and process understanding that assures reproducible product quality and process performance. These controls may encompass critical process parameters, material attributes related to drug substance or quality attributes pertaining to finished product, components, facility, finished product specifications, the associated methods and frequency of monitoring. Process Analytical Technology is invariably a part of the control strategy in a QbD approach. Fishbone or the Ishikawa diagram is found to be an effective tool to identify potential process parameters that influence the quality of the finished product. Mapping the process flow diagram is used to define the scope of risk management and to identify the critical process parameters[13]. The fishbone diagram depicting potential process parameters that may potentially influence the performance of drug-in-adhesive TPS is shown in Figure 5.8.

### 5.3.4 PRODUCT PERFORMANCE AND FINISHED PRODUCT QUALITY TESTING

Product performance testing evaluates the drug release from patch systems and other quality attributes that have profound effects on the patch performance. In vitro drug release testing is performed using a paddle over disk method (Apparatus 5), rotating cylinder method (Apparatus 6) and reciprocating holder method (Apparatus

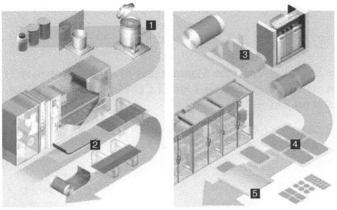

Manufacturing method dor drug-in-adhesive
type matrix patches

1. Mixing and weighing of all ingredients as liquid drug-containing adhesive solution

2. Coating, drying and lamination of liquid mass to result in drug-in-adhesive layer

3. Slitting of the laminate into daughter rolls

4. Punching of the patch contoures

5. Single patches are scaled into pouches

**FIGURE 5.6** General process flow graphic of a drug-in-adhesive transdermal patch development. (Reproduced with kind permission from Acino Pharma, Switzerland.)

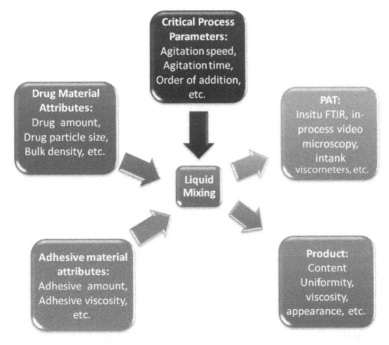

**FIGURE 5.7** The process parameters and material attributes including the PAT involved in the liquid mixing step.

**TABLE 5.8**

**List of Processes Involved in the Manufacture of drug-in-adhesive TPS, Various Processing Parameters that Affect CQA and Effective Control Strategy Based on PAT**

| Pharmaceutical Unit Operation | Critical Process Parameters | Critical Quality Attributes | Control Strategy (PAT Tools used for Process Monitoring) |
|---|---|---|---|
| **Mixing** Compounding process of adhesive, enhancer, API and other excipients | Product temperature Order of addition Agitation speed Agitation time | Drug identification Drug content Appearance Viscosity Particle size | FTIR Inline viscometers Laser-based detection systems Video microscopy |
| **Coating, Drying and Laminating** Process of forming drug-in-adhesive layer from liquid compound | Drying air flow Drying temperature Machine speed Laminator roll pressure Laminator roll size | Drug identification Drug content Polymorphism Patch thickness | Infrared sensors Temperature sensors Web thickness sensors Moisture sensors Data collection and feedback systems |
| **Filling, Laminating and Sealing** Process of filling reservoir blend onto multilayer film, laminating and sealing | Fill volumes Sealing station temperature Time Pressure | Patch fill weight Seal integrity Drug identification Liquid presence | On-line vision systems Check weight systems Leak detectors Data collection and feedback systems Online vision systems for checking patch size |
| **Die cutting and Pouching** Final stage in which patch is cut to pre-determined size and shape and placed in primary package | Web tension Die temperature Sealing temperature Sealing time Sealing pressure | Patch shape Primary packing Output size Pouch seal integrity Drug identification | Feedback systems for monitoring pouch seal integrity |

7) as described in USP 34/NF29, General Chapter <724>, *Drug Release*. This test is an indicator of a residual drug in "drug-in-adhesive TPS" and is known to identify "faulty" reservoir type TPS that may sensitize the skin or dump the entire dose. The in vitro flux study is used to assess drug delivery/flux rate from the patch system and to evaluate the effects of material properties on critical quality attributes of the patch system. The study is also a discriminative test for identifying robust formulations and tests such effects as API particle size/polymorphism, effects of penetration enhancers and effect of adhesive ratios/contents. The test is highly critical to evaluate TPS performance and helps to better define and continuously monitor its critical quality attributes. Critical conditions to be considered for the flux study are type of diffusion cell, type of biological membrane (human cadaver skin, animal skin or synthetic membranes), receptor fluid, stirring speed, temperature, etc[10]. TPS is subjected to a list of other important finished product quality analysis tests which

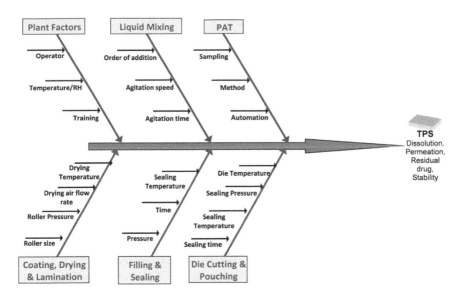

**FIGURE 5.8** Fishbone (Ishikawa) diagram for the manufacture of drug- in-adhesive TPS.

is summarized in Table 5.9. It is often desired that these tests are quantitative in nature and help to establish the lower and upper limits for acceptance criteria for product performance.

### 5.3.5 PROCESS VALIDATION AND FILING

Once the product design, process design and appropriate control strategy have been identified, the process will then be validated to demonstrate if it consistently yields the product with desired quality attributes when operated within the design space. Process validation also confirms whether the research scale pharmaceutical development report used to create the design space can accurately model the manufacturing scale process. The PAT tools described in the control strategy on p. 178 will be pivotal to design and carry out the process validation study. The approach towards process validation for TPS manufacturing is identical to that of oral solid dosage forms and involves the following key steps:

1. Developmental work that is capable of establishing manufacturing targets.
2. Demonstration of capability of in-process and final product control criteria and overall product quality by manufacture and testing of validation batches.
3. Periodic confirmation of the finished product quality throughout the product life cycle by means of tracking and trending.

Regulatory filing is then pursued in which several key technical specifics of the pharmaceutical developmental work are detailed. Such specifics are product design space, process design space, acceptable ranges of the design space, control strategy

**TABLE 5.9**
**List of Finished Product Quality Testing Performed on the Transdermal Patch System**

| S. No. | Quality tests | Description |
|---|---|---|
| 1. | Product description, identification, assay | Visual examination, qualitative description that includes shape, size, color, drug content, packaging details. |
| 2. | Impurities | Assess process impurities, synthetic by-products and residual solvents. |
| 3. | Content uniformity | Assess drug content uniformity in patch and migration of drug from active patch layer to other inactive layers upon storage. |
| 4. | Polymorphism | Test drug polymorphic changes due to manufacturing process and storage conditions. |
| 5. | Residual solvent levels | The test performed as per the ICH Q3C (R4) guidelines helps to determine the residual solvent levels in TPS. |
| 6. | Creep resistance (cold flow property) | Cold flow is a unique quality aspect of pressure sensitive adhesive patches. The adhesive layers flow out of the patch edges either upon storage or during usage. Creep resistance test is measurement of resistance to cold flow. |
| 7. | Adhesion evaluation test i. Peel adhesion test ii. Release liner peel test iii. Probe tack test iv. Rolling ball method | Testing include several patch characteristics like the ease of removal of the release liner, satisfactory adherence to skin for intended period of use and the ease of removal post application duration. |
| 8. | Particle size | Particle size testing is recommended for patch systems that contain API dispersed in it. A change in API particle size, appearance, shape, aggregation may occur either during processing or on storage. |
| 9. | Crystal formation | When amorphous form of API is formed in carrier matrix in patch systems, potential recrystallization may be observed during storage. Crystal seeding studies performed during product development may reveal valuable information. |
| 10. | Leak test | Leak testing is applicable to certain types of matrix and reservoir patch systems. Patch systems may exhibit leaking due to perforations, cuts, faulty seals and other defects caused during the manufacturing process. It is ideal to evaluate the manufacturing process by utilization of PAT and in-process testing, which may prove beneficial to identify these defects. |
| 11. | Microbial test | Even though certain type of TPS may not support microbial growth, bioburden is important for product validation if any post approval changes are made. |
| 12. | In Vitro Release Testing (IVRT) | In vitro release testing is a critical quality control test to evaluate batch-to-batch consistency of TPS performance (with minimal clinical relevance). |

for yielding final product within the design space, outcomes of validation of manufacturing processes and plan for continuous process monitoring. In the QbD model, the filing also details possibly a pre-approved criterion, agreed by the applicant and regulatory agency, concerning post-approval changes within the design space. After successful regulatory approval of the product (approval of design space under the QbD paradigm), a change within the design space does not mandate additional review or approval by the regulators. The routine manufacturing process is then undertaken with continually monitoring and ensuring, if required, the CQA of the product are met and if the process is performed within the acceptable variability that represents the design space. However, any change made to the design space post-approval requires extensive characterization, validation and further approval of the regulatory agency.

### 5.3.6 STATISTICAL APPROACHES FOR DESIGN OF EXPERIMENTS (DoEs), MULTIVARIATE DATA ANALYSIS AND PROCESS ANALYTICAL TECHNOLOGY (PAT)

A fair number of excipients along with multiple process parameters in each unit process are likely to affect the quality of TPS. Thus, overall understanding of the effects of variable material properties and process parameters on the performance of TPS is not practically feasible. In this context, undertaking a combined approach of performing risk assessment and statistically designed experiments has contributed significantly to develop a quality product. Moreover, use of multivariate data analysis has inevitably emerged as a diagnostic tool to support product manufacturing, process scale-up and scale-down, and process troubleshooting. This enables root cause analysis and to efficiently build process knowledge and enhance process understanding. Thus statistical design of experiments and multivariate data analysis has become a fundamental tool to implement QbD.

Controlling the product variability during the pharmaceutical manufacturing still remains the biggest challenge in inculcating QbD into routine practice. This could be attributed to the fact that the current practices still revolve around the conventional pharmaceutical development which relies primarily on the validated batch data and ignores continuous monitoring of the subsequent manufacturing. However, enabling PAT technologies in the manufacturing phase has offered a continuous window for process monitoring which allows real-time data acquisition and avoids potential process drifts to move out of the design space. PAT can be viewed as a facilitator of QbD implementation and has been defined as "a system for designing, analyzing, and controlling manufacturing through timely measurements (i.e., during processing) of critical quality and performance attributes of raw and in-process materials and processes, with the goal of ensuring final product quality"[4].

## 5.4 CONCLUDING REMARKS

In the current scenario, transdermal patch delivery systems constitute a niche therapeutic area with only a few approved products. Despite its prevalence in clinical usage for over three decades, quality issues are continually widespread and pose potential risks concerning therapeutic efficacy and patient safety. Manufacturers involved in

**TABLE 5.10**
**Generalized Key Challenges and Roadblocks Impeding QbD Implementation and Possible Solutions**

| Issue | Possible steps |
|---|---|
| Limited understanding of relationship between quality attributes and their impact on the clinical safety and efficacy of a product. | 1. Increased use of non-clinical studies to enhance knowledge about the impact of a quality attribute on the clinical safety and efficacy of a product. |
| | 2. Sharing of best practices in this rapidly evolving field will greatly benefit the entire community. |
| | 3. According to the FDA critical path initiative, standardization of data collection and reporting to the regulatory authorities will facilitate more across-product and across-sponsors analysis by the regulatory agencies. |
| Challenges due to the large number of process variables and raw materials used in manufacturing processes. | 1. Use of process and analytical platforms will enable sponsors to invest more time and resources to understand the impact of the process on the product because the results can be applied to other processes and products. |
| | 2. Use of sophisticated statistical tools will facilitate data acquisition, analysis and modeling of unit operations. |
| | 3. Use of high-throughput analytical and process methodologies will enable sponsors to gather more information using limited time and resources. |
| Lack of harmonization across regulatory agencies worldwide discourages early adoption of QbD. | 1. Regulatory agencies need to engage more aggressively in discussions to facilitate harmonization. |

developing transdermal patches should aggressively implement QbD-based developmental practices. Due to lack of appropriate case studies in literature, the roadmap outlined in this chapter is only a concise review for QbD implementation for transdermal patch development. A few major concerns that impede QbD inculcation are limited knowledge resources available for the innovators (Table 5.10), scarcity of PAT enabled equipment and data management systems in current manufacturing plants. Academia, industry and regulatory agencies need to work hand-in-hand to facilitate and share best practices in research and development, scale-up, manufacturing and regulatory areas for successful adoption of QbD in the transdermal drug products domain.

## REFERENCES

1. Stericycle Expert Recall. Recall Index – First Quarter (2013). Pharmaceutical Recalls. ed.
2. Kweder SL, Dill S (2013). Drug shortages: the cycle of quantity and quality. *Clinical Pharmacology and Therapeutics* 93(3):245–251.
3. Yu LX (2008). Pharmaceutical quality by design: product and process development. *Understanding and Control* 25(4):781–791.

4. Department of Health and Human Services, Food and Drug Administration (2004). PAT Guidance for Industry – A Framework for Innovative Pharmaceutical Development, Manufacturing and Quality Assurance.
5. International Conference on Harmonization of Technical Requirements for Registration of Pharmaceuticals for Human Use (2009). ICH Harmonised Tripartite Guideline: Q8(R2) Pharmaceutical Development.
6. International Conference on Harmonization of Technical Requirements for Registration of Pharmaceuticals for Human Use (2005). ICH Harmonised Tripartite Guideline: Q9 Quality Risk Management.
7. International Conference on Harmonization of Technical Requirements for Registration of Pharmaceuticals for Human Use (2008). ICH Harmonised Tripartite Guideline: Q10 Pharmaceutical Quality System.
8. Rathore AS (2009). Roadmap for implementation of quality by design (QbD) for biotechnology products. *Trends in Biotechnology* 27(9):546–553.
9. Pastore MN, Kalia YN, Horstmann M, Roberts MS (2015). Transdermal patches: history development and pharmacology. *British Journal of Pharmacology* 172:2179–2209.
10. Van Buskirk GA, Arsulowicz D, Basu P, Block L, Cai B, Cleary GW, Ghosh T, Gonzalez MA, Kanios D, Marques M, Noonan PK, Ocheltree T, Schwarz P, Shah V, Spencer TS, Tavares L, Ulman K, Uppoor R, Yeoh T (2012) Passive transdermal systems whitepaper incorporating current chemistry, manufacturing and controls (CMC) development principles. *AAPS PharmSciTech* 13(1):218–230.
11. Sharma PK, Panda A, Pradhan A, Zhang J, Thakkar R, Whang C-H, Repka MA, Murthy SN (2018). Solid-state stability issues of drugs in transdermal patch formulations. *AAPS PharmSciTech* 19(1):27–35.
12. Strasinger C, Raney SG, Tran DC, Ghosh P, Newman B, Bashaw ED, Ghosh T, Shukla CG (2016). Navigating sticky areas in transdermal product development. *Journal of Controlled Release* 233:1–9.
13. McCurdy V. (2011). 'Quality by Design' In Housan I (Ed). *Process Understanding: For Scale-up and Manufacture of Active Ingredients.* 1st Edn., VCH Verlag GmbH & Co. Wiley Pg 1–16. e
14. Department of Health and Human Services, Food and Drug Administration (2011). Guidance for Industry – Residual Drug in Transdermal and Related Drug Delivery Systems (www.fda.gov/downloads/Drugs/Guidances/UCM220796pdf).

# 6 Microneedles for Drug Delivery
## *Industrial and Regulatory Perspectives*

*Lisa A. Dick, Daniel M. Dohmeier,*
*Ann M. Purrington and Scott A. Burton*

## CONTENTS

## 6.1   INTRODUCTION TO INTRADERMAL DELIVERY WITH MICRONEEDLES

The skin has been a favorite application site for various pharmaceutical preparations, and medicines have been delivered through the skin for many years. Since the first transdermal patch was introduced by Alza more than 30 years ago, patients have enjoyed the comfort of the noninvasive, painless and simple application of transdermal drug delivery. However, the number of drugs amenable to passive transdermal delivery is limited to lipophilic small molecules that can be readily transported through the stratum corneum, epidermis and dermis layers of the skin. Biologic drugs in particular are not amenable to traditional passive transdermal delivery with drug-in-adhesive or reservoir systems. The stratum corneum is such an extremely good barrier to molecular diffusion that it must be breached in order to deliver therapeutic amounts of hydrophilic and large molecular weight drugs.

Intramuscular and subcutaneous injections, established via hypodermic syringe in the 1850s, effectively bypass the skin barrier for delivery of drugs, and remain primary routes of delivery for many classes of compounds. In particular, biologic drugs – vaccines, therapeutic proteins and peptides, and monoclonal antibodies – which represent a significant proportion of drugs currently under development, are easily degraded in the digestive tract and, therefore, must be administered by injection using a syringe and hypodermic needle. Usually such injections are made beneath the dermis to the subcutaneous, intramuscular and intravenous spaces.

Alternate delivery methods have been developed to break the barrier of the outer layers of the skin, but not go so deep as subcutaneous injection. Methods such as transdermal iontophoresis (Kalia & Naik, 2004), sonophoresis (using ultrasound to cavitate the stratum corneum) (Doukas & Kollias, 2004) and the needle-free liquid jet injector gun (U.S. Patent No. 3,057,349, 1962) (Mitragotri, 2006) were developed. Additional delivery methods such as a dry powder injector (Burkoth & Bellhouse, 1999), thermal ablation of the stratum corneum followed by transdermal patch application (Bramson & Dayball, 2003), and radiofrequency ablation of the stratum corneum followed by transdermal patch application have followed (Levin & Gershonowitz, 2005). Among the newest of these, microneedle technology opens the range of molecules which are available for delivery through the skin, by providing shallow physical channels through which drugs can be delivered directly to the epidermis and dermis. Using this approach, the convenience of a transdermal patch can be applied to the delivery of biologic drugs.

Many recent efforts have targeted intradermal delivery of drugs using microneedles for local or systemic delivery (Harvey, et al., 2011; Burton, et al., 2011; Daddona, Matriano, Mandema, & Maa, 2011; Norman, Brown, Raviele, Prausnitz, & Felner, 2013; Spierings, et al., 2018). Microneedles are much narrower and shorter than a hypodermic syringe, with drug delivery terminating in the dermis, out of range of many nerve endings, for limited pain upon needle insertion. In addition, the limited length of the needles is less intimidating and the risk of accidental needle sticks is greatly reduced.

In addition to the patient convenience factor of transdermal patches, delivery of drugs directly into the dermal space can provide therapeutic advantages for some drugs. There is potential for improved bioavailability and faster absorption of biologics (Gupta, Felner, & Prausnitz, 2009; Daddona, Matriano, Mandema, & Maa, 2011; Burton, et al., 2011; Harvey, et al., 2011; Norman, Brown, Raviele, Prausnitz, & Felner, 2013; Korkmaz, et al., 2015; Yao, et al., 2017) and potential for improved immune response for vaccines (Arnou, et al., 2009; Quan, Kim, Compans, & Prausnitz, 2013). Additionally, there is potential for rapid, efficient local delivery of drugs (Duan, et al., 2011; Jain, Lee, & Gill, 2016).

This book chapter aims to address major considerations of microneedle technology development, from technical, manufacturing and regulatory points of view. Foundational information with respect to skin physiology specific to microneedles and microneedle types sets the stage. Next, common technical, design and manufacturing issues are discussed. Following development of specific types of microneedle systems, preclinical and tolerability aspects are highlighted. Finally, quality and regulatory considerations are presented in the context of developing products for global approval. As microneedle and delivery system technology matures, technical, regulatory, quality and manufacturing will all come together for successful commercialization of this promising dosage form.

### 6.1.1 BACKGROUND – SKIN PHYSIOLOGY

Human skin is comprised of three layers: the epidermis (up to approximately 150 microns thick), dermis (~1,500–4,000 microns thick) and subcutaneous layers (U.S. National Institutes of Health, N. C., 2019a). The outer layer of the epidermis, the stratum corneum, consists of several layers of dead skin cells which serve as a protective barrier between the body and the outside world while retaining water. The epidermis contains lipids for chemical barriers, Langerhans cells for an immunological barrier and cells that absorb UV light for an oxidative barrier. The dermal layer contains a dense network of blood capillaries for thermoregulation, wound repair and cell nutrition; and a network of lymphatic vessels which transport interstitial fluid and feed local lymph nodes. The dermal layer also contains a high concentration of potent immune cells that play a key role to initiate the immune response following vaccinations. The subcutaneous layer is comprised of adipose and connective tissues along with blood vessels and nerves and is an insulating layer.

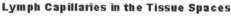

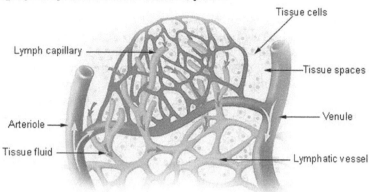

**FIGURE 6.1** Illustration of lymphatic and blood capillaries.

Skin cells and interstitial fluid from the dermis are co-located with lymphatic and blood capillaries, as shown in Figure 6.1 (U.S. National Institutes of Health, N. C., 2019b).

The dermal interstitial space, or interstitium, is comprised of two phases: the interstitial fluid, consisting of interstitial water and its solutes, and the structural molecules of the extracellular matrix. Normally interstitial fluid transports nutrients, peptides, proteins and dermal waste products through prelymphatic channels to the lymphatic capillaries (Wiig & Swartz, 2012). Fluid in the dermis is exchanged into the lymph and circulatory capillaries directly in the interstitium, and then transported; these capillaries also provide the systemic absorption mechanism of drugs delivered intradermally.

### 6.1.2 MICRONEEDLE TYPES

Scientists have creatively designed microneedles for drug delivery in a variety of ways. Representative designs are outlined in Figure 6.2, where the hardware of a microneedle system is indicated by a solid portion and the active pharmaceutical ingredient is shown as partially shaded regions.

In (A), the drug is incorporated in the microneedle matrix, forming a solid drug + excipient microneedle structure. In (B), solid microneedles may be used to penetrate the stratum corneum in a first step, and followed by topical application of a drug in a gel, cream or patch presentation. Solid microneedles, shown in (C), are manufactured and a drug formulation is then allowed to dry in a hard coat on the surface. In (D), hollow microneedles are designed to transport fluid from a drug reservoir to the intradermal space, delivering liquid formulations of drug into the dermis. Any of these microneedle types can be grouped together in an array format to increase the number of holes created in the stratum corneum and increase drug delivery capacity.

Dissolvable microneedles are constructed by depositing a drug-containing formulation into a microneedle mold, and allowing the formulation to dry (Singh,

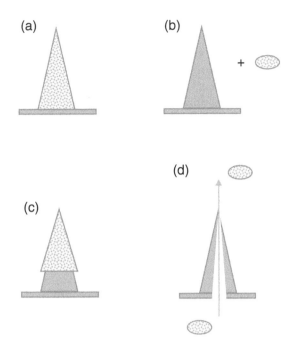

**FIGURE 6.2** Microneedle types.

Chen, & Worsham, 2013; Chu, Choi, & Prausnitz, 2010). The shape of the mold then determines the physical dimensions of the microneedle. The dissolvable microneedle formulation must be strong enough to maintain integrity during storage and application, yet also be water soluble such that once applied to the skin it dissolves in the interstitial fluid for drug delivery during the prescribed wear time. These restrictions on the physical properties of the dissolvable microneedles limit the amount of drug that can be incorporated into the microneedle matrix without negatively impacting the microneedle strength and rigidity; this, combined with restrictions in the length and density of microneedles, limits the deliverable dose of drug from dissolvable microneedle arrays to one milligram or less.

Solid microneedles may be made from a variety of materials, including metal, glass, silicon and plastic. These solid microneedles may be used directly on the skin to poke holes in the stratum corneum. Drug is then administered in a second step where a liquid, gel, cream or patch is allowed to sit on the skin and passively penetrate through the resulting holes for delivery (Henry, McAllister, Allen, & Prausnitz, 1998; Duan, et al., 2011; Milewski, Brogden, & Stinchcomb, 2010). Alternatively, solid microneedles may also be coated with a drug-containing formulation that is then allowed to dry on the surface of the microneedles. The drug is administered by applying the coated microneedles to the skin and during the wear time, the drug dissolves in the interstitial fluid for drug delivery (Matriano, et al., 2002; Tas, et al., 2012; Zhang, et al., 2012a; Daddona, Matriano, Mandema, & Maa, 2011). Again, due to restrictions in the length and density of the microneedles on the array, coated solid microneedle applications are typically limited to delivery of drug doses of 0.5 milligram or less.

Like solid microneedles, hollow microneedles may be constructed from metal, glass, silicon or plastic (Burton, et al., 2011; Harvey, et al., 2011; Gupta, Felner, & Prausnitz, 2009). Once inserted into the skin, these short needles provide a direct conduit for a liquid drug formulation from a reservoir to the interstitial dermal space. Because the drug is delivered in a liquid form, higher doses are possible. In order to increase the rate of intradermal drug delivery, multiple hollow microneedles can be grouped together on an array so that when inserted into the skin, intradermal delivery can occur through more than one microneedle at the same time, thus increasing the delivery rate.

Many microneedle systems are in development, with global efforts in both academia and industry. Representative systems that deliver therapeutic agents intended for systemic administration are presented in Table 6.1. These systems have been commercialized or are approaching regulatory consideration, as evidenced by preclinical or clinical studies.

### TABLE 6.1
### Representative Microneedle Systems in Development for Systemic Delivery of Therapeutic Agents

| Name | Company | Microneedle Type | Description |
|---|---|---|---|
| Micro-Cor® | Corium International, Inc. | Dissolvable | Patch of Biodegradable microneedles containing drug |
| Microneedle Patch | Micron Biomedical, Inc. | Dissolvable | Patch of dissolvable microneedles containing vaccine |
| Nanopatch™ | Vaxxas Inc. | Solid | Microneedle array patch coated with vaccine |
| ZP Patch | Zosano Pharma Inc. | Solid | Microneedle array patch coated with drug |
| 3M™ Solid Microstructured Transdermal System (sMTS) | 3M Company, Drug Delivery Systems Division | Solid | Microneedle array patch coated with drug |
| BD Soluvia™ | Becton Dickinson and Co. | Hollow | Hand-held microinjection system, single needle |
| BD Libertas™ Microinfuser | Becton Dickinson and Co. | Hollow | Patch system with single needle for various volumes and viscosities |
| 3M Hollow Microstructured Transdermal System (hMTS) | 3M Company, Drug Delivery Systems Division | Hollow | Patch system with a 12 microneedle array, various volumes and viscosities |
| MicronJet600™ | Nanopass Technologies Ltd. | Hollow | Hand-held adapter with three microneedles, used with syringe |
| Debioject™ | Debiotech S.A. | Hollow | Hand-held single or three-needle device |

## 6.2 COMMON CONSIDERATIONS FOR MICRONEEDLE DELIVERY SYSTEMS

Whether microneedles are dissolvable, solid or hollow, there are several common considerations for any product in development.

### 6.2.1 MATERIALS OF CONSTRUCTION

A first key consideration is the material used to make the microneedle array (and for dissolvable microneedles, the base support).

For all configurations, a primary concern is the safety and biocompatibility of the microneedle array material. Development is eased if a material of proven biocompatibility can be used; concepts which require new materials can add significantly to the time and cost of development. A consensus standard commonly utilized in the determination of acceptable biocompatibility is ISO 10993-1:2018 (ISO, 2018).

For dissolvable microneedles, the material must maintain its shape during storage, be non-irritating to the skin, and must not leave behind polymer matrix material that accumulates in the skin. Solid and hollow microneedles need to be strong enough to avoid fracture during needle insertion and not leave behind fragments after the microneedles are removed from the skin. Finally, in order to be a viable long-term marketed product, the microneedles must be manufacturable according to quality, stability and cost requirements.

Possible materials of construction include dissolving polymers (Chu, Choi, & Prausnitz, 2010), metal (Daddona, Matriano, Mandema, & Maa, 2011), glass (Gupta, Felner, & Prausnitz, 2009), silicon (Haq, et al., 2009) and plastic (Zhang, et al., 2012a).

An example of a durable medical grade plastic which may be used for solid and hollow microneedles is shown in Figure 6.3. Liquid crystal polymer, or LCP, can

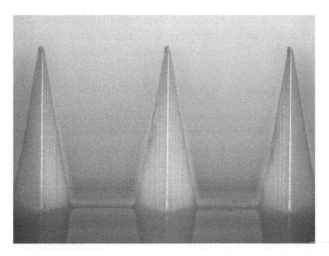

**FIGURE 6.3** Optical micrograph of uncoated microneedles on array (100x magnification). (From Dick, 2016a.)

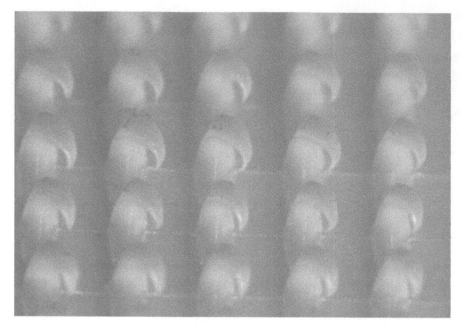

**FIGURE 6.4** LCP microneedles after subjecting to 250 N of static force. (From Dick, 2016a.)

be molded into microneedles that are stiff enough to penetrate the skin, but when subjected to extreme mechanical stress, bend rather than fracturing. The LCP material can be molded with very sharp tips, and at economical commercial scale, as illustrated in Figure 6.3.

As a demonstration of the resistance to fracture of the LCP material, the image in Figure 6.4 shows a microneedle array after being subjected to 250 Newtons(N) of force which is significantly higher than the force an array would be subjected to during insertion into skin. The needles bend rather than break.

### 6.2.2 Microneedle Shape and Array Design

The geometry of particular microneedles should be designed to penetrate to the desired delivery depth but not lacerate the skin. For epidermal and dermal delivery, the ideal depth of penetration is somewhere between 50 and 1,500 microns. The target site of administration and associated skin physiology may be a consideration in determining the selected microneedle length (Laurent, 2007a). The number of microneedles must be sufficient to provide effective delivery of the necessary dose.

For formulations associated with solid microneedles, there is a balance between drug loading, the number of microneedles, the geometric arrangement of microneedles and efficient delivery of the dose. If the microneedles are too closely packed, a "bed of nails" effect may prohibit microneedles from penetrating to the necessary depth.

An optimized geometry is critical to skin penetration (Kochhar, et al., 2013; Olatunji, Das, Garland, Belaid, & Donnelly, 2013).

For liquid formulations of a large volume, it may be desirable to use multiple microneedles instead of a single needle in order to enlarge the delivery space. The dermal interstitial channels are narrow and provide resistance to drug fluid flow. During an intradermal injection, in order to inject a large volume of fluid in a reasonable amount of time – to overcome the inherent dermal interstitial resistance to fluid flow – a combination of high injection pressure, number of and arrangement of microneedles can be used.

### 6.2.3 APPLICATION PROCESS

Another critical consideration for development of a microneedle system is the means of applying the microneedle array to the skin. There are two possibilities: hand application or use of an application device to supply the energy required for microneedle insertion.

Hand application is possible, especially for relatively shallow delivery to the epidermis. Depth of penetration through hand application is limited, in large part, due to the viscoelastic properties of skin –when an array is pressed into the skin, the skin has the ability to move away from the microneedles and resist penetration (Larraneta, et al., 2014). In addition, variability in individual skin thickness, as well as variability in the force individuals would use for application, suggests that hand application may result in significant variability in drug delivery if the dermis, rather than the epidermis, were the target (Norman, et al., 2014).

Other approaches have focused on the use of a force-based or spring-driven applicator to reproducibly apply the microneedle array into the skin. With an applicator, the microneedles are driven into the skin at a defined velocity. This velocity overcomes the skin's ability to react and flex away from the array, and as a result the penetration of the microneedles is increased (Wu, Qiu, Zhang, Qin, & Gao, 2008; Verbaan, et al., 2008).

The primary goal of an applicator is to ensure complete delivery of the drug dose to the target tissue. To ensure successful delivery, each microneedle must be inserted into the skin to a proper depth. Multiple factors affect microneedle penetration: needle length, needle sharpness (tip radius), needle strength, needle geometry (for example, diameter), needle density, and other factors (Davis, Prausnitz, & Allen, 2003; Kochhar, et al., 2013; Bal, et al., 2010; Olatunji, Das, Garland, Belaid, & Donnelly, 2013).

### 6.2.4 DEPTH OF PENETRATION

Recognizing that depth of penetration (DOP) into the skin, and the reproducibility of that depth of penetration is a critical quality attribute (Lutton, et al., 2015), it is necessary to measure DOP during development of a microneedle drug product. Several methodologies may be used. For example, a histological approach may be undertaken using animal skin models as surrogates for human skin. Following microneedle application, the skin surrounding the application site is excised, then

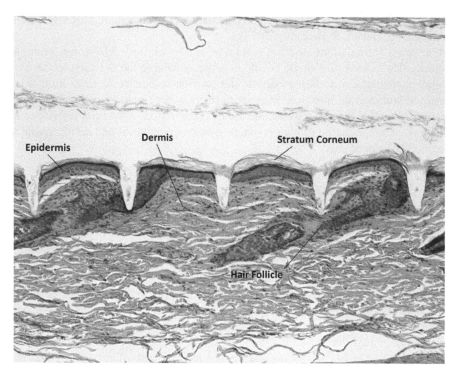

**FIGURE 6.5** Depth of penetration by histology. (From Dick, 2016a.)

fixed and stained. The skin sample may be sectioned horizontally or vertically, in order to visualize DOP. An example image following application of 250 micron (μm) microneedles to hairless guinea pig skin is shown in Figure 6.5.

This method of measuring DOP is quite labor intensive, and provides relatively small sample sizes, so alternative methods such as optical coherence tomography (Donnelly, et al., 2010) or dye dissolution may also be used.

DOP measurements are critical to development not only of the microneedle arrays, but also of the applicator. The chart in Figure 6.6 shows the effect of changing aspects of applicator design on the measured DOP. A similar plateau in DOP has been observed for other application sources as well (Larraneta, et al., 2014). By measuring depth of penetration during applicator development, the applicator design can be optimized to maximize the amount of drug that can be delivered into the skin.

### 6.2.5 MICRONEEDLE ARRAY ADHESION

Once the microneedles have been inserted into the dermis, they must remain in place during drug delivery (for example, as the formulation dissolves from solid microneedles or as fluid is delivered via hollow microneedles into the dermis). Medical adhesive can be employed to hold the microneedles in place. Figure 6.7 shows the importance of choosing the appropriate adhesive. It shows the results of a

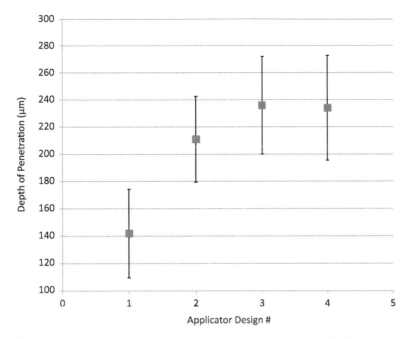

**FIGURE 6.6** Depth of penetration vs applicator design. (From Dick, 2016b.)

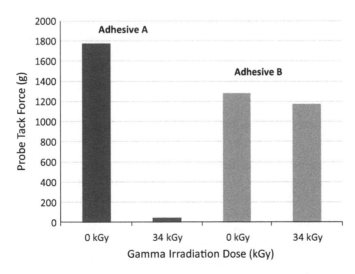

**FIGURE 6.7** Adhesive tack following gamma irradiation. (From Dick, 2016a.)

test to measure the "tack" or "stickiness" of two different adhesives following sterilization with gamma irradiation. The first adhesive shows high tack force initially, but following irradiation with a 34 kilogray (KGy) dose of gamma rays the tack drops significantly. The second adhesive, on the other hand, shows much less sensitivity to gamma irradiation.

### 6.2.6 SKIN MODELS

Another key consideration for development of a microneedle-based system is the skin model used for technology, formulation and drug product development.

Historically, measurement of drug diffusion through human cadaver skin has been a primary tool for development and optimization of the formulation for transdermal and topical drug products. In order to use this same approach for development of microneedle-based systems, a number of questions should be considered: What type of cadaver skin should be used (e.g., neonatal porcine skin, human cadaver skin)? Is full-thickness skin the best model? Or should the skin be dermatomed to a defined thickness? Will the skin be strong enough to withstand application of the microneedles, including when applied with an applicator? Is the physiological difference between live and cadaver skin important for the outcome of the experiment?

Preclinical testing in live animal models may be an alternative to cadaver skin. However, it is important to understand the impact of the animal model as a predictor for clinical studies during early phase research and development studies. If an in vivo model is chosen, the preclinical species is a significant choice due to skin physiology, handling and available skin area (Barbero & Frasch, 2009). Based on the similarities to human skin thickness and physiology, swine is often a preferred species (Meyer, Schwarz, & Neurand, 1978; Simon & Maibach, 2000).

In addition, there are efforts aimed at developing artificial membranes and other skin simulants that may be particularly useful in testing microneedle array penetration and other fundamental aspects of microneedle development (Koelmans, et al., 2013; Ranamukhaarachchi, Hafeli, & Stoeber, 2014; Larraneta, et al., 2014).

### 6.2.7 APPLICATION OF HUMAN FACTORS TO DESIGN (OF SOLID AND HOLLOW MICRONEEDLES)

The design of the microneedle delivery system should take into consideration the intended user population, the expected indications for use and the environment of use through human factors design testing. Useful references for considering these factors are offered by the FDA on a delivery system specific basis (Food and Drug Administration, 2013) and also in regard to general principles (Food and Drug Administration, 2016). A microneedle delivery system should be configured to ensure that the user can safely and successfully apply the microneedle delivery system with few steps.

An example design cycle including human factors testing is shown in Figure 6.8. The user-device interface is typically studied with several rounds of formative human factors testing. The user needs to feel comfortable with the size, shape and weight of the delivery system. The shape of the injector/applicator can be designed to assist in

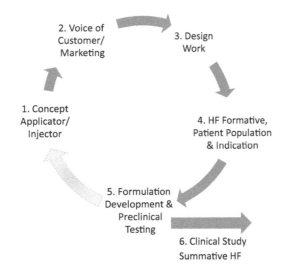

**FIGURE 6.8** Development cycle with human factors (HF) testing.

proper use. Early in the design process, models of various sizes, shapes and weights can be designed and tested to facilitate selection of an optimum configuration. Factors such as height, profile, footprint, conformability, weight and adhesion of microneedles to the skin will be taken into account.

To evaluate safety and ease of use, human factors studies investigate each user task involved in applying the microneedle system, which may include tasks such as removal of the microneedle system from packaging, preparation of the delivery system for administration of the drug, administering the dose, removing the system from the administration site and, finally, disposal of the unit. Tasks unique to administration of fluid formulations may include inspection of the formulation, and observing the dose completion indicator. Visual as well as auditory cues help the user know when the injection is complete. For all systems, instructions need to be clear and concise. The optimum design will intuitively allow the user to use the microneedle delivery system properly.

Once the shape and general usability requirements of the microneedle injector/applicator are established, the functionality of the microneedle delivery system can be optimized with the assistance of an initial hazard and risk analysis to reduce risk. In the risk analysis, each function and action is considered, and ways to ameliorate errors and hazards are incorporated. The nature and extent of safety measures will be determined after a through risk analysis. Sharps injury prevention is a common topic in risk analyses. There may be an opportunity to reduce or eliminate completely the sharps injury protection features in microneedle delivery systems due to the shorter needles and the reduced restick potential for some systems.

Following the risk analysis and any needed redesign, the microneedle delivery system is tested in a formative human factors study. Subjects perform mock deliveries while following written instructions. Tasks such as system preparation, positioning, actuation and device removal can be monitored for user errors. Additional intradermal delivery elements including skin adhesion, application sites, application duration and application frequency may also be evaluated. User actions and feedback are noted during the study, the results are analyzed and any significant design deficiencies are again addressed using hazard/risk analysis. The results are used to further optimize the microneedle delivery system and instructions for use.

After a risk analysis, redesign and following formative trials, the delivery system is evaluated in a summative human factors validation study. This may be conducted concurrently or in a separate time sequence to the continuing formulation development, preclinical evaluations and human clinical trials. Ultimately, the human factors processes, evaluation and results of successful validation testing confirm that the users are able to use the delivery system properly.

### 6.2.8 MANUFACTURING, SUPPLY CHAIN

For microneedle products to become approved for use in the marketplace, their manufacture must be possible at different stages of development. In early stages of development, arrays and devices are made on a limited basis with labor-intensive efforts. This is often sufficient to support preclinical and some phase I clinical studies. As development to phase II clinical studies is approached, there is increasing automation, capacity and control over the manufacturing process. Finally, by phase III clinical studies, supplies would progress with the most automation, reasonable capacity and better process control.

The optimal product design will take the following manufacturing issues into consideration: availability of raw materials, component complexity, assembly step complexity, number of assembly steps, and the ability to use existing manufacturing processes. Further, the application system design must accommodate target manufacturing volumes and costs.

The scale-up of manufacturing processes to produce cGMP (current good manufacturing practice)-compliant drug products will present significant technological, infrastructure and aseptic processing challenges. For coated solid microneedles, for example, optimizing coating efficiency and the scale-up of array manufacturing will be crucial to the success of this technology in the drug delivery space.

### 6.2.8.1 Precision Molding

The ability to reproducibly make thousands of microneedle arrays with high shape fidelity is challenging. An example of the high shape fidelity that can be obtained with a well-controlled molding process was shown previously in Figure 6.3. Figure 6.9 presents an example dataset demonstrating the reproducibility that is possible with such a molding process. A histogram of the average microneedle height for 140 arrays randomly sampled from a batch of over 35,000 arrays is shown. The heights of 40 individual microneedles distributed across the approximate 1 cm$^2$ area of each array were measured with a microscope, and the average microneedle height was calculated for each array. For this batch of molded arrays, the average microneedle height was distributed over a narrow range of 502–508 µm, indicative of a robust molding process. The relative standard deviation of the average microneedle height for the 140 array sample set was 0.25%, while the

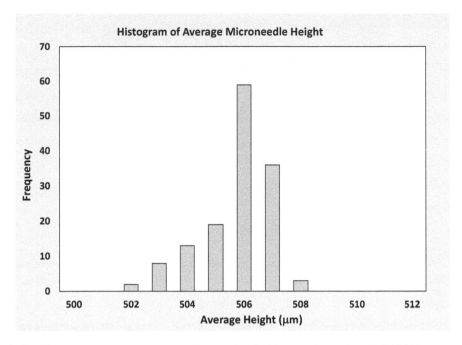

**FIGURE 6.9** Average needle height for sample of 140 arrays from a batch of 35,000. (From Hansen, 2013.)

pooled within-array relative standard deviation of the height for the 40 measured microneedles on individual arrays was 1.4% (i.e., the variability in the average height between arrays was less than the variability in height within each individual array) (Hansen, 2013).

### 6.2.8.2 Control of Material Flow

Materials used in the manufacture of the drug product must be tracked from as far back in the supply chain as possible, in order to ensure consistent handling, appropriately clean environments and adequate control over the entire manufacturing process. Once materials have been received, processes should be designed with appropriate environmental controls to be capable of aseptic manufacture for those drug products that require sterility.

### 6.2.8.3 Consistency of Dose

Consistency of drug delivery is critical for the safety and efficacy of a therapeutic treatment, and this starts with a consistent drug product. The drug must be able to be routinely incorporated into the microneedle matrix, filled into a mold and subsequently dried into dissolvable microneedles. For solid microneedles, the drug must be reproducibly coated. For a hollow system, the drug must be consistently delivered via hollow microneedles with a carefully designed injector. Void volume in the fluid flow pathway should be minimized and, in order to avoid leaks, fluid pressurization of the drug reservoir should begin after microneedle insertion. The injector needs to

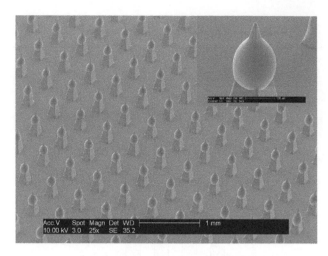

**FIGURE 6.10**   Scanning electron micrograph of coated microneedle array. Inset: Individual coated microneedle. (From Hansen, 2013.)

be designed to produce adequate injection pressure and also to achieve dose accuracy after various storage conditions (ISO, 2014).

Transitioning from a manual manufacturing operation to a more automated operation incorporating, for example, robotic execution of various steps in the manufacturing operation will lead to a more reproducible manufacturing process. An example of robotically coated solid microneedles is shown in Figure 6.10, as a scanning electron microscope image (Hansen, 2013). The repeatability and control of the coating process limits the coated formulation to the upper half of the microneedle, resulting in a uniform appearance of the coated microneedles across the array. This uniformity presumably aids in consistent delivery of the drug from the coated formulation into the skin.

The coating process also results in consistent drug content on each array. An example of the coating precision obtained during a manufacturing optimization run lasting about three hours is shown in Figure 6.11 where drug content was measured for 100 arrays out of a total of approximately 1,300 arrays (Dick, 2016a). For this run, the measured relative standard deviation in content was 5.5%, with no trending observed upward or downward over time, indicating a well-controlled process.

Increased automation in all steps of the manufacturing process, including array molding, microneedle height measurement for quality control, assembly of the array onto the adhesive patch, and coating of the drug formulation onto the microneedle arrays is key to not only increase capacity, but also to improve the control of the process to ensure the quality of the final coated drug product.

### 6.2.8.4   Product Distribution: Stability Considerations

Another key consideration for any drug product, including one based on microneedle delivery technology, is the stability of the drug product. Stability and shelf life

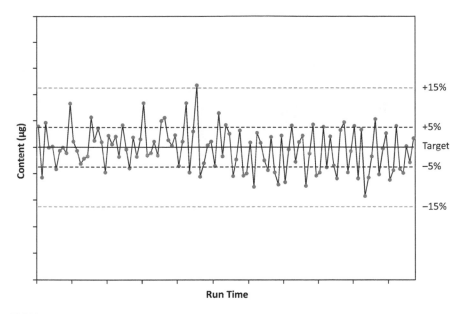

**FIGURE 6.11** Average coated content from arrays during a process development coating run. (From Dick, 2016a.)

considerations impact the required storage conditions for the drug product, including the potential for cold chain requirements during shipping and storage in distribution centers, pharmacies and patient homes. A potential advantage for microneedle delivery of biotherapeutics and vaccines by solid or dissolvable microneedles is the potential for improved stability. For example, Ameri et al. demonstrated a parathyroid hormone (1–34)-coated solid microneedle system with 18 months of storage stability at ambient temperature (25°C), compared to the marketed PTH(1–34) liquid injectable formulation, which requires refrigerated storage for long-term stability (Ameri, Daddona, & Maa, 2009).

In another example, solid arrays coated with a trivalent flu vaccine were subjected to three freeze/thaw cycles. Arrays coated with influenza hemagglutinin (HA) antigen were frozen at −15°C for a minimum of 24 hours, then passively equilibrated to ambient temperature (approximately 25°C) for three hours. This cycle was repeated up to three times, and the HA was desorbed from the patches and assayed by single radial immunodiffusion (SRID). At the end of the three freeze/thaw cycles, all three strains of influenza antigen retained roughly 85–90% of their reactivity in the SRID assay (Figure 6.12). The 10–15% reactivity loss observed in the study was reported to be within the variability of SRID analysis and thus does not represent a significant change in the antigen potency (Kommareddy, et al., 2013).

While many of the considerations for design and development of a microneedle delivery system are applicable to any of the described microneedle formats, there are also aspects of product design and development that are specific to the particular microneedle format being used. Some of those specific considerations are discussed in the following sections of this chapter.

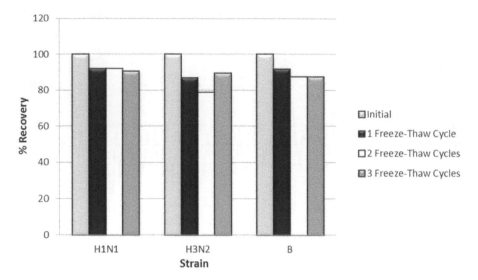

**FIGURE 6.12** Freeze-thaw stability of influenza antigens coated on solid microneedle arrays. The graph shows percent recovery of HA after zero to three freeze-thaw cycles. (From Kommareddy, et al., 2013, with permission from Elsevier.)

## 6.3 SOLID MICRONEEDLES: FORMULATION, COATING AND RELEASE CONSIDERATIONS

A key consideration for the development of coated solid microneedles is the necessity to design coating formulations that coat the microneedle tips evenly without wasting a significant amount of drug-containing formulation on the array base (which does not penetrate the stratum corneum; a drug coated on the base thus will not be delivered into the skin), and which will maintain their physical integrity over the product's shelf life. Coating formulations typically contain excipients that aid in localizing the drug on the microneedles rather than the array base, and also help to ensure that the coating droplets maintain their physical shape and location on the microneedles during storage. Figure 6.13 shows an example of a very stable formulation containing a model protein drug with a single coating excipient added to the formulation. After three years of storage at ambient conditions, the coated formulation droplets maintained their location at the tips of the microneedles (the drug-containing droplets did not slide down the needle towards the array base or migrate to one side of the microneedles), and maintained their shape.

While the formulation used to coat the microneedles must ensure the chemical and physical stability of the coated drug, it must also allow release of the drug off of the microneedles into the skin once the microneedle array has been applied. The release of the drug from the microneedle array determines the wear time of the microneedle delivery system, and must be characterized during formulation and product development. Examples of release profiles, measured in vivo in swine skin, are shown in Figure 6.14. The data in these graphs were generated by putting a number of coated microneedle arrays on a swine, then removing subsets of the

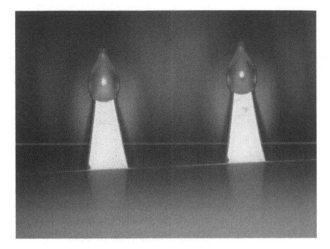

**FIGURE 6.13** Microscopic image of stable protein formulation coated on solid microneedles after three years of storage at ambient conditions. (From Dick, 2016a.)

arrays at various times and analyzing the amount of drug remaining on the arrays at each time point to determine how much drug was released from the array into the skin during that wear time.

The top graph in the figure shows an example of a drug formulation that released from the microneedle array very rapidly, so that over 90% of the drug was released in the first five minutes of wear. The bottom graph shows a drug formulation that released more gradually, and less completely, with only 75–80% of the drug released in 60 minutes of wear. The bottom graph also shows the impact of different formulation excipients on drug release for the same drug, with formulation G releasing more slowly than formulation D.

In general, release from coated solid microneedle arrays is rapid relative to traditional drug-in-adhesive patches or reservoir transdermal patches which are designed to provide drug delivery over the course of hours or days, and so coated solid microneedle delivery system wear times are typically short, on the order of five to 30 minutes. But as shown in Figure 6.14, drug release is dependent on both the characteristics of the specific drug and on the coating formulation, and should be assessed during preclinical development of the drug product.

Similar considerations for formulation design apply to dissolvable microneedles, with the added requirement that the matrix in which the drug or vaccine is incorporated must be strong enough to be formed into microneedles that can penetrate the skin and maintain integrity during application, yet also be water soluble to allow dissolution and delivery of the drug into the skin during application.

## 6.3.1 Preclinical Solid Microneedle Studies

While there are currently no approved drug products utilizing microneedle delivery technologies, numerous proof-of-concept studies have been conducted to demonstrate

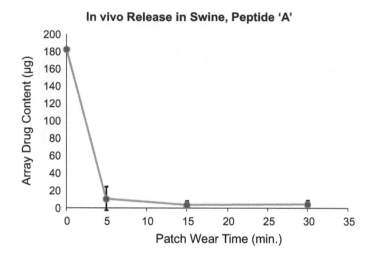

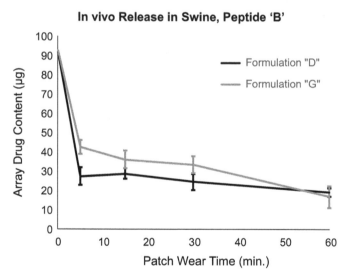

**FIGURE 6.14** Examples of in vivo release profiles of experimental peptide drugs from coated solid microneedles, obtained in swine. (From Dick 2016a.)

the potential for delivery of a large number of therapeutic agents, including small molecule drugs, therapeutic peptides and vaccines.

An example of the delivery of a small molecule using microneedles to provide a potential therapeutic advantage is the rapid delivery of lidocaine as a local anesthetic for pretreatment prior to minor vascular access procedures like venipuncture and IV insertion. A current standard of care for such local anesthetic pretreatment is the use of EMLA cream, which is a eutectic mixture of lidocaine and prilocaine. Because this is a topical application, 60 minutes is needed for enough drug to diffuse

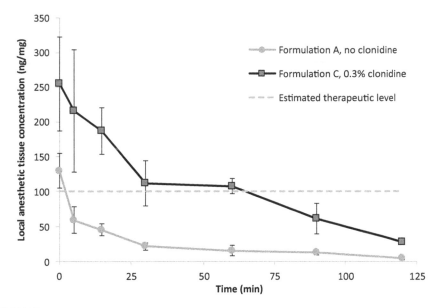

**FIGURE 6.15** Skin concentrations of lidocaine delivered via sMTS alone (A) or co-formulated with clonidine (C). The estimated therapeutic level is based on the lidocaine + prilocaine levels resulting from a one-hour exposure to EMLA. (From Zhang, et al., 2012b, with permission from Elsevier.)

through the stratum corneum and to develop the full anesthetic effect with EMLA. In a proof of concept study for delivery of a local anesthetic using microneedles, a combination of lidocaine and clonidine was coated onto 3M's solid microstructured transdermal system (sMTS), and applied to swine skin for one minute (Zhang, et al., 2012b). Skin was biopsied at the application site and the local tissue concentration of lidocaine was measured as a function of time following the coated microneedle array application. The results of the study are shown in Figure 6.15. A 60-minute application of EMLA was used as a benchmark for anesthetic effect in the study. After one hour, the swine skin tissue contained 100 ng/mg of lidocaine and prilocaine at the EMLA application site. When lidocaine was co-formulated with clonidine, the microneedle system delivered lidocaine immediately to the skin, and the tissue concentration stayed above the 100 ng/mg level for more than 50 minutes. These results suggest that microneedle delivery of a local anesthetic could be a way to provide rapid and long-lasting local anesthetic effect.

Intradermal delivery of vaccines can lead to enhanced immune responses to a variety of vaccines (Lambert & Laurent, 2008), but accurate and repeatable injection into the intradermal space using a needle and syringe requires a skilled clinician. As a result, a great deal of effort has been devoted to investigating the delivery of vaccines via both dissolving and solid microneedles, including vaccines for influenza (Koutsonanos, et al., 2009; Kommareddy, et al., 2012; Seok, et al., 2017; Rouphael, et al., 2017; Fernando, et al., 2018), measles (Edens, Collins,

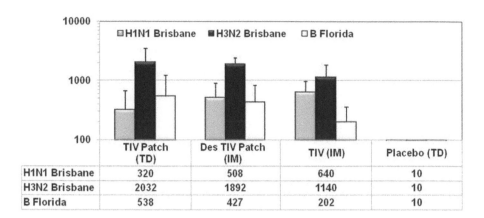

| | TIV Patch (TD) | Des TIV Patch (IM) | TIV (IM) | Placebo (TD) |
|---|---|---|---|---|
| H1N1 Brisbane | 320 | 508 | 640 | 10 |
| H3N2 Brisbane | 2032 | 1892 | 1140 | 10 |
| B Florida | 538 | 427 | 202 | 10 |

**FIGURE 6.16** Serum hemagglutinin inhibition titers against strains H1N1 A/Brisbane, H3N2 A/Brisbane, and B/Florida in guinea pigs two weeks after the second immunization. Results are shown as geometric mean titers and error bars represent one standard deviation. (From Kommareddy, et al., 2013, with permission from Elsevier.)

Ayers, Rota, & Prausnitz, 2013), human papilloma virus (Corbett, Fernando, Chen, Frazer, & Kendall, 2010), hepatitis B (Andrianov, et al., 2009), hepatitis C (Gill, Soderholm, Prausnitz, & Sallberg, 2010), West Nile and chikungunya (Prow, et al., 2010), diphtheria (Schipper, et al., 2017) and bacillus Calmette-Guerin (Hiraishi, et al., 2011). The majority of these studies were proof-of-concept demonstrations of vaccine delivery in preclinical animal models; in some instances, initial clinical studies in humans have progressed.

As just one example of vaccine delivery using coated solid microneedles, a trivalent influenza vaccine was delivered to guinea pigs either by intramuscular injection or by coated solid microneedles, and Serum Hemagglutinin Inhibition (HI) titers against influenza strains H1N1 A/Brisbane, H3N2 A/Brisbane, and B/Florida were measured two weeks after the second immunization (Kommareddy, et al., 2013). Figure 6.16 shows the HI titers for guinea pig groups treated with the trivalent vaccine coated on solid microneedles (labeled TIV Patch [TD] in the figure), the trivalent vaccine desorbed from the microneedles and subsequently injected intramuscularly (Des TIV Patch [IM]), and the trivalent vaccine injected intramuscularly as a control (TIV [IM]).

Overall, the titers elicited by immunization with coated microneedles were comparable to the titers elicited by intramuscular injection in this study, with slight variations between influenza strains – titers for H3N2 and B Florida strains were higher for microneedle delivery, while the response for H1N1 was lower for microneedle delivery compared to intramuscular injection. None of the differences were statistically significant, however. These results are comparable to those reported by others in mice (Koutsonanos, et al., 2009; Chen, et al., 2011; Kommareddy, et al., 2012), indicating the potential for effective, convenient and patient-friendly immunization with microneedle delivery systems.

### 6.3.2 DERMAL TOLERANCE OF SOLID MICRONEEDLES

A potential concern for microneedle delivery in which the stratum corneum is breached is the possibility of dermal irritation or reaction. The safety of microneedle delivery has been assessed in several human studies.

Bal et al. measured the skin irritation of volunteers following application of uncoated stainless steel microneedles of varying lengths using a chromameter (Bal, Caussin, Pavel, & Bouwstra, 2008). This study reported minimal irritation for microneedle application compared to tape stripping (an accepted noninvasive means of disrupting the stratum corneum), and the irritation was of short duration.

In a six-month clinical study of the microneedle delivery of teriparatide, microneedle delivery was well tolerated, with no delayed hypersensitivity or skin infection reported, and only mild to moderate erythema at the application site for both the placebo and the active drug product. A few incidents of swelling, bruising and pinpoint bleeding at the site of administration were reported (Cosman, et al., 2010).

In a phase II clinical study of abaloparatide, a new peptide drug under investigation for the treatment of osteoporosis, subjects self-administered the coated solid microneedle drug product daily for up to 24 weeks, providing an opportunity to assess the patient tolerance to repeated delivery via coated solid microneedles. Study results indicated that none of the adverse events reported in the small percentage (3.6%) of patients were considered to be related to study drug or route of administration (Brenner, et al., 2013). In addition, treatment compliance during the 24-week study was greater than 95% for microneedle delivery, consistent with an overall favorable skin tolerance profile.

Through these studies and others, the dermal tolerability of microneedle delivery has been assessed. Dermal tolerance when using microneedles has been demonstrated, with mild erythema as the primary observation.

## 6.4   HOLLOW MICRONEEDLE DELIVERY SYSTEMS

### 6.4.1 FORMULATION CONSIDERATIONS

The intradermal formulation envelope can accommodate many drug formulations. As with other parenteral drugs, when formulating a safe and effective drug for intradermal administration, one must consider multiple factors including formulation drug concentration, excipients, pH, tonicity, dose volume and viscosity. In addition, the formulation must be sterile and pyrogen-free.

Skin tolerability of the intradermal drug formulation should be addressed early in the development program. During administration, intradermal formulations displace the normal interstitial fluid surrounding the microneedles for the duration of the injection, typically from one to five minutes for low viscosity formulations. Intradermal injection rate is inversely proportional to formulation viscosity; thus, it is anticipated that delivery of viscous solutions may take even longer. Further, during injection, it is anticipated the blood flow is restricted in the capillaries near the microneedles due to the high injection pressure of the drug solution and the low pressure in the dermal capillaries. Depending on the inherent biocompatibility of the specific drug, these three factors (high local drug concentration, injection duration and decreased local blood flow during injection) may become important factors.

### 6.4.2 COMPONENTS OF A HOLLOW MICRONEEDLE INJECTOR

A hollow microneedle injector is composed of a number of components that work in concert to administer an intradermal injection. The microneedle injector contains one microneedle or an array of hollow microneedles. The needles need to be strong enough to maintain their shape during insertion and long enough to stay beneath the epidermis during fluid delivery. The applicator needs to have a means to actuate it. Following actuation, the microneedle insertion means may be a gas cartridge or a spring.

After microneedle insertion, the drug reservoir is fluidically connected to the array; and then the fluid in the drug reservoir is pressurized (often with spring force) to force the drug fluid from the drug reservoir through the hollow microneedles and into the skin. A cartridge or a syringe are often chosen for the drug reservoir, however some designs use bladder reservoirs.

The microneedle(s) must be held in place with a force such as hand pressure or pressure sensitive adhesive. Intradermal drug delivery using hollow microneedles occurring at high pressure (20 to 40 pounds per square inch) requires a strong seal between the needle and the skin for a minute or more. If this seal is breached, the drug formulation will leak onto the surface of the skin rather than remain in the body. The liquid pressure pushes against the microneedles during the injection and can force the needles back out of the skin unless they are held in place. The injection pressure may be provided by a spring, a gas cartridge or other physical means.

### 6.4.3 PRECLINICAL HOLLOW MICRONEEDLE STUDIES

Several research groups and companies have investigated hollow microneedles to deliver a variety of small molecules, vaccines, antibodies and proteins to preclinical models. Many classes of drugs have also been successfully delivered into swine skin intradermally using a single microneedle including antibodies, hormones and dyes (Harvey, et al., 2011). Multiple hollow microneedles have been used to deliver insulin, naloxone, equine anti-tetanus IgG, and human growth hormone (Burton, et al., 2011), and DNA delivery (Dul, et al., 2017).

#### 6.4.3.1 Human Growth Hormone Intradermal Delivery

Researchers at Becton Dickinson have reported administration of human growth hormone (approximately 22 kDa) using an array of three 1mm-long microneedles. In this study the injection volume was 100 uL and an injection rate of 45 uL/min resulted in a 2.2min infusion duration. The unique PK profile of somatropin (recombinant human growth hormone, rhGH) after ID, SC and IV administration to eight Yucatan mini pigs showed that ID delivery of somatropin gave a higher $C_{max}$ and an earlier $T_{max}$ compared to SC delivery (Harvey, et al., 2011).

Separately, 3M Company used an hMTS Injector with an array of 12 microneedles to deliver 0.75 mL of hGH. The PK profile of hGH after ID and SC administration

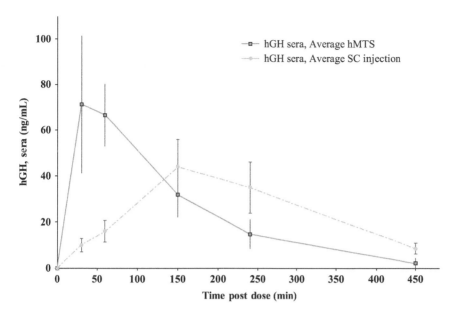

**FIGURE 6.17** PK Results of hGH in swine. (From Burton, et al., 2011, with permission from Springer.)

to female domestic swine showed a higher $C_{max}$ and an earlier $T_{max}$ compared to SC delivery as shown in Figure 6.17 (Burton, et al., 2011).

### 6.4.3.2 Methotrexate

Methotrexate is used to treat cancer, severe psoriasis and rheumatoid arthritis. At clinically relevant doses it has adverse side effects such as hair loss and severe nausea. In order to understand the potential for lower dosing, the concentration of methotrexate in plasma as a function of administration route was studied in swine. Figure 6.18 shows the results of a PK study of methotrexate delivered via intravenous, intradermal and oral administration (Hansen, et al., 2012).

Intradermal delivery of methotrexate using 3M's hollow microneedle injector (3M™ hMTS) produced blood levels nearly identical to intravenous administration. Both intravenous and intradermal delivery had significantly higher bioavailability than oral administration.

### 6.4.3.3 Adalimumab Preclinical

Adalimumab, a large 150kDa protein, has been successfully delivered intradermally with hollow microneedles and an intradermal injector. Figure 6.19 shows the results from an adalimumab PK study in swine (n=3) using the 3M hMTS injector (Johnson, et al., 2012). Intradermal delivery with the 3M hMTS injector in swine demonstrated approximately 20% higher bioavailability compared to subcutaneous injection. Further, after microneedle delivery there was very good skin site tolerability.

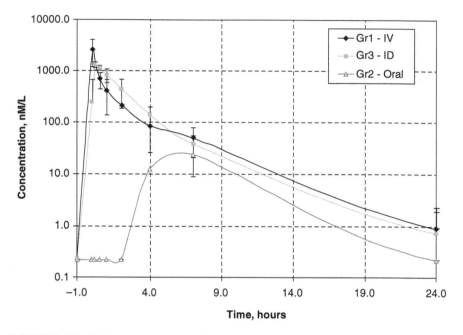

**FIGURE 6.18** Methotrexate concentration in plasma after IV, ID and oral administration. (From Hansen, et al., 2012.)

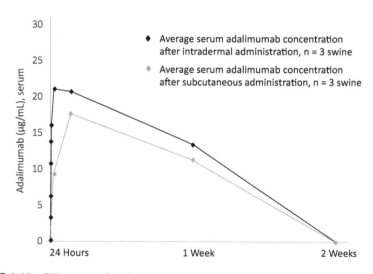

**FIGURE 6.19** PK results of adalimumab in swine. (From Johnson, 2012.)

### 6.4.4 CLINICAL HOLLOW MICRONEEDLE STUDIES

Becton Dickinson (BD) conducted clinical trials to demonstrate that the BD Microneedle system was safe and easy to use (Laurent, 2007b). Also, clinical testing showed that the BD Microneedle was barely perceptible when it entered the skin and ensured the administration of the injected solution to the dermal layer irrespective of the subject's gender, age, ethnicity and body mass (Laurent, 2007b).

In a study completed in 2012, 3M researchers investigated the performance of intradermal delivery versus the currently marketed subcutaneous autoinjector for delivery of HUMIRA® in the context of a physician conducted phase I clinical study using hollow microneedles as in "D" of Figure 6.2 (Dick, 2014). The full dose was successfully delivered. The results demonstrate the capability of 3M's hMTS intradermal delivery device to successfully deliver a therapeutic dose of a large biologic (144kDa) molecule.

In a non-significant risk device clinical study completed in 2015, the same researchers investigated the performance of intradermal delivery devices for 2 mL of 5% dextrose fluid (Bohlke, 2015). Data collected in 30 healthy volunteers age 18+ demonstrated that intradermal self-administration of a full 2 mL volume via the hMTS device was achieved. Delivery times were site dependent: average delivery time on the lower thigh (near knee) was 106 seconds, whereas the average delivery time to the upper thigh was faster, at 52 seconds. Pain, erythema and edema scores were in the mild–moderate range and pain was reduced close to the baseline by the end of the fluid administrations. These results demonstrate the capability of a hollow microneedle intradermal delivery device to successfully deliver 2 mL of liquid formulation.

A phase I study reported by Troy et al. studied the immune response to inactivated polio vaccine (IPV) delivered intradermally using the MicronJet600™ hollow microneedle system in HIV-infected adults (Troy, et al., 2015). The study found that intradermal administration of 40% of the standard dose of IPV produced an immune response comparable to delivery of the standard dose administered intramuscularly. Intradermal administration showed a higher incidence of local side effects including redness and itching, but a similar incidence of systemic side effects, and study participants reported a preference for intradermal administration over intramuscular administration.

## 6.5 REGULATORY ASPECTS OF MICRONEEDLE PLATFORM

Several disciplines are employed in the development and control of microneedle systems, including chemistry, toxicology, biopharmaceutics, skin physiology, materials science, human factors and mechanical engineering. All of these are underpinned by the unique quality system used for drug-device combination products to ensure appropriate considerations are evaluated at the right time in a microneedle product's development.

### 6.5.1 DRUG-DEVICE COMBINATION PRODUCT CATEGORIZATIONS

Drug–device combination products are common for targeted delivery of therapeutic agents. In many regions of the world, the therapeutic agent, e.g., drug or biologic, defines the drug–device combination products as a medicinal product. In the USA, a unique categorization is available as defined in 21 CFR 3.2(e) (Federal Register, 1991). The combination product categorization originated in 1991 with four types of combination products:

1. A product comprised of two or more regulated components, i.e., drug/device, biologic/device, drug/biologic or drug/device/biologic, that are physically, chemically or otherwise combined or mixed and produced as a single entity.
2. Two or more separate products packaged together in a single package or as a unit and comprised of drug and device products, device and biological products or biological and drug products.
3. A drug, device or biological product packaged separately that according to its investigational plan or proposed labeling is intended for use only with an approved individually specified drug, device or biological product where both are required to achieve the intended use, indication or effect and where upon approval of the proposed product the labeling of the approved product would need to be changed, e.g., to reflect a change in intended use, dosage form, strength, route of administration or significant change in dose.
4. Any investigational drug, device or biological product packaged separately that according to its proposed labeling is for use only with another individually specified investigational drug, device or biological product where both are required to achieve the intended use, indication or effect.

Combination product designations for these systems are likely defined as either single integrated [3.2(e)(1)] or co-packaged [3.2(e)(2)] combination products or a combination of these two types. Microneedle systems utilize the component or device constituent to administer the agent for the desired effect by the drug or biologic. The primary mode of action of these combination products is the drug or biologic. In the case of solid microneedle systems where the therapeutic agent is coated on the microneedle array and delivery is assisted by a power-supplied applicator, the array component is a primary packaging component with a delivery function, when used in concert with the applicator. The array component is integrated in the adhesive patch, all of which are supported with the use of a backing. The applicator is a device which is designed for the specific use with the microneedle patch and for the identified drug product. Due to the unique characteristics of the applicator in relation to its usage with only the planned coated microneedle patch, the applicator would gain market authorization in the NDA or BLA of the complete combination product. It is likely in this example that the solid microneedle combination product would be categorized 3.2(e)(2), when the applicator would be co-packaged with the coated microneedle patch. Some interpretations may consider the patch containing the microstructures a 3.2(e)(1) product on its own, however as described earlier in this chapter, solid microneedle systems benefit from inclusion of an applicator for uniform delivery.

The hollow microstructured systems described earlier in this chapter are also considered combination products; however, the products which use a microneedle delivery device for administration could be assigned either a designation of 3.2(e)(1) or 3.2(e)(2), dependent on how the system is assembled for final market presentation.

Considering the complexity of some hMTS devices and the assurance needed for proper assembly of the drug constituent part into the device, some manufacturers may decide to assemble the completed combination product at their manufacturing facility(ies), making the unit ready to use by the patient or health care provider upon opening the packaging. This type of combination product is considered a 3.2(e)(1) or single integrated product where the drug constituent part and device constituent part are designed to be provided in one single finished unit to the user. If the device constituent part is designed for insertion of a drug filled ampule by the patient or health care provider, the product may be considered co-packaged where the drug filled vial is co-packaged with the device.

### 6.5.2 Quality Systems Considerations: cGMP Expectations

As combination products, the development and manufacture of these systems is governed by the cGMP system described in 21 CFR 4 in the United States (Federal Register, 2013). In other regions, cGMP systems would be defined by the discrete or combined characteristics of the product(s) used to deliver the medicinal agent. In the USA, cGMP may follow a streamlined approach, blending the requirements of drug cGMP found in 21 CFR 210/211 with device cGMP found in 21 CFR 820 by selecting a base set of requirements from one of the core cGMP systems and adding the 21 CFR 4 specified elements of the other cGMP system. If the product is a combination product which incorporates a biologic, the relevant provisions of 21 CFR 600–680 apply to the biologic constituent and throughout the product's manufacturing after the biologic constituent has been incorporated. These cGMP rules across all of these product types mean that during development of the microneedle delivery systems, design controls (21 CFR 820.30) are to be utilized. In addition to applying design controls to the discrete device, e.g., applicator, the firm designing the combination product also needs to apply design controls to the product *in its combination* (Federal Register, 2013; Food and Drug Administration, 2017). This means the interaction of the drug constituent part, e.g., the patch with the integrated microneedles, and the co-packaged device, e.g., the applicator, is to be characterized. Additionally, primary packaging components which perform a delivery function are to be characterized in terms of the requirements for primary packaging for suitability, compatibility, safety, performance, functionality and drug delivery (Food and Drug Administration, 1999). Functionality and drug delivery are addressed through design and testing appropriate to the dosage form. The European Medicines Agency also recommends characterization of formulation and product design influences on active substance permeation through the skin for transdermal products, thereby requesting the study of drug and delivery system interaction (European Medicines Agency, 2014).

### 6.5.3 Data Packages Expectations: Leveraging Standards

Microneedle systems blend drug and device benefits into one delivery system. Data packages that justify appropriate chemistry, manufacturing and control of these systems may leverage requirements from the source drug and device standards. For example, intradermal delivery systems utilize patches for support of the microneedle component and assurance of delivery of the drug. It is useful to consider the expectations of USP <3>, Topical and Transdermal Products and assess if they may be appropriate to the specific patch of the combination product under development (United States Pharmacopeia – National Formulary, 2019). As defined in USP <3>:

> Topically applied drug products fall into two general categories: those applied to achieve local action and those applied to achieve systemic effects after absorption through the skin into the blood circulation. Local action can occur at or on the surface of the application site (e.g., stratum corneum), in the underlying tissues (e.g., epidermis and/or dermis), and in subcutaneous tissues (e.g., muscle or joint). Topically applied drug products include but are not restricted to creams, gels, ointments, pastes, suspensions, lotions, foams, sprays, aerosols, solutions, and transdermal delivery systems (TDS).

Although microneedle products cross the stratum corneum through the use of the microneedles rather than solely absorb from intact skin, aspects related to the physical integrity of the patch and some aspects related to chemical stability of the patch still apply. Table 6.2 lists some of the quality attributes from USP <3> and whether that product quality test may be applicable to a patch which incorporates a microneedle component which includes a drug. An analysis for each specific product would define which elements of USP <3> might apply.

Other specific tests for transdermal delivery systems are related to the adhesive layer and ensuring contact with the skin to allow the delivery of the dosage. Examples of tests discussed in USP <3> include peel adhesion test, release liner peel test and tack test. Evaluations of applicability and specifics of the method need to be assessed on a case-by-case basis for the desired microneedle patch product.

**TABLE 6.2**
**Consideration of USP <3> Product Quality Tests for Solid Microneedle Patches**

| Product Quality Tests from USP <3> | Comment on applicability to solid microneedle patch systems |
|---|---|
| Description | Yes |
| Identification | Yes |
| Assay | Yes, dependent on product and assay sensitivity |
| Impurities | Yes, dependent on product and assay sensitivity |
| Uniformity of dosage units | Product dependent, <905> criteria may not apply |
| Water content | Formulation dependent |
| Microbial Limits | Discussion beyond scope of this book chapter |
| Antimicrobial preservative content | Applicable to multi-dose products, generally not applicable to solid microneedle patch systems due to single dose |
| Antioxidant content | Formulation dependent |
| Sterility | Discussion beyond scope of this book chapter |
| pH | Product dependent, may not apply |
| Particle size | Formulations typically solutions, hence likely not applicable |

**TABLE 6.3**
**Potential Consensus Standards for Microneedle Applicator Devices**

| Device Aspect | Applicable Standard | Timeframe |
|---|---|---|
| Materials of construction | USP Class VI for plastics that have patient/product contact. Biocompatibility – ISO 10993-1 (ISO, 2018) | Prior to phase I |
| Human Factors | Guidance for Industry and FDA Staff: Applying Human Factors and Usability Engineering to Optimize Medical Device Design (Food and Drug Administration, 2016) IEC 62366-1 (IEC, 2015) | Phased approach; summative prior to or during phase III |
| Applicator packaging | ASTM D4169-16: Standard Practice for Performance Testing of Shipping Containers and Systems (ASTM, 2016) | Phased approach |
| Sterility & Sterile Barrier* | ISO 11137: Sterilization of Health Care Products – Radiation (ISO, 2006–2017) ISO 11607: Packaging for Terminally Sterilized Medical Devices (ISO, 2019) | Phased approach |
| Device Performance | ISO 11608: Needle Based Injection Systems for Medical Use (ISO, 2014) | Phase III |

* Sterile barrier needs determinant with patient, therapy and product requirements.

Several standards are applicable when designing an applicator for a microneedle delivery system. Example standards which can be leveraged in the development of the device constituent or stand alone device of a microneedle system are offered in Table 6.3. Example product aspects for consideration, potential standards to apply and timeframe of preparation of the data packages in relation to the development and clinical plans are provided in Table 6.3.

The materials of construction and risk analysis in accordance with ISO 10993 are constraints that must be fulfilled early on in a device configuration's development. In contrast, some device aspects may be a consideration in early applicator design but not verified until later in a combination product's development and, hence, a phased approach is applied to that aspect. Technical requirements from ISO 11608 may be applicable to microneedle delivery systems on a case-by-case basis. The selected bench tests further leverage relevant existing standards. These requirements are to be assigned against the desired and required product characteristics for the delivery system.

The International Council for Harmonization of Technical Requirements for Pharmaceuticals for Human Use (ICH) provides recommendations on interpretation and application of technical guidelines and requirements in the longstanding effort towards global data package harmonization. The effort includes members and observers across the globe from industry and regulatory bodies. The primary mode of action for microneedle combination products is the drug or biologic. Therefore, as pharmaceutical products, the following ICH Quality Guidances (ICH, multiple) offer relevant recommendations in planning for microneedle products chemistry, manufacturing and controls (CMC) data packages. Table 6.4 reviews several quality guidelines and recommends relevant topics to microneedle products.

**TABLE 6.4**
**ICH Quality Guidelines for Microneedle Products CMC Data Packages**

| ICH Quality Guidance | Title of Guidance(s) | Scope of Guideline | Relevance to Microneedle Products |
|---|---|---|---|
| *ICH Q1* | *Stability Testing:* | | |
| A(R2): | New Drug Substances and Products | Recommendations on stability testing protocols including temperature, humidity and trial duration | Basis for combination products' stability protocol design for determination of expiry |
| B: | Photostability of New Drug Substances and Products | Annex to main stability guideline; evaluation protocol for light sensitivity | Applicability is product specific |
| C: | New Dosage Forms | Annex to main stability guideline; new dosage form stability requirements when same API is in a different product type | Potential for reduced stability database at submission time if API used in previous dosage form |
| D: | Bracketing and Matrixing Designs | General principles for reduced stability testing, bracketing & matrixing designs | If multiple strengths of products, pull point matrices may reduce testing, can add risk to expiry prediction |
| E: | Evaluation of Stability Data | Statistical methodology for stability data analysis and expiry prediction | Guideline is applicable |
| *ICH Q3* | *Impurities:* | | |
| A(R2): | New Drug Substances | Thresholds for reporting, identification and qualification | Same base requirements as other dosage forms |
| B(R2): | New Drug Products | Degradation products arising from interactions | Analogous to other dosage forms for interactions of drug substance, excipients and components of primary packaging materials |
| C(R7): | Guideline for Residual Solvents | Sets pharmaceutical limits for residual solvents in drug products | Analogous to other dosage forms, high dependency on API and excipients. |
| D(R1)*: | Guideline for Elemental Impurities | Control of elemental impurities in drug products and Permitted Daily Exposures (PDEs) for oral, parenteral and inhalation. | |

**TABLE 6.4**
**ICH Quality Guidelines for Microneedle Products CMC Data Packages (Cont.)**

| ICH Quality Guidance | Title of Guidance(s) | Scope of Guideline | Relevance to Microneedle Products |
|---|---|---|---|
| *ICH Q6* | *Specifications: Test Procedures and Acceptance Criteria:* | | |
| A: | New Drug Substances and New Drug Products: Chemical Substances | Process of selecting tests/ methods and setting specifications | General guidance offered for specification setting for tests, as applicable |
| B: | Biotechnological/ Biological Products | Justifying and setting of specifications for proteins and polypeptides | Specifications as a component of the product's control strategy |
| *ICH Q8(R2)* | *Pharmaceutical Development* | Guidance on contents of Module 3.2.P.2 Pharmaceutical Development and Quality by Design (QbD) approaches | Analogous to other dosage forms, opportunity to uniquely define quality target product profile (QTPP) and critical quality attributes (CQA) for microneedle products |

* The ICH Q3D(R2) Maintenance Expert Working Group is undertaking maintenance of the Guideline to develop Permitted Daily Exposure (PDE) levels for cutaneous and transdermal products.

The blending of CMC requirements from pharmacopeia, device expectations and ICH illustrates analysis that can be used to evaluate if existing standards on related products are appropriate and justify the safety and control of the product as it is being developed. Microneedle system specifics have been discussed by FDA scientists at technical forums that focus on microneedle products (Strasinger, 2014; Ghosh, 2014; Cole, 2014). Additional focus and clarifications have been offered with respect to biopharmaceutics, nonclinical, mechanical aspects, stability, sterility and patient use considerations. Example studies include an evaluation and characterization of the mechanical properties of the microneedles and packaging of the finished product. Properties such as resilience against breaking and ability to withstand a minimum force before deformation are critical attributes for the mechanical performance of the microneedles. Additionally, the chemical stability of the materials and potential for interaction with the formulation in the form of extractables/leachables is a consideration for data packages involving microneedles and associated product packaging. An example of an interaction study concerning the physical stability of the combination product which has been recommended by the FDA scientists is an evaluation of the placement of the coated drug on the microneedle over time. The scientific considerations for a clearly defined Quality Target Product Profile (QTPP) early in development and related process features has also been presented (Norman & Strasinger, 2016).

### 6.5.4 REGULATORY SUMMARY

Data packages need to be established for all disciplines utilized in the development of microneedle products, within the framework of an appropriate quality system for these drug–device combination products. Combination product development and data package preparation requires careful consideration of the elements of each part of the product on its own and also the crucial interactions. A product's registration status may vary based upon region of the world, but the intent is the same, to deliver a drug or biologic with the assistance of a delivery system.

## 6.6 CONCLUSION

Microneedle delivery systems have been in development for a relatively short time, in comparison to transdermal systems which have been commercially available for over 30 years and in comparison to deeper tissue injection systems which have been used for over a century. The unique blending of transdermal with microneedles has many benefits in the delivery of agents unable to cross the stratum corneum, such as proteins, peptides and biological molecules. The microneedle delivery systems in development have amassed significant preclinical data, and in some cases, clinical trials with microneedles have demonstrated similar PK profiles to existing injection systems. The systems are developed with patients' needs in mind with a focus on human factors and usability engineering. Technical considerations leverage the large amount of knowledge available on modern transdermal and injection systems. Unique considerations also arise which are addressed as a product's definition is identified and refined. Delivery with these systems offers great potential. As the technology matures, further advances and opportunities are to be realized for these microneedle dosage forms.

## BIBLIOGRAPHY

Ameri, M., Daddona, P., & Maa, Y. (2009). Demonstrated solid-state stability of parathyroid hormone PTH(1–34) coated on a novel transdermal microprojection delivery system. *Pharm. Res.*, (11) pp. 2454–2463.

Andrianov, A., DeCollibus, D., Gillis, H., Kha, H., Marin, A., Prausnitz, M., Babiuk, L. Townsend, H., & Mutwiri, G. (2009). Poly[di(carboxylatophenoxy)phosphazene] is a potent adjuvant for intradermal immunization. *Proc. Nat. Acad. Sci.*, (106) pp. 18936–18941.

Arnou, R., Icardi, G., DeDecker, M., Ambrozaitis, A., Kazek, M., Weber, F., & VanDamme, P. (2009). Intradermal influenza vaccine for older adults: a randomized controlled multicenter phase III study. *Vaccine*, (52) pp. 7304–7312.

ASTM. (2016). ASTM D4169-16. *Standard Practice for Performance Testing of Shipping Containers and Systems*. West Conshohocken, PA: ASTM International, www.astm.org.

Bal, S., Caussin, J., Pavel, S., & Bouwstra, J. (2008). In vivo assessment of safety of microneedle arrays in human skin. *Eur. J. Pharm. Sci.*, (35) pp. 193–202.

Bal, S., Kruithof, A., Zwier, R., Dietz, E., Bouwstra, J., Lademann, J., & Meinke, M. (2010). Influence of microneedle shape on the transport of a fluorescent dye into human skin in vivo. *J. of Controlled Release*, (147) pp. 218–224.

Bohlke, A. (2015). Development and Scale-Up of Microneedle-based Drug Delivery Systems for Drugs and Biologics. *Transdermal and Intradermal Drug Delivery Systems Conference*. Philadelphia, PA.

Barbero, A., & Frasch, H. (2009). Pig and guinea pig skin as surrogate for human in vitro penetration studies: a quantitative review. *Tox. In Vitro*, (23) pp. 1–13.

Bramson, J., & Dayball, K. (2003). Enabling topical immunization via microporation: a novel method for pain-free and needle-free delivery of adenovirus-based vaccines. *Gene Ther.*, (10) pp. 251–260.

Brenner, L., Hansen, K., Clarkin, M., Haraldsen, K., Riis, B., Bolognese, M., & Miller, P. (2013). Safety and tolerability of BA058 Transdermal, a novel analog of hPTHrP delivered via microneedle path: results of a Phase 2 clinical trial. *American Society for Bone and Mineral Research Annual Meeting* (pp. LB-SA29). Baltimore, MD: ASBMR.

Burkoth, T., & Bellhouse, B. (1999). Transdermal and transmucosal powdered drug delivery. *Crit Rev Ther Drug Carrier Syst*, (16) pp. 331–384.

Burton, S., Ng, C., Simmers, R., Moeckly, C., Brandwein, D., Gilbert, T., Johnson, N., Brown, K., Alston, T., Prochnow, G., Siebenaler, K., & Hansen, K. (2011). Rapid intradermal delivery of liquid formulations using a hollow microstructured array. *Pharm. Res.*, (28) pp. 31–40.

Chen, X., Corbett, H., Yukiko, S., Raphael, A., Fairmaid, E., Prow, T., Brown, L., Fernando, G., & Kendall, M. (2011). Site-selectively coated, densely-packed microprojection array patches for targeted delivery of vaccines to skin. *Adv. Funct. Mat.*, (21) pp. 464–473.

Chu, L., Choi, S., & Prausnitz, M. (2010). Fabrication of dissolving polymer microneedles for controlled drug encapsulation and delivery: bubble and pedestal designs. *J. Pharm. Sci.*, (99) pp. 4228–4238.

Cole, J. (2014). Product Quality Microbiology Evaluation of CDER Regulatory Submissions. *Third International Conference on Microneedles*. Baltimore, MD: U of MD, School of Pharmacy.

Corbett, H., Fernando, G., Chen, X., Frazer, I., & Kendall, M. (2010). Skin vaccination against cervical cancer associated human papillomavirus with a novel micro-projection array in a mouse model. *PLoS One*, 5, e13460.

Cosman, F., Lane, N., Bolognese, M., Zanchetta, J., Garcia-Hernandez, P., Sees, K., Matriano, J., Gaumer, K., & Daddona, P. (2010). Effect of transdermal teriparatide administration on bone mineral density in postmenopausal women. *J. Clin. Endocrinol. Metab.*, (95) pp. 151–158.

Daddona, P., Matriano, J., Mandema, J., & Maa, Y. (2011). Parathyroid hormone(1–34)-coated microneedle patch system: clinical pharmacokinetics and pharmacodynamics for treatment of osteoporosis. *Pharm. Res.*, (28) pp. 159–165.

Davis, S., Prausnitz, M., & Allen, M. (2003). Fabrication and characterization of laser micromachined hollow microneedles. *Proceedings of Transducers*, pp. 1435–1438.

Dick, L. (2014). Pointing the way. *Innovations in Pharmaceutical Technology*, (50).

Dick, L. (2016a). Considerations for Commercialization of a Microneedle Product. *Fourth International Conference on Microneedles*. London, England: GSK House.

Dick, L. (2016b). Phase-Based Development for a Commercializable Microneedle Product. *Transdermal and Intradermal Drug Delivery Systems Conference*. Philadelphia, PA.

Donnelly, R., Garland, M., Morrow, K., Migalska, K., Singh, T., Majithiya, R., & Woolfson, A. (2010). Optical coherence tomography is a valuable tool in the study of the effects of microneedle geometry on skin penetration characteristics and in-skin dissolution. *J. Control Release*, (147) pp. 333–41.

Doukas, A., & Kollias, N. (2004). Transdermal drug delivery with a pressure wave. *Adv. Drug Deliv. Rev.*, (56) pp. 559–579.

Duan, D., Moeckly, C., Gysbers, J., Novak, C., Prochnow, G., Siebenaler, K., Albers, L., & Hansen, K. (2011). Enhanced delivery of topically applied formulations following skin pre-treatment with a hand-applied, plastic microneedle array. *Current Drug Delivery*, (8) pp. 1–9.

Dul, M., Stefanidou, P., Porta, P., Serve, J., O'Mahony, C., Malissen, B., Henri, S., Levin, Y., Kochba, E., Wong, F., Dayan, C., Coulman, S., & Birchall, J. (2017). Hydrodynamic gene delivery in human skin using a hollow microneedle device. *J. Contr. Release*, (265) pp. 120–131.

Edens, C., Collins, M., Ayers, J., Rota, P., & Prausnitz, M. (2013). Measles vaccination using a microneedle patch. *Vaccine*, (31) pp. 3403–3409.

European Medicines Agency. (2014, October). *European Medicines Agency: Guideline on quality of transdermal patches*. Retrieved from EMA/CHMP/QWP/608924/2014: www.ema.europa.eu/docs/en_GB/document_library/Scientific_guideline/2014/12/WC500179071.pdf

Federal Register. (1991, November 21). Assignment of Agency Component for Premarket Review of Applications. 56 FR 58754.

Federal Register. (2013, January 22). Current Good Manufacturing Practice Requirements for Combination Products. 78 FR 4307.

Fernando, G., Hickling, J., Jayashi Flores, C., Griffin, P., Anderson, C., Skinner, S., Davies, C., Witham, K., Pryor, M., Bodle, J., Rockman, S., Frazer, I., & Forster, A. (2018). Safety, tolerability, acceptability and immunogenicity of an influenza vaccine delivered to human skin by a novel high-density microprojection array patch (NanopatchTM). *Vaccine*, (36), pp. 3779–3788.

Food and Drug Administration. (1999, May). *Food & Drug Administration: Container Closure Systems for Packaging Human Drugs and Biologics: Chemistry, Manufacturing, and Controls Documentation, Guidance for Industry*. Retrieved from www.fda.gov/media/70788/download

Food and Drug Administration. (2013, June). *Guidance for Industry and FDA Staff-Technical Considerations for Pen, Jet and Related Injectors for Use with Drugs and Biological Products*. Retrieved from www.fda.gov/media/76403/download

Food and Drug Administration. (2016, February). *Guidance for Industry and FDA Staff - Applying Human Factors and Usability Engineering to Optimize Medical Device Design*. Retrieved from www.fda.gov/media/80481/download

Food and Drug Administration. (2017, January). *Guidance for Industry and FDA Staff: Current Good Manufacturing Requirements for Combination Products*. Retrieved from www.fda.gov/media/90425/download

Ghosh, T. (2014). Biopharmaceutics and Clinical Pharmacology Aspects of Microneedle Product Development. *Third International Conference on Microneedles*. Baltimore, MD: U of MD, School of Pharmacy.

Gill, H., Soderholm, J., Prausnitz, M., & Sallberg, M. (2010). Cutaneous vaccination using microneedles coated with hepatitis C DNA vaccine. *Gene Therapy*, (17) pp. 811–814.

Gupta, J., Felner, E., & Prausnitz, M. (2009). Minimally invasive insulin delivery in subjects with type 1 diabetes using hollow microneedles. *Diabetes Technol. Ther.*, (11) pp. 329–337.

Hansen, K. (2013). Development and Scale-up of a Coated Microneedle Patch for Delivery of Vaccines and Biotherapeutics. *Skin Vaccination Summit*. Seattle, WA.

Hansen, K., Chu, L., Schafer, S., Burton, S. (2012). Hollow Microneedle Delivery of a therapeutic dose of Methotrexate and Humira advantages of intradermal delivery over conventional routes. *American Association of Pharmaceutical Scientists (AAPS) Conference*. Chicago, IL.

Haq, M., Smith, E., John, D., Kalavala, M., Edwards, C., & Anstey, A. (2009). Clinical administration of microneedles: skin puncture, pain and sensation. *Biomed. Microdev.*, (11) pp. 35–47.

Harvey, A., Kaestner, S., Sutter, D., Harvey, N., Mikszta, J., & Pettis, R. (2011). Microneedle based intradermal delivery enables rapid lymphatic uptake and distribution of protein drugs. *Pharm. Res.*, (28) pp. 107–116.

Henry, S., McAllister, D., Allen, M., & Prausnitz, M. (1998). Microfabricated microneedles: a novel method to increase transdermal drug delivery. *J. Pharm. Sci.*, (87) pp. 922–925.

Hiraishi, Y., Nandakumar, S., Choi, S., Lee, J., Kim, Y., Posey, J., Sable, J., & Prausnitz, M. (2011). Bacillus Calmette-Guirin vaccination using a microneedle patch. *Vaccine*, (29) pp. 2626–2636.

ICH. (multiple). *Quality Guidelines*. Retrieved from International Council for Harmonisation of Technical Requirements for Pharmaceuticals for Human Use: www.ich.org/products/guidelines/quality/article/quality-guidelines.html

IEC. (2015). IEC 62366-1: 2015. *Medical devices — Part 1: Application of usability engineering to medical devices*. Geneva, Switzerland: International Electrotechnical Commission, www.iec.ch.

Ismach, A. (1962). *US Patent No. 3,057,349*.

ISO. (2006–2017). ISO 11137. *Sterilization of Health Care Products – Radiation, Parts 1–3*. Geneva, Switzerland: International Organization for Standardization, www.iso.org.

ISO. (2014). ISO 11608-1: 2014. *Needle Based Injection Systems for Medical Use – Requirements and Test Methods – Part 1: Needle based injection systems*. Geneva, Switzerland: International Organization for Standardization, www.iso.org.

ISO. (2018). ISO 10993-1: 2018. *Biological Evaluation of Medical Devices — Part 1: Evaluation and Testing Within a Risk Management Process*. Geneva, Switzerland: International Organization for Standardization, www.iso.org.

ISO. (2019). ISO 11607. *Packaging for Terminally Sterilized Medical Devices, Parts 1 and 2*. Geneva, Switzerland: International Organization for Standardization, www.iso.org.

Jain, A., Lee, C., & Gill, H. (2016). 5-Aminolevulinic acid coated microneedles for photodynamic therapy of skin tumors. *J. Contr. Release*, (239) pp. 72–81.

Johnson, P., Burton, S., Chu, L., Brandwein, D., Hansen, K. (2012). A Portal to the Lymphatic System: Intradermal Drug Delivery by 3M Microstructured Transdermal Systems. *Well Characterized Biopharmaceuticals Conference*. San Francisco, CA..

Kalia, Y., & Naik, A. (2004). Iontophoretic drug delivery. *Adv. Drug Deliv. Rev.*, (56) pp. 619–658.

Kochhar, J., Quek, C., Soon, W., Choi, J., Zou, S., & Kang, L. (2013). Effect of microneedle geometry and supporting substrate on microneedle array penetration into skin. *J. Pharm. Sci.*, (102) pp. 4100–4108.

Koelmans, W., Krishamoorth, G., Heskamp, A., Wissink, J., Misra, S., & Tas, N. (2013). Microneedle characterization using a double-layer skin simulant. *Mechanical Engineering Research*, (3) pp. 51–63.

Kommareddy, S., Baudner, B., Bonificio, A., Gallorini, S., Palladino, G., Determan, A. S., Dohmeier, D., Kroells, K., Sternjohn, J., Singh, M., Dormitzer, P., Hansen, K., & O'Hagan, D. T. (2013). Influenza subunit vaccine coated microneedle patches elicit comparable immune responses to intramuscular injection in guinea pigs. *Vaccine*, (31) pp. 3435–3441.

Kommareddy, S., Baudner, B., Oh, S., Kwon, S., Singh, M., & O'Hagan, D. (2012). Dissolvable microneedle patches for the delivery of cell-culture-derived influenza vaccine antigens. *J. Pharm. Sci.*, (101) pp. 1021–1027.

Korkmaz, E., Friedrich, E., Ramadan, M., Erdos, G., Mathers, A., Burak Ozdoganlar, O., Washburn, N., & Falo Jr., L. (2015). Therapeutic intradermal delivery of tumor necrosis factor-alpha antibodies using tip-loaded dissolvable microneedle arrays. *Acta Biomater.*, (24) pp. 96–105.

Koutsonanos, D., Martin, M., Zarnitsyn, V., Sullivan, S., Compans, R., Prausnitz, M., & Skountzou, I. (2009). Transdermal influenza immunization with vaccine-coated microneedle arrays. *PLoS One*, 4: e4773.

Lambert, P., & Laurent, P. (2008). Intradermal vaccine delivery: will new delivery systems transform vaccine administration? *Vaccine*, (26) pp. 3197–3208.

Larraneta, E., Moore, J., Vicente-Perez, E. M., Gonzalez-Vasquez, P., Lutton, R., Woolfson, A. D., & Donnelly, R. F. (2014). A proposed model membrane and test method for microneedle insertion studies. *Int. J. Pharmaceut.*, (472) pp. 65–73.

Laurent, P. (2007a). Echographic measurement of skin thickness in adults by high frequency ultrasound to assess the appropriate microneedle length for intradermal delivery of vaccines. *Vaccine*, (25) pp. 6423–6430.

Laurent, P. (2007b). Evaluation of the clinical performance of a new intradermal vaccine administration technique and associated delivery system. *Vaccine*, (25) pp. 8833–8842.

Levin, G., & Gershonowitz, A. (2005). Transdermal delivery of human growth hormone through RF-microchannels. *Phar. Res*, (22) pp. 550–555.

Lutton, R., Moore, J., Larraneta, E., Ligett, S., Woolfson, A., & Donnelly, R. (2015). Microneedle characterisation: the need for universal acceptance criteria and GMP specifications when moving towards commercialization. *Drug Deliv. and Transl. Res.*, (5) pp. 313–331.

Matriano, J., Cormier, M., Johnson, J., Young, W., Buttery, M., Nyam, K., & Daddona, P. (2002). Macroflux microprojection array patch technology: a new and efficient approach for intracutaneous immunization. *Pharm. Res.*, (19) pp. 63–70.

Meyer, W., Schwarz, R., & Neurand, K. (1978). The skin of domestic mammals as a model for the human skin, with special reference to the domestic pig. *Curr. Probl. Dermatol.*, (7) pp. 39–52.

Milewski, M., Brogden, N., & Stinchcomb, A. (2010). Current aspects of formulation efforts and pore lifetime related to microneedle treatment of skin. *J Drug Targ*, (7) pp. 617–629.

Mitragotri, S. (2006). Innovation–Current status and future prospects of needle-free liquid jet injectors. *Nat. Rev. Drug Discov.*, (5) pp. 543–548.

Norman, J., & Strasinger, C. (2016). Scientific Considerations for Microneedle Drug Products: Product Development, Manufacturing and Quality Control. *Fourth International Conference on Microneedles.* London, England: GSK House.

Norman, J., Arya, J., McClain, M., Frew, P., Meltzer, M., & Prausnitz, M. (2014). Microneedle patches: usability and acceptability for self-vaccination against influenza. *Vaccine*, (32) pp. 1856–1862.

Norman, J., Brown, M., Raviele, N., Prausnitz, M., & Felner, E. (2013). Faster pharmacokinetics and increased patient acceptance of intradermal insulin delivery using a single hollow microneedle in children and adolescents with type 1 diabetes. *Pediatr. Diabetes*, (14) pp. 459–465.

Olatunji, O., Das, D., Garland, M., Belaid, L., & Donnelly, R. (2013). Influence of array interspacing on the force required for successful microneedle skin penetration: theoretical and practice approaches. *Journal of Pharmaceutical Sciences*, 102(4) pp. 1209–1221.

Prow, T., Chen, X., Prow, N., Fernando, G., Tan, C., Raphael, A., Chang, D., Ruutu, M., Jenkins, D., Pyke, A., Crichton, M., Raphaelli, K., Goh, L., Frazer, I., Roberts, M., Gardner, J., Khromykh, A., Suhrbier, A., Hall, R., & Kendall, M. A. (2010). Nanopatch-targeted skin vaccination against West Nile virus and Chikungunya virus in mice. *Small*, (6) pp. 1776–1784.

Quan, F., Kim, Y., Compans, R., & Prausnitz, M. (2013). Dose sparing enabled by skin immunization with influenza virus-like particle vaccine using microneedles. *Journal of Controlled Release*, (147) pp. 326–332.

Ranamukhaarachchi, S., Hafeli, U., & Stoeber, B. (2014). Development of an artificial skin model for microneedle insertion profiling. *Third International Conference on Microneedles* (p. 37). Baltimore, MD: U of MD, School of Pharmacy.

Rouphael, N., Paine, M., Mosley, R., Henry, S., McAllister, D., Kalluri, H., Pewin, W., Frew, P., Yu, T., Thornburg, N., Kabbani, S., Lai, L., Vassilieva, E., Skountzou, I., Compans, R., Mulligan, M., & Prausnitz, M. (2017). The safety, immunogenicity, and acceptability of inactivated influenza vaccine delivered by microneedle path (TIV-MNP 2015): a randomised, partly blinded, placebo-controlled phase 1 trial. *Lancet*, (390) pp 649–658.

Schipper, P., van der Maaden, K., Groeneveld, V., Ruigrok, M., Romeijn, S., Uleman, S., Oomens, C., Kersten, G., Jiskoot, W., & Bouwstra, J. (2017). Diphtheria toxoid and N-trimethyl chitosan layer-by-layer coated pH-sensitive microneedles induce potent immune responses upon dermal vaccination in mice. *J. Contr. Release*, (262) pp. 28–36.

Seok, H., Noh, J., Lee, D., Kim, S., Song, C., & Kim, Y. (2017). Effective humoral immune response for a H1N1 DNA vaccine delivered to the skin by microneedles coated with PLGA-based cationic nanoparticles. *J. Contr. Release*, (265), pp. 66–74.

Simon, G., & Maibach, H. (2000). The pig as an experimental animal model of percutaneous permeation in man: qualitative and quantitative observations – an overview. *Skin Pharmacol. Appl. Skin Physiol.*, (13) pp. 229–234.

Singh, P., Chen, G., & Worsham, W. (2013). MicroCor Transdermal Delivery System: A Safe, Efficient, and Convenient Transdermal System for Vaccine Administration. In *Novel Immune Potentiators and Delivery for Next Generation Vaccines* (pp. 233–244). US: Springer.

Spierings, E., Brandes, J., Kudrow, D., Weintraub, J., Schmidt, P., Kellerman, D., & Tepper, S. (2018). Randomized, double-blind, placebo-controlled, parallel-group, multi-center study of the safety and efficacy of ADAM zolmitriptan for the acute treatment of migraine. *Cephalalgia*, (38) pp. 215–224.

Strasinger, C. (2014). Scientific Considerations for Microneedle Product Development. *Third International Conference on Microneedles*. Baltimore, MD: U of MD, School of Pharmacy.

Tas, C., Mansoor, S., Kalluri, H., Zarnitsyn, V. G., Choi, S., Banga, A. K., & Prausnitz, M. R. (2012). Delivery of salmon calcitonin using a microneedle patch. *Int. J. Pharm.*, (423) pp. 257–263.

Troy, S., Kouiavskaia, D., Siik, J., Kochba, E., Beydoun, H., Mirochnitchenko, O., Levin, Y., Khardori, N., Chumakov, K., & Maldonado, Y. (2015). Comparison of the immunogenicity of various booster doses of inactivated polio vaccine delivered intradermally versus intramuscularly to HIV-infected adults. *J. Infect. Dis.*, (211) pp. 1969–1976.

U.S. National Institutes of Health, N. C. (2019a, Aug 5). *SEER Training Modules: Layers of the Skin*. Retrieved from National Cancer Institute: http://training.seer.cancer.gov/melanoma/anatomy/layers.html

U.S. National Institutes of Health, N. C. (2019b, Aug 5). *SEER Training Modules: Components of the Lymphatic System*. Retrieved from National Cancer Institute: http://training.seer.cancer.gov/anatomy/lymphatic/components/

United States Pharmacopeia – National Formulary. (2019). *<3> Topical and Transdermal Drug Products – Product Quality Tests*. Rockville, Maryland: United States Pharmacopeial Convention, Inc.

Verbaan, F., Bal, S., van den Berg, D., Dijksman, J., van Hecke, M., Verpoorten, H., van den Berg, A., Luttge, R., & Bouwstra, J. (2008). Improved piercing of microneedle arrays in dermatomed human skin by an impact insertion method. *J. Controlled Release*, (128) pp. 80–88.

Wiig, H., & Swartz, M. (2012). Interstitial fluid and lymph formation and transport: physiological regulation and roles in inflammation and cancer. *Physiol. Rev*, (92) pp. 1005–1060.

Wu, Y., Qiu, Y., Zhang, S., Qin, G., & Gao, Y. (2008). Microneedle-based drug delivery: Studies on delivery parameters and biocompatibility. *Biomed. Microdevices*, (10) pp. 601–610.

Yao, G., Quan, G., Lin, S., Peng, T., Wang, Q., Ran, H., Chen, H., Zhang, Q., Wang, L., Pan, X., & Wu, C. (2017). Novel dissolving microneedles for enhanced transdermal delivery of levonorgestrel: in vitro and in vivo characterization. *Int. J. Pharm.*, (534) pp. 378–386.

Zhang, Y., Brown, K., Siebenaler, K., Determan, A., Dohmeier, D., & Hansen, K. (2012a). Development of lidocaine-coated microneedle product for rapid, safe, and prolonged local analgesic action. *Pharm. Res.*, (29) pp. 170–177.

Zhang, Y., Siebenaler, K., Brown, K., Dohmeier, D., & Hansen, K. (2012b). Adjuvants to prolong the local anesthetic effects of coated microneedle products. *Int. J. Pharmaceut.*, (439) pp. 187–192.

# 7 Biopharmaceutics Aspects of Dermally Applied Drug Delivery Systems

*Tapash K. Ghosh*

## CONTENTS

## 7.1   INTRODUCTION TO DIFFERENT DERMAL DRUG DELIVERY SYSTEMS (DDS)

Development of dermal delivery systems (DDS) is one of the most exciting and challenging areas of pharmaceutical research. DDS fall under two major categories: (A) Transdermal delivery systems (TDS) designed to deliver an active ingredient (drug substance) across the skin and into systemic circulation, and (B) Topical delivery systems designed to deliver the active ingredient to local tissue.

While topical delivery systems range from solutions, aerosols, suspensions, emulsions, powder, gels, etc., TDS are mostly available as matrix and liquid or gel reservoir type delivery systems. However, with the combination of high permeability of the drug substances and choice of drug product formulation, a topical product can be formulated as a semisolid also for systemic use. Therefore, TDS can be matrix, reservoir and semisolid types.

The site of local action for topical products could be: External (on the surface of the physiological barrier), Internal (at and about the physiological barrier) and Regional (beyond the physiological barrier in adjacent tissues). A variety of prescription and over-the-counter dermal semisolid products are currently marketed as lotions, gels, creams and ointments mostly distinguished by their composition, thermal behavior and rheological properties. Based on these findings, new definitions and a decision tree was published by Buhse et al. in 2005 to assist in the determination of the appropriate nomenclature for a topical dosage form [1].

This chapter will focus on the biopharmaceutics evaluation of matrix/reservoir and semisolid type TDS for systemic use only which are described at Drugs@ FDA [2] and Orange Book [3] websites as topical or transdermal delivery systems (Tables 7.1 and 7.2). However, some commonalities in the biopharmaceutics evaluation do exist between the DDS for systemic use and local use, especially for the semisolid dosage forms.

## 7.2   BIOPHARMACEUTICS EVALUATION OF DERMAL PRODUCTS

Tests for dermal drug products are divided into two categories: (1) those that assess general *product quality* attributes, and (2) those that assess *product performance*, e.g., in vitro release of the drug substance from the drug product. Quality tests assess the integrity of the dosage form, and performance tests, such as drug release, assess attributes that relate to in vivo drug performance. Taken together, quality and performance tests are intended to ensure the identity, strength, quality, purity, comparability and performance of dermal drug products.

The United States Pharmacopeia (USP) has an advisory panel charged with developing appropriate product quality tests and product performance tests for topical dosage forms. Following regulatory approval of a drug product by the regulatory authority, e.g., U.S. Food and Drug Administration (FDA), the product performance tests are used to monitor the ongoing performance of the dosage form.

For information to the readers, USP general chapter *Topical and Transdermal Drug Products – Product Quality Tests* <3> provides information related to product

**TABLE 7.1**

**U.S. Approved Brand Topical Gels for Systemic Use (Transdermal Gels)**

| Trade Name | API | Dosage Form | Indication |
|---|---|---|---|
| Gelnique | Oxybutynin chloride | 3% and 10% Gel | Treatment of overactive bladder |
| Anturol | Oxybutynin | 3% Gel | Treatment of overactive bladder |
| Divigel | Estradiol | 0.1% Gel | Treatment of moderate to severe vasomotor symptoms associated with menopause |
| Elestrin | Estradiol | 0.06% Gel | Treatment of moderate to severe vasomotor symptoms associated with menopause |
| Estrogel | Estradiol | 0.06% Gel | Treatment of moderate to severe vasomotor symptoms associated with menopause |
| Testim | Testosterone | 1% Gel | Testosterone replacement therapy in adult males for conditions associated with a deficiency or absence of endogenous testosterone |
| AndroGel | Testosterone | 1% Gel | Testosterone replacement therapy in males for conditions associated with a deficiency or absence of endogenous testosterone |
| AndroGel | Testosterone | 1.62% Gel | Testosterone replacement therapy in males for conditions associated with a deficiency or absence of endogenous testosterone |
| FORTESTA™ | Testosterone | 2% Gel | Testosterone replacement therapy in males for conditions associated with a deficiency or absence of endogenous testosterone |
| VOGELXO | Testosterone | 50 mg gel | Testosterone replacement therapy in males for conditions associated with a deficiency or absence of endogenous testosterone |

quality tests for topical and transdermal dosage forms [4]. The chapter *Drug Release* **<724>** [5] provides procedures and details for drug release testing from matrix/reservoir transdermal delivery systems (TDS), whereas the chapter *Semisolid Drug Products – Performance Tests* **<1724>** provides general information about performance testing of semisolid products including the theory and applications of such testing, availability and choice of appropriate equipment and procedures for determining drug release from semisolid dosage forms [6].

The *product quality* attributes include the following: description, identification, assay (strength), impurities, physicochemical properties, uniformity of dosage units,

**TABLE 7.2**
**U.S. Approved Brand Transdermal Delivery Systems (TDS)**

| Proprietary Name | Established Name | Type | Indication |
|---|---|---|---|
| Butrans | Buprenorphine Transdermal System | Systemic | Management of chronic pain |
| Qutenza | Capsaicin patch | Topical | Management of neuropathic neuragia |
| Catapres-TTS | Clonidine Transdermal System | Systemic | Hypertension |
| Flector Patch | Diclofenac Epolamine Patch | Topical | Management of topical pain |
| Climara | Estradiol Transdermal System | Systemic | To treat vasomotor symptoms with menopause |
| Esclim | Estradiol Transdermal System | Systemic | To treat vasomotor symptoms with menopause |
| Estraderm | Estradiol Transdermal System | Systemic | To treat vasomotor symptoms with menopause |
| FemPatch | Estradiol Transdermal System | Systemic | To treat vasomotor symptoms with menopause |
| Menostar | Estradiol Transdermal System | Systemic | To treat vasomotor symptoms with menopause |
| Minivelle (Estradiol) | Estradiol Transdermal System | Systemic | To treat vasomotor symptoms with menopause |
| Vivelle | Estradiol Transdermal System | Systemic | To treat vasomotor symptoms with menopause |
| Vivelle-Dot | Estradiol Transdermal System | Systemic | To treat vasomotor symptoms with menopause |
| Alora | Estradiol Transdermal Systems | Systemic | To treat vasomotor symptoms with menopause |
| ClimaraPro | Estradiol/Levonorgestrel Transdermal System | Systemic | To treat menopause symptoms |
| CombiPatch | Estradiol/Norethindrone Acetate Transdermal System | Systemic | To treat menopause symptoms |
| Xulane | Ethinyl Estradiol/Norelgestromin Transdermal System | Systemic | Contraception |
| Duragesic | Fentanyl Transdermal System | Systemic | To relieve chronic or acute pain |
| Sancuso | Granisetron Transdermal System | Systemic | To treat chemotherapy induced nausea and vomiting |
| Synera | Lidocaine 70 mg/ Tetracaine 70 mg Topical Patch | Topical | Local anaesthetic |
| Lidoderm | Lidocaine Transdermal System | Topical | Local anaesthetic |
| Daytrana | Methylphenidate Transdermal System | Systemic | To treat attention deficit hyperactivity disorder |
| Habitrol | Nicotine Transdermal System | Systemic | For smoking cessation |
| NicoDerm CQ and NicoDerm CQ Clear | Nicotine Transdermal System | Systemic | For smoking cessation |

*(continued)*

## TABLE 7.2
## U.S. Approved Brand Transdermal Delivery Systems (TDS) (Cont.)

| Proprietary Name | Established Name | Type | Indication |
|---|---|---|---|
| Nicotrol Patch | Nicotine Transdermal System | Systemic | For smoking cessation |
| Nicotrol Patch | Nicotine Transdermal System | Systemic | For smoking cessation |
| Prostep | Nicotine Transdermal System | Systemic | For smoking cessation |
| NitroDisc | Nitroglycerin Microsealed Drug Delivery System (MDD-NG) | Systemic | Prophylaxis of Angina and Hypertension |
| Nitro-Dur | Nitroglycerin Transdermal Infusion System | Systemic | For prophylaxis of Angina and Hypertension |
| Nitro-Dur II | Nitroglycerin Transdermal Infusion System | Systemic | For prophylaxis of Angina and Hypertension |
| Nitro-Dur; Nitro-Dur 30 cm²; Nitro-Dur 20 cm² | Nitroglycerin Transdermal Infusion System | Systemic | For prophylaxis of Angina and Hypertension |
| Deponit | Nitroglycerin Transdermal System | Systemic | For prophylaxis of Angina and Hypertension |
| Nitrol Patch | Nitroglycerin Transdermal System | Systemic | For prophylaxis of Angina and Hypertension |
| NTS-5/NTS-15 | Nitroglycerin Transdermal System | Systemic | For prophylaxis of Angina and Hypertension |
| Transderm-Nitro | Nitroglycerin Transdermal Therapeutic System | Systemic | For prophylaxis of Angina and Hypertension |
| Ortho Evra | Norelgestromin and Ethinyl Estradiol Transdermal System | Systemic | Contraceptive |
| Oxytrol | Oxybutynin Transdermal System | Systemic | For treatment for overactive bladder |
| Oxytrol for Women | Oxybutynin Transdermal System | Systemic | For treatment for overactive bladder |
| Exelon | Rivastigmine Transdermal System | Systemic | For Alzheimer's and Parkinson's disease |
| Neupro | Rotigotine Patch | Systemic | For Parkinson's disease and RLS |
| Transderm Scop | Scopolamine Transdermal System | Systemic | For motion sickness |
| Emsam | Selegiline Transdermal System | Systemic | For treatment of depression |
| Androderm | Testosterone Transdermal System | Systemic | For endogenous testosterone replacement |
| Testoderm TTS | Testosterone Transdermal System | Systemic | For endogenous testosterone replacement |
| Testoderm; Testoderm with Adhesive | Testosterone Transdermal System | Systemic | For endogenous testosterone replacement |
| Salonpas Pain Relief Patch | 10% Methyl salicylate and 3% l-Menthol Transdermal System | Topical | For topical pain relief |

water content, pH, apparent viscosity, cold flow, adhesion, microbial limits, antimicrobial preservative content, antioxidant content, sterility, if applicable, and other tests that may be product specific. On the contrary, *Product performance* testing assesses drug release and other attributes that affect drug release from the finished dosage form.

### 7.2.1 PRODUCT QUALITY TESTS

Product quality tests generally do not belong under biopharmaceutics evaluation; therefore, they are not covered in detail here. Details of these tests can be found in the currently official USP 41 [4]. An outline is given in the following sections.

These tests are categorized under the following categories:

- Universal tests which are applicable to all types of topical and transdermal drug products.
- Specific tests which are applicable to a specific type of dosage form.

#### 7.2.1.1 Universal Tests

Universal tests (see ICH Guidance Q6A—Specifications: Test Procedures and Acceptance Criteria for New Drug Substances and New Drug Products: Chemical Substances, available at www.ich.org) are applicable to all dermally applied drug products. They include:

- Description
- Identification
- Assay
- Impurities

#### 7.2.1.2 Specific Tests

In addition to the universal tests listed previously, the following specific tests are considered on a case-by-case basis:

- Uniformity of Dosage Units
- Water Content
- Microbial Limits
- Antimicrobial Preservative Content
- Antioxidant Content
- Sterility
- pH
- Particle Size Distribution
- Crystal Formation [4*]
- In vitro Drug Release Test for matrix/reservoir type TDS (for semisolid dosage forms, in vitro drug release testing is currently not required for batch release.) [4*]

In addition, the following specific tests are applicable only for *Dermally Applied Semisolid Drug Products*:

- Apparent viscosity
- Uniformity in containers

The following specific tests are applicable only for matrix/reservoir-type *Transdermal Delivery Systems (TDS)*:

- Peel adhesion
- Release liner peel
- Tack
- Cold flow
- Shear

In addition to this physical testing, there is also Leak Test applicable to form-fill-seal-type (reservoir or pouched) TDS and a pouch seal test to ensure integrity of the packaged film/patch.

## 7.2.2 PRODUCT PERFORMANCE TESTS

These tests for dermally applied drugs fall directly under biopharmaceutics evaluation and will be discussed in the following section.

The degrees to which formulation and product design may influence active substance permeation through the skin are characterized by conducting biopharmaceutics studies. They include (a) drug release testing using a synthetic membrane and (b) drug permeation testing using animal or human skin. Each has advantages and disadvantages.

The results of drug release and skin permeation can together inform about the contribution of the formulation and the skin in controlling absorption.

A performance test for topical drug products must have the ability to measure drug release from the finished dosage form for a quality control purpose. It must be reproducible and reliable, and although it is not a measure of bioavailability, the performance test should be capable of detecting changes in drug release characteristics from the finished product. The latter have the potential to alter the biological performance of the drug in the dosage form. Those changes may be related to active or inactive/inert ingredients in the formulation, physical or chemical attributes of the finished formulation, manufacturing variables, shipping and storage effects, aging effects, and other formulation factors critical to the quality characteristics of the finished drug product.

Product performance tests can serve many useful purposes in product development and in post-approval drug product monitoring. They provide assurance of equivalent performance for products that have undergone post-approval raw material changes, relocation or change in manufacturing site, and other changes as detailed in the FDA SUPAC – SS Guidance for Industry [7].

### 7.2.2.1   In Vitro Release Testing (IVRT) of Matrix/Reservoir-Type TDS

IVRT is utilized as a quality control measure for TDS performance from batch to batch analogous to a dissolution test for a solid oral dosage form but generally with no clinical relevance. The IVRT methodology for Matrix and Reservoir Type TDS is well-described in USP 41 General Chapter <724> [5]. IVRT for Matrix and Reservoir-Type TDS is typically performed using specific, qualified USP apparatus: Paddle over Disk (Apparatus 5), Cylinder (Apparatus 6) or Reciprocating Holder (Apparatus 7). In general, it has been found that Apparatus 5, a modified paddle method, is simpler and is applicable for most of these dosage forms.

Given the complexity of the transdermal dosage form, changes in release rate can result from a wide variety of scenarios including but not limited to: changes in the source, type or quality of active and/or inactive ingredients, change in manufacturing process, manufacturing site, batch size, or equipment, shipping, storage, and/or age of the drug product. The selected method should be able to differentiate the release profiles of TDS that are different in regard to critical process parameters and formulation components.

When properly developed and validated, IVRT can serve as a quality control test for product performance during both pre-approval and product life-cycle phases of the TDS.

The final method would be adequate to support a batch release as well as stability specification. Examples of such IVRT method parameters include the selection of the equipment or USP apparatus, the choice of dissolution/receptor medium, the rotation or agitation speed, temperature, pH, analytical assay, sink conditions, use of a surfactant, discriminating ability and other such technical aspects of the test. Of particular importance, potential study designs to support an IVRT method's discrimination sensitivity may involve a comparison between drug release profiles of the target (reference) product and test products that have been manufactured by intentionally varying potentially critical manufacturing parameters by 10 to 20% outside the specified control limits.

An IVRT method development for matrix and reservoir-type TDS should focus on the rationale for the selection of the following (but not limited to) parameters:

- Equipment/apparatus
- Media composition and pH, speed, temperature
- Assay
- Sampling time
- Sink conditions, etc.

Once an IVRT method is developed, it needs to be properly validated for the following (but not limited to):

- Linearity and range
- Precision, accuracy and reproducibility
- Robustness
- Dose proportionality

- Discriminating ability to detect changes in:
  - o Excipient type
  - o Amount of excipient
  - o Size of batch
  - o Method of manufacture
- Selectivity and specificity
- Analytical
- Dependence of release rate on temperature
- Receptor solution solubility
- Apparatus qualification

The IVRT method validation report is not to be confused with the validation of the analytical (e.g., high-performance liquid chromatography [HPLC]) sample analysis method. The IVRT method validation report, instead, focuses on the validation of the IVRT method itself (i.e., the measurement of the rate of drug release from the TDS). The report should describe the validation of the analytical method's linearity and range, reproducibility, specificity, accuracy, recovery, precision, sensitivity selectivity and robustness. However, it is equally important to demonstrate the validation of the range and sensitivity of the IVRT method, itself, across different strengths of TDS. The selectivity of the IVRT method to discriminate similar or different release profiles for equivalent and nonequivalent strengths of the TDS product, the reproducibility of the IVRT method across different runs, and the robustness of the IVRT method to changes in receptor medium temperature, paddle rate or other method parameters are just a few items that assist in validation of the IVRT method. Ultimately, an appropriately developed and validated IVRT provides a practical method to monitor for variations in product quality that may affect the performance of the TDS and to verify the consistent quality of each batch of the drug product.

Based on sound scientific principles, product performance tests can be used for bridging pre- and post-manufacturing changes and as a basic quality control tool for demonstrating product similarity.

**In Vitro Release Acceptance Criteria for Matrix/Reservoir TDS**: To set the acceptance criteria for the in vitro drug release test, a complete drug release profile encompassing initial, middle and terminal phases should be considered by collecting data until there is no increase in drug release over three consecutive time points. The format and content of the data collection and reporting and rules to setting of the Acceptance criteria may vary among different Agencies.

Unless otherwise specified in the individual monograph, the requirements are met if the quantities of the active ingredients released from the system conform to Acceptance Table 1 under Dissolution <711> for transdermal drug delivery systems, or as specified in the individual monograph. Continue testing through the three levels unless the results conform at either L1 or L2.

### 7.2.2.2 In Vitro Release Testing (IVRT) of Semisolids

Product performance tests for semisolid drug products are conducted to assess drug release from the pharmaceutical dosage forms. It can reflect the combined effect of several factors as shown in Figure 7.1.

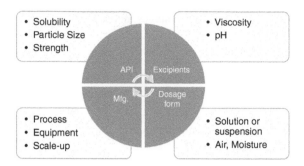

**FIGURE 7.1**  Several factors affecting performance of semisolid drug products.

It does not, however, directly predict the in vivo performance of drugs. The primary factor that impacts bioavailability and clinical performance are the barrier properties of the epithelia to which the product is applied (epidermal). Although product performance tests do not directly measure bioavailability and relative bioavailability (bioequivalence), they can be used as a quality control tool to ensure batch-to-batch product quality, and to monitor the effect of formulation or manufacturing related changes such as minor differences in formulation composition, changes in particle size and changes in manufacturing site. These changes may arise from changes in physicochemical characteristics of the drug substance and/or excipients or to the formulation itself, changes in the manufacturing process, shipping and storage effects, aging effects, and other formulation and/or process factors.

The IVRT methodology is well-described in USP 41 General Chapter <1724> [6] and SUPAC-SS guidance [7]; however, the validation of this performance test (which is not addressed in USP <1724>) is briefly discussed here along with special considerations for the IVRT method design.

At present, IVRTs are used in the pharmaceutical industry as product performance tests for creams, ointments, lotions and gels using several different types of equipment, including the Franz cell, the enhancer cell and a special cell used with USP Apparatus 4 (flow through cell) as shown in Figure 7.2.

In these methods, a thick layer of the semisolid product under evaluation is placed in contact with a dissolution (receptor) medium in a reservoir via an inert, highly permeable support membrane. Membranes are chosen to offer the least possible diffusional resistance and not to be rate controlling. The formulation can either be occluded or non-occluded and the amount applied may be a finite dose or an infinite dose. The amount of drug released from the formulation into a receptor medium maintained at a constant temperature is monitored over a period of time. The amount of drug released generally over six hours is plotted against the square root of time following the Higuchi's equation, as shown in the following equation, and release rate specifications are prepared around the variation in slopes and intercepts [8]:

$$M = \sqrt{2 \times Q \times D_m \times C_s \times t}$$

where M is the cumulative amount of drug released/depleted at time t per unit area of matrix ($cm^2$), $C_s$ is the solubility of the drug in the releasing matrix in mass unit per $cm^3$, $D_m$ is the diffusion coefficient of the drug ($cm^2$/sec) in the semisolid matrix and Q is the total amount of drug, both dissolved and undissolved in per $cm^3$.

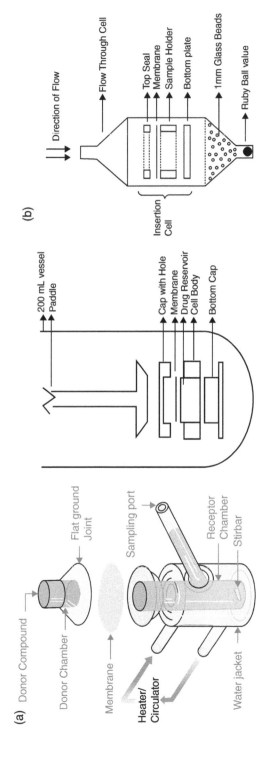

**FIGURE 7.2** Different types of diffusion cells.

The synthetic membrane, receptor media and the equipment should be validated for a particular formulation. The method used for in vitro release and the analytical method used for assaying the drug should be simple, reliable, reproducible, sensitive and specific.

**Development of IVRT:** The major components of the development of an IVRT are described in Figure 7.3.

An IVRT needs to be developed keeping in mind that the test should assure batch-to-batch uniformity and be applicable to all the batches that are (and will be) marketed. It also should be discriminating enough to detect product or process related changes that (may) influence product performance and where possible, should have proven relevance to in vivo product performance. An IVRT Development Report generally describes the rationale for the selection of the following (but not limited to) parameters:

- Equipment/apparatus
- Membrane
- Media composition and pH, speed, temperature
- Assay
- Sampling time
- Sink conditions, etc.

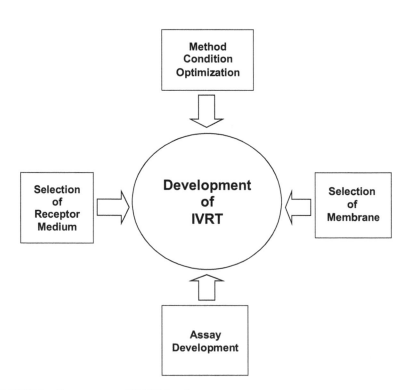

**FIGURE 7.3**   Components of IVRT development.

Once an IVRT method is developed, it needs to be properly validated for the following (but not limited to):

- Linearity and range
- Precision, accuracy and reproducibility
- Robustness
- Dose proportionality
- Sensitivity to changes in:
  ○ Excipient type
  ○ Amount of excipient
  ○ Size of batch
  ○ Method of manufacture
- Selectivity and specificity
- Recovery, mass balance and dose depletion
- Analytical
- Back diffusion of alcohol in the dosage form
- Dependence of release rate on temperature
- Differences in instrumentation
- Membrane inertness
- Receptor solution solubility
- Apparatus qualification

Overall IVRT can be utilized in various areas including product development, quality control, post-approval changes and other areas as mentioned in Figure 7.4. IVRT results are mostly used to bridge minor process and/or formulation changes and stability testing in approved semisolid dosage forms in which any difference in delivery rate is not expected. IVRT results may not provide meaningful results to evaluate large formulation changes, unless extensive validation is performed to select test parameters that ensure that the sensitivity of the test is meaningfully correlated with in vivo performance.

While conducting and interpreting results of an IVRT study, it is important to keep in mind that a failure does not necessarily signal that the formulation is clinically unsatisfactory (not efficacious or even different from the control product). Rather it should prompt one to look into the situation to identify the reason for the discrepant behavior as it may simply be an artifact of the test.

There are some concerns regarding IVRT including but not limited to: 1) IVRT is not clinically meaningful and therefore does not add value to existing specifications; 2) IVRT is imprecise and unreliable and therefore unnecessary; 3) IVRT expectations/criteria need clarity to define acceptance criteria for release and stability; 4) IVRT does not add value to existing specifications, therefore, IVRT specs will disrupt drug product supply, which in turn will harm industry's financial health.

While some of these concerns have justifiable basis, some may need a further look. While it can be argued that IVRT is not clinically meaningful and IVRT expectations/criteria need clarity, it is difficult to argue against IVRT as a quality test claiming that it is imprecise, unreliable and redundant. For a semisolid product development, a properly developed and validated IVRT can be sensitive to changes

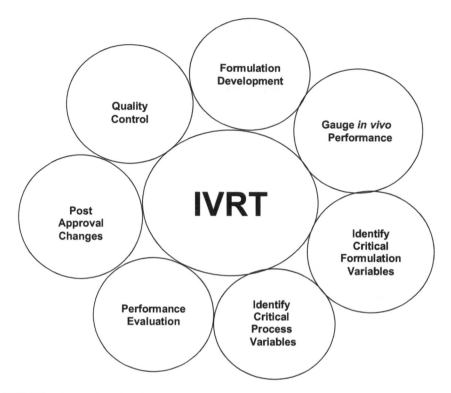

**FIGURE 7.4**  Utility of IVRT.

in Q3 quality attributes, and can provide performance verification to help mitigate risks associated with potential failure modes and as such adds value to quality control measures. It is important to emphasize that IVRT need not be perfect, or provide in vitro/in vivo correlation (IVIVC), to be highly valuable for quality risk management.

In summary, while IVRT is a useful test to assess product "sameness" under scale-up and post-approval changes for semisolid products, it is neither as convincing as that for in vitro dissolution test as a surrogate for in vivo bioavailability of solid oral dosage forms, nor alone, it can be a surrogate test for in vivo bioavailability or bioequivalence for topical products. Also, IVRT results should not be used for comparing different formulations across manufacturers. Nevertheless, it will be good for all semisolid products to have a properly developed and validated in vitro release method with appropriate specification for routine batch-to-batch quality control test of drug products. The same method can be used for future post-approval changes; this may also save time and trouble of developing a new method to bring back a discontinued product.

Recently, FDA issued draft guidance for acyclovir ointment where two options (in vitro and in vivo) are proposed to demonstrate bioequivalence (BE) [9]. According to the guidance, to qualify for the in vitro option for this drug product pursuant to 21 CFR 320.24 (b)(6), under which "any other approach deemed adequate by FDA to measure bioavailability or establish bioequivalence" may be acceptable for determining the bioavailability or BE of a drug product, all of the following criteria must be met:

1. The test and reference listed drug (RLD) formulations are qualitatively and quantitatively the same (Q1/Q2).
2. Acceptable comparative physicochemical characterization of the test and RLD formulations.
3. Acceptable comparative in vitro drug release rate tests of acyclovir from the test and RLD formulations.

The last two requirements state that generic product and its RLD need to be microstructurally the same (Q3) as demonstrated by the similarities of release rates, polymorphic form, particle size, viscosity, molecular weight distribution, etc. This advancement is deemed as a new initiative of BE assessment by the FDA relying on physicochemical evaluation and in vitro release test [9].

Draft Guidance on Cyclosporine ophthalmic emulsion [10] and Draft Guidance on Benzyl Alcohol topical lotion [11] also mentioned in vitro options.

### 7.2.2.3 In Vitro Skin Permeation Testing (IVPT)

In vitro skin permeation refers to the diffusion of active ingredients across the animal or human skin. Because the human skin is structurally and functionally different compared to the skin of other mammals, substantial differences in permeability characteristics may exist among skins of different species. Therefore, to characterize the rate and extent of transdermal or topical drug delivery, use of excised human skin is preferred. IVPT studies are routinely performed using two common diffusion cell systems, the vertical diffusion cell (VDC) and the flow-through diffusion cell, often referred to as a Franz cell and the Bronaugh cell, respectively. In conducting an IVPT, the formulation is applied to the skin surface maintained at a physiological temperature of 32°C and in a state of hydration after ensuring the barrier integrity of the skin (before and after application) through pulse dose of tritiated water, Transepidermal Water Loss (TEWL) or electrical resistance. The amount of drug that permeates over time through the skin is measured by collecting samples from the receptor phase at different time intervals and assaying the samples. At the end of the experiment, the amount of drug remaining on the skin can be extracted and determined.

Like IVRT, the following factors (including but not limited to) need to be considered during IVPT model development:

- Selection of the diffusion apparatus and the operating conditions like the receptor solution composition, stirring rate or flow rate, sampling time points, as well as temperature control.
- Source of the skin, skin storage conditions, choice of skin type (i.e., age range, gender, race and consistent anatomical region), skin thickness, the skin preparation technique (e.g., full-thickness, dermatomed, isolated epidermis) and barrier integrity.

The regulatory utility of IVPT in the approval of new or generic drug products in the USA has not been fully established. However, the importance of IVPT characterization of formulation performance is exemplified by its inclusion as an essential component in the EMA Guideline on quality of transdermal patches [12]. Section 4.2.6.2. of EMA **"Guideline on quality of transdermal patches"** indicates that in vitro permeation studies are not normally expected to correlate to in vivo release, but may be considered a valuable measure of product quality, reflecting the thermodynamic activity of the active substance in the product. In vitro skin permeation studies are principally used during product development and are not currently used for product approval and/or for routine batch testing. For the following hypothetical example, IVPT data from six different prototype formulations of a compound can help the formulator to screen formulation/s for further development and in vivo testing based on clinical relevance (Figure 7.5).

Franz et al. compared seven approved generic topical drug products with their corresponding reference listed drug (RLD) via IVPT conducted with human cadaver skin and Franz diffusion cell. The results suggested that six out of seven cases are in good agreement with clinical data, emphasizing the predictive power of IVPT, and its usefulness in in vivo BE studies [13]. In another study, Lehman and Franz demonstrated the BE of dermatological corticosteroids via IVPT with cryopreserved human skin and compared the outcome with vasoconstrictor assay results. The results showed that IVPT was more sensitive and less variable than pharmacodynamic study in assessing clobetasol bioavailability, which supported the application of IVPT in determining BE of certain topical products [14].

In summary, while IVPT may not be suitable for a routine Quality Control test, it is a good tool for formulation development and screening and has the potential to be useful in stability assessments.

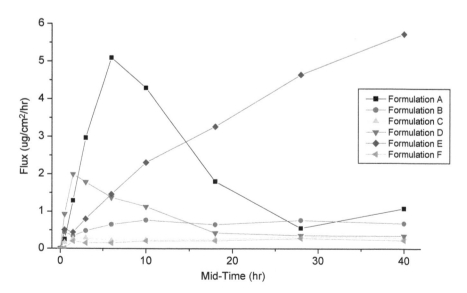

**FIGURE 7.5**   IVPT data from six different prototype formulations.

### 7.2.2.4 In Vitro Release Testing (IVRT) versus In Vitro Skin Permeation Testing (IVPT)

This section clarifies the specific differences between these methods. As the name implies, IVPT is a "skin permeation" study where a skin sample is mounted between the donor and the receptor compartment to conduct the transfer of dug molecules from the donor side to the receptor side. The source of skin is generally human cadaver skin; however, during early screening or product development, appropriate animal skin can be used. In contrast, an IVRT study evaluates the release of a drug molecule across a "synthetic membrane" for semisolid or directly in the release medium for matrix/reservoir TDS. Other than this basic difference, other characteristic features of IVPT are as follows: it is conducted with a finite dose in an un-occluded condition where the receptor solution is generally a physiological medium. The amount permeated can be measured in a nanogram (ng) to picogram (pg) range. The product applied on the skin stays dry as it does not come in contact with the receptor medium. An in vitro/in vivo correlation (IVIVC) may be established if the method can be validated properly. However, inter- and intra-person variability is fairly high when calculating the flux Profile ($J_{max}$, etc.). In comparison, characteristic features of IVRT for semisolids include application of an infinite dose in an occluded condition where receptor solution is generally a hydro-alcoholic medium. The amount released is generally measured in a microgram (µg) to milligram (mg) range. The product applied on the membrane may have a product-media interface. The method is used mainly as a quality control tool to evaluate batch-to-batch consistency, to bridge various pre- and post-approval product changes as per SUPAC-SS guidance and recently as an additional matrix (Q3) for approval of a few semisolid dermal products [9, 10, 11]. As release across synthetic membrane is measured, the calculated release rate (slope) is fairly consistent.

### 7.2.2.5 Other Performance Tests

Other performance tests including Dermatopharmacokinetics (DPK), Dermal microdialysis (DMD), Pharmacokinetic study (PK) and Pharmacodynamic (PD) responses have been described in detail in Chapter 2. A short description on them and some additional techniques have been described in the following section:

*Dermatopharmacokinetics*: Dermatopharmacokinetics (DPK), also known as "tape stripping" or "skin stripping" involves sequentially removing microscopic layers (0.5–1.0 micrometers) of the stratum corneum (SC) by repeatedly placing strips of adhesive tape onto the skin surface and then removal by a sharp upward movement, theoretically removing the uppermost layer of the skin. Due to serious consideration of this method to be a surrogate test for bioequivalence of topical products, the FDA did publish a draft guidance in 1998 [15]. In this draft guidance, the detailed methodology and calculation procedure was explained. However, there have been issues and limitations surrounding this method including issues of reproducibility due to variability between subjects, operators and types of tapes used. Amidst all these limitations, the FDA draft guidance was withdrawn in 2002.

*Dermal Microdialysis*: Dermal microdialysis or DMD is a continuous in vivo sampling technique that is used to measure endogenous and exogenous compounds in the interstitial fluid (ISF) of the dermal tissue. The method causes minimal tissue trauma and involves the implantation of an "ultrathin hollow fiber," called a probe, that resembles semi-permeable membrane systems, at specific regions in the dermis. Dermal microdialysis has many advantages that could favor its use in determining bioequivalence. Since more than one probe can be used, and multiple skin sites can be studied during a study on a single patient, this can reduce the number of subjects needed to be employed in the study. Also, the DMD method can be employed to evaluate drug permeation across both normal and diseased skin and may have the potential to quantify a biomarker for therapeutic activity. Even though there are many advantages for the use of DMD, there are several limitations also [16].

*Pharmacokinetic (PK) study*: In the draft guidance for generic lidocaine patches in 2006, the FDA recommended a pharmacokinetic approach in BE establishment – despite the target being topical and not systemic [17]. Of note, the dosage form discussed in the guidance is not semisolid but a matrix system. Based on the fact that the plasma level of lidocaine is proportional to its presence at the site of action, and it is feasible to measure lidocaine in plasma, plasma level is recommended for establishment of BE. For other topical patches, in absence of measurable plasma level, methods other than plasma level are recommended. In summary, in some special cases of topical dermatological products, where the systemic absorption is significant and the drug level in plasma can be correlated with its presence at target organ, a PK study may be used to determine their BE.

*Spectroscopy*: In order to develop more noninvasive methods to assess BE of dermal products, spectroscopy study seems to be a suitable method in terms of safety, time and ease of application. Various methods such as attenuated total reflectance-Fourier transform infrared (ATR-FTIR) spectroscopy, near infrared spectroscopy, Raman spectroscopy, and terahertz scanning reflectometry have been employed to detect permeation of active drug across the SC. It is important to remember that not all pharmaceutically active drug molecules have quantifiable spectral properties. In order to use a specific type of spectroscopic method, the active drug molecule of interest should have distinct spectral features of intensity to differentiate it from the skin spectrum. This could very well be a limitation of these methods. Near-infrared spectrometry (NIRS) and confocal Raman spectroscopy (CRS) are two major advanced noninvasive in vivo approaches for real-time monitoring of drug penetration across the skin. However, both NIRS and CRS require that the molecule of interest should possess distinct spectral peaks with sufficient intensity. NIR wave is capable of penetrating the skin to a depth of several centimeters. Thus, by measuring the IR spectrum and combining with linear multivariate statistics, the drug diffusion through skin can be quantified. In addition, some NIR approaches are capable of real-time monitoring the rate and quantity of chemical penetration through the skin. NIR is superior to other methods due to its nondestructive, rapid, simple (without sample preparation) and quantitative properties; therefore the possibility of drug diffusion during scanning process can be eliminated, which is favorable for the analysis of volatile drugs [18].

Confocal Raman spectroscopy (CRS) has been used in research widely in the determination of SC thickness, water content in SC and effect of percutaneous penetration enhancers. Like NIR, CRS is a completely noninvasive and rapid approach, which provides real-time in vivo signal to measure the penetration of chemicals through skin. However, like other spectroscopic methods, Raman spectroscopy requires that there should be sufficient concentration and spectral intensity of active drug molecules of interest in order to differentiate the tested spectra from the spectra of the skin. Also, CRS can only determine relative, instead of absolute, concentrations of active drug within the skin. Nonetheless, when designed properly, CRS can be a noninvasive tool for dermatopharmacokinetic evaluation of topical pharmaceutical formulations [19].

Another type of spectrometric method that has been developed recently is terahertz scanning reflectometry. Terahertz (THz) imaging is a nondestructive, label-free, rapid imaging technique which gives the possibility of a real-time tracing of spatial distribution and penetration of drugs within the skin. It can quantitatively measure permeation kinetics and concentration profiles of drug molecules in the skin. The terahertz spectrometer is a powerful tool that has the potential to diagnose specific disease states as well. The machine is able to use frequencies from 100 GHz to over 30THz in order to receive topographic information of the tissue [20].

In summary, there is a need to have more noninvasive analytical methods capable of assessing dermal permeation and topical bioequivalence. The spectroscopic methods serve as a simpler tool to analyze and image skin drug concentrations within the dermis. However, validation of the methods to serve as a Regulatory tool needs further evaluations.

*Pharmacodynamic Responses*: A pharmacodynamic response can be used as a method for certain drugs to differentiate different formulations and to establish bioequivalence. Based on the published FDA guidance, the Stoughton-McKenzie vasoconstrictor assay has been used to evaluate the pharmacodynamic response for glucocorticoids that are used topically to treat skin inflammation such as atopic dermatitis or psoriasis [21]. The assay uses the correlation between the skin blanching produced by the topical steroid and clinical efficacy. Although this method may seem subjective, improvements have been made to accurately quantify blanching response by the use of a chromameter.

*Skin Suction Blister*: Suction blister is a procedure where one applies a partial negative pressure to the skin to disrupt the epidermal and dermal junction which results in a blister. The blister is consequently filled with interstitial fluid and serum, which may provide a pharmacokinetic compartment to determine active drug concentration of a topically applied formulation. The use of a hypodermic needle makes this method invasive. Concentration vs time profiles can be obtained also with this method if multiple blisters are raised on the same subject. Highly lipophilic and tissue binding drug molecules may limit this method to appropriately quantify drug concentrations [22].

*Skin Biopsy*: Skin biopsy is probably the most invasive method to quantify permeation of active drug after the application of a topical formulation. It is generally performed under local anesthesia. Therefore, the use of this method has not been favored for tissue sampling and analysis of in vivo drug concentration. Two forms of skin biopsies have been explored. Shave biopsy involves removal to the level of the dermis, and Punch biopsy involves tissue removal to the subcutaneous level. This method provides a "snapshot" of drug disposition in the various skin levels; however, it involves a lot of trauma to the skin [22].

In a nutshell, there are other methods that have been explored to evaluate performance and bioequivalence for topical dermatological products. Unfortunately, none except the vasoconstrictor assay for glucocorticoids has been accepted by regulatory agencies, such as the FDA, to serve as surrogate measures for bioequivalence and clinical efficacy. It will be nearly impossible to find a universal solution to evaluate performance and to demonstrate bioequivalence for all topical formulations. Instead, different methods may have to be used for different therapeutically active products. Until alternate methods are accepted by the FDA and other agencies, clinical studies still remain a gold standard to evaluate efficacy, safety and bioequivalence. Of note, recent Draft Guidances on Acyclovir Ointment [9], Cyclosporine ophthalmic emulsion [10] and Benzyl Alcohol topical lotion [11] did mention about alternate in vitro options which may open up the prospect for other in vitro options in future.

### 7.2.3 IN VITRO/IN VIVO CORRELATION (IVIVC)

In the absence of quantifiable systemic level, traditional IVIVC from topical dosage forms for local therapy is not feasible. For TDS (be it matrix, reservoir or semisolid type), establishment of an IVIVC may be possible. Transdermal dosage forms are designed for extended release; however, the drug release and permeability mechanism from these systems are more complicated than oral extended release dosage forms. Transdermal IVIVC generally uses drug permeability data whereas oral drug IVIVC uses dissolution data. In order to obtain in vitro permeability data, excised human skin or animal skin are used to conduct an in vitro test using a diffusion cell. Some studies used artificial membrane to conduct permeability tests. A few studies employed USP apparatus, including the use of Apparatus 5 (Paddle over Disk Method), Apparatus 6 (Rotating Cylinder Method) and Apparatus 7 (Reciprocating Holder Method) as described in USP General Chapter <724> describing Drug Release for transdermal systems (TDS) and other dosage forms to obtain drug release data from TDS [5]. However, drug release data might not be appropriate to be used to simulate the process of in vivo drug penetration through the skin.

Difficulties for transdermal IVIVC in humans might come from intra- and interpersonal skin permeability variability. Also, permeability of the skin at different anatomical sites might be different. Generally difference in the permeability based on race, gender and age (except not fully matured neonatal skin which may have higher permeability) is not usual [23]. Besides the known fact that different types of molecules (hydrophilic vs hydrophobic) might have different permeability pathways across skin, the same molecule may permeate differently across animal skin and human skin. This can bring problems for IVIVC if animal skin is used to replace human skin for in vitro permeability tests. So far, porcine ear skin is shown to be the best animal skin as a surrogate of human skin to conduct in vitro permeability tests because of its structural resemblance to human skin [24]. In spite of these potential issues to establish IVIVC for transdermal products, it may still be possible to develop correlation between in vitro permeability and in vivo absorption for some products if the best approaches and test conditions are carefully chosen as described by some noteworthy works in the following section.

In the work reported by Venkateschwaran on the development of transdermal testosterone (Androderm ®) and estradiol (Alora®), the rate of absorption (when expressed as average cumulative absorption) profiles obtained in vitro for both drugs were strikingly similar to those obtained in vivo (Figure 7.6) [25]. Although the data for estradiol showed divergence in absorption after 48 hours, this difference was explained by the authors due to the conditions of the experiment in which the area available for diffusion in vitro was only 67% of the total TDS area. This led to a lower rate of drug depletion from the patch in vitro than in vivo since part of the patch was not in contact with the skin.

In another significant work by Franz et al., a total of 92 datasets were collected from 30 published studies [26]. The average IVIV ratio across all values was 1.6, though for any single dataset there could be a nearly 20-fold differences between the in vitro and in vivo values. In 85% of the cases, however, the difference was less than three-fold.

The correlation was significantly improved when data were excluded from studies in which the protocols for both studies were not fully harmonized. For harmonized datasets, the average IVIV ratio was 0.96 and there was a less than two-fold difference between the in vitro and in vivo results for any one compound, with IVIV ratios

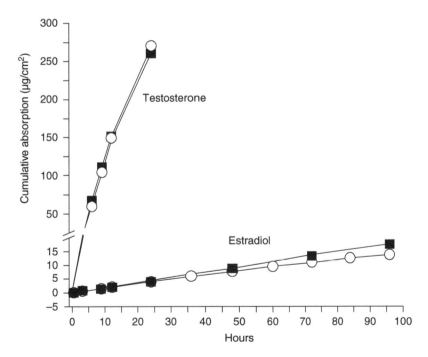

**FIGURE 7.6** Comparison of the rate of absorption of estradiol and testosterone from separate transdermal systems as measured in vitro (■) in excised skin and in vivo (○) in human subjects. The in vivo rate was determined by measuring drug loss from the patch [25].

ranging from 0.58 to 1.28. The dominant factors leading to exclusion of data were the use of skin from different anatomical sites and vehicles of differing composition. The authors concluded that percutaneous absorption data obtained from the excised human skin model closely approximate those obtained from living man when the two study protocols are appropriately matched [26].

### 7.2.4 ASSESSING THE EFFECTS OF HEAT

Heat is expected to enhance the transdermal delivery of various drugs by increasing skin permeability, body fluid circulation, blood vessel wall permeability, rate-limiting membrane permeability, and drug solubility. Heat from external sources such as a heating blanket or sauna and potentially from a rise in internal body temperature due to strenuous exercise or fever, may affect the rate of drug release from the TDS. External heating also induces changes in hemodynamics, body fluid volume and blood flow distribution, which in turn may affect the absorption of drug into and through the skin altering the pharmacokinetics or bioavailability of a transdermally administered drug. Therefore, the impact of an elevated temperature on the delivery profile of TDS needs to be evaluated in a properly designed study. However, currently, there is no standard in vitro test method to evaluate and compare the performance of TDS under the influence of elevated temperature. Therefore, the applicant of a regulatory submission should contact the appropriate Regulatory Agency to seek help in designing such a study.

## 7.3 BIOWAIVERS

### 7.3.1 BIOWAIVERS FOR THE MATRIX/RESERVOIR TRANSDERMAL DELIVERY SYSTEMS (TDS)

As per Title 21 of the Code of Federal Regulations (CFR) Part 320 Section 320.22 (i.e., 21 CFR 320.22), the term biowaiver refers to a regulatory waiver of the requirement for evidence of in vivo bioavailability (BA) or bioequivalence (BE). A biowaiver for a TDS generally refers to granting waiver for different size and strength of a particular TDS. However, biowaiver may not be applicable for all transdermal systems. For example, in reservoir or semisolid systems in which varying strengths of a product are dependent on differing concentration of drug in the reservoir, a change in surface area may not exhibit dose proportionality. Conversely, for matrix-type systems, one or more lower strengths can sometimes be granted a waiver as long as the different strengths of the transdermal products can be manufactured from the same laminate and the strengths are proportional to surface area. In this case, various strengths are considered proportionally similar in their active and inactive ingredients and it is assumed that the change in bioavailability is proportional to the change in the TDS size. Therefore, acceptable results from the proposed pivotal BA/BE study from the highest strength in combination with in vitro drug release profile comparison studies demonstrating similarity (using the f2 approach) to the highest strength typically support such biowaiver requests. The principles of modified-release dosage forms are typically applied for matrix type transdermal products in terms of demonstrating in vitro release profile similarity requirements [27] provided that a discriminating IVRT method has been properly developed and that all batches manufactured are of adequate and consistent quality [28].

A biowaiver may be for pre- and post-approval site and minor process related changes. However, formulation changes, such as a change in adhesive or adhesive supplier, generally require special consideration because even slight modifications in a formulation can change adhesion, irritation and potentially the delivery of the drug substance. In comparative BA/BE studies, the systemic exposure profile of a reference drug product (pre-change) is compared to that of a test drug product (post-change). The regulatory definitions and the procedures for determining the BA or BE of drug products are provided in Subparts A and B, respectively, of 21 CFR 320. For the products to demonstrate equivalent BA or BE, the active drug ingredient or active moiety in the test product must exhibit the same rate and extent of absorption as the reference drug product.

### 7.3.2 BIOWAIVERS FOR THE TOPICAL SEMISOLID DERMAL PRODUCTS

The onset, duration and magnitude of therapeutic response for any semisolid formulation depend on the relative efficiency of three sequential processes: release of the active drug substance from the dosage form, penetration/diffusion of the drug through the stratum corneum and other layers of skin, and finally eliciting the desired pharmacological effect at the site of action. The variability associated with these processes give rise to challenges in the determination of bioequivalence (BE) of semisolid products for both systemic and local use. Therefore, biowaiver requests for the semisolid products (except for solution, e.g., eye drop solutions, nasal spray solutions or cutaneous solutions) are not that common as different strengths (e.g., 1% vs 5% API) of the product do not generally produce linear pharmacokinetics (PK), or pharmacodynamic (PD) relationship for semisolid products (for local as well as systemic formulations). However, a biowaiver may be requested for pre- and post-approval site and/or process and/or formulation changes based on IVRT data which will be subjected to the Agency's review.

In the absence of a measurable systemic level of the active ingredient, measurement of bioavailability at the site of action of a semisolid product for local action is not feasible most of the time due to absence of a standardized technique (unlike systemic pharmacokinetic measurement from a transdermal product). Therefore, clinical trials are mostly used to demonstrate therapeutic equivalence for topical products; however, other models as described in the previous section may be used to provide convincing evidence to predict therapeutic equivalence, if adequately validated with accuracy, sensitivity, reproducibility and robustness.

Therefore, development of acceptable generic formulations of topical products by the pharmaceutical industry and their approval by regulatory authorities remains a hurdle.

In the USA, a generic product is required to be both pharmaceutically equivalent (PE) and bioequivalent (BE). Currently, comparative clinical endpoint trials are used to establish BE for most local dermatological drug products except for glucocorticoids which are tested via an established pharmacodynamic test [21]. These trials with a large number of patients are often tedious, expensive and associated with a high degree of variability and low sensitivity to formulation factors. As a result, they often turn out to be less efficient and in some cases not conclusive. Of note, the FDA has recently issued three draft guidances for generic acyclovir ointment [9], Cyclosporine ophthalmic emulsion [10] and Benzyl Alcohol topical lotion [11] respectively where alternate in vitro options to establish BE relying on comparative physicochemical evaluation of topical semisolids and in vitro release (IVR) testing have been described.

### 7.3.3 Concept of Topical Classification System (TCS) Based Biowaivers for the Topical Semisolid Dermal Products

Keeping in vitro option to establish BE in mind and using the concept of the Biopharmaceutics Classification System (BCS) for immediate release solid oral dosage form, recently the concept of developing a "Topical Drug Classification System (TCS)" has been proposed in the literature by Shah et al. (Figure 7.7) [29].

In parallel to BCS which is based on the properties of the active pharmaceutical ingredient (API), its aqueous solubility and intestinal permeability [30], TCS has been proposed by the authors of the article to grant biowaivers for topical semisolid dosage forms as per the schematics described in Figure 7.8.

The concept of TCS is based on science-based principles of SUPAC-SS [7] combined with the use of IVR methods. It utilized qualitative and quantitative equivalence of composition (Q1 and Q2) and on the similarity of IVR rates (as estimator of microstructural sameness, Q3) between a generic product and RLD. The IVR (Q3) reflects the microstructure, arrangement of the matter and the state of aggregation of the dosage form. According to 21 CFR 314.94, for topical dosage forms, apart from being in the same dosage form with the same API concentration, the generic product will need to have the same excipients and be qualitatively (Q1) and quantitatively (Q2) the same as the RLD in terms of both active and excipients. The authors of the article hypothesized that if all three parameters, Q1, Q2 and Q3, are the same

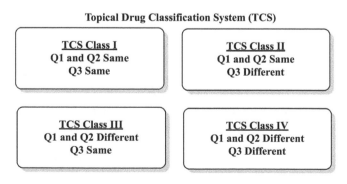

**FIGURE 7.7**  Topical drug classification system, TCS forms proposed by Shah et al. (Redrawn from Ref 29.)

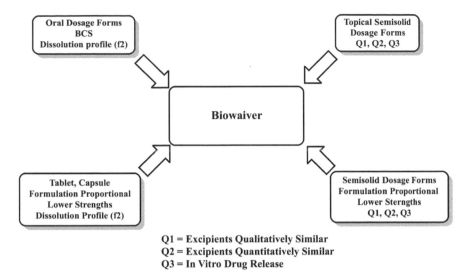

Q1 = Excipients Qualitatively Similar
Q2 = Excipients Quantitatively Similar
Q3 = In Vitro Drug Release

**FIGURE 7.8** Schematics of biowaiver for oral immediate release and topical semisolid dosage forms proposed by Shah et al. (Redrawn from Ref 29.)

between the RLD and the generic product, the generic product may be suitable for a biowaiver. If they are not the same, then of course, biowaiver cannot be granted and additional studies or a biostudy will be required. Using these scientific principles, a decision tree (Figure 7.9) in granting biowaivers for topical dosage forms is proposed by the authors Shah et al. [29].

TCS may facilitate generic product development, reduce the regulatory burden, assure product quality and ultimately availability of topical semisolid generic products to patients and consumers at a more reasonable cost. However, it needs to be emphasized that the concept is still in its infancy and needs further research and validation. As of now, it is purely a concept proposed by the authors Shah et al. [29]. The FDA and/or any other regulatory body has not vetted on it.

European Medicines Agency (EMA) published a "Concept paper on the development of a guideline on quality and equivalence of topical products" aimed to develop a systematic approach to describe methods or combinations of methods for the prediction of therapeutic equivalence. According to EMA, the new guideline should address the quality requirements of topical products, containing new or known active substances, throughout their marketing life cycle [31]. It also proposed that the guideline should consider the application of an extended pharmaceutical equivalence with alternative in vitro and in vivo models and methods to predict therapeutic equivalence with reference to medicinal products, in lieu of therapeutic equivalence studies in patients. A concept of extended pharmaceutical equivalence could be developed based on appropriate comparative quality data with the relevant reference topical product, including qualitative and quantitative composition, microstructure, physical properties, product performance and administration and additional measures. The additional measures of equivalence currently available include

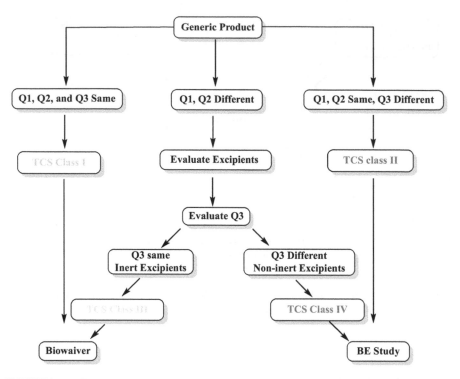

**FIGURE 7.9** Proposed decision tree in granting biowaivers for topical dosage forms by Shah et al. (Redrawn from Ref 29.)

in vitro drug release through an artificial membrane and/or human skin membrane to determine the rate and extent of drug release or permeation, in vivo tape stripping to determine dermatopharmacokinetics and possibly microdialysis. Furthermore, when drug absorption to the blood compartment from the site of application is sufficiently high, then comparative pharmacokinetic studies should be supportive of equivalence. Other methods might also be valid for some specific medicinal products.

The scientific rationale as to how these methods may be used to support a claim of therapeutic equivalence needs to be developed, taking account of the site of action of the active substance(s). The advantages and disadvantages of each method, considering method limitations, variability, sensitivity and discrimination power, need to be evaluated [32].

As mentioned earlier, the FDA's draft guidances for generic acyclovir ointment [9], Cyclosporine ophthalmic emulsion [10] and Benzyl Alcohol topical lotion [11] respectively are based on these thought processes.

Other useful parameters for the evaluation of matrix/reservoir TDS performance include but are not limited to in vivo skin adhesion, residual drug analysis, strength, anatomical placement, impact of heat, and skin irritation and sensitization, and they have been described in various guidances [33, 34, 35, 36, 37], literature [38] and other chapters in this book.

## 7.4 CONCLUSION

Whether it is topical or transdermal, effectiveness of the formulation depends on the release of the active drug from its dosage form to the skin surface. Once the drug is presented to the skin surface, either it stays mostly on the skin surface or penetrates through the stratum corneum to other cutaneous layers all the way up to systemic circulation to manifest its pharmacological action depending on the location of the disease to be treated. Therefore, development of the right product with the drug molecule with appropriate physical-chemical and pharmacokinetic properties as well as optimization of the product performance throughout the shelf life is very important. This chapter outlined the general product development principles and performance evaluation of different DDS mainly from a biopharmaceutics perspective. This combined knowledge can be helpful in developing a dermal product for the patients and the care givers.

## ACKNOWLEDGMENTS

The comments and technical help provided by Drs. Kaushalkumar Dave, Caroline Strasinger, Hansong Chen, Sameersingh Raney, Amit Mitra and Okponanabofa Eradiri of CDER, FDA are gratefully acknowledged.

## REFERENCES

1. Lucinda Buhse et al., Topical drug classification, *International Journal of Pharmaceutics*, vol. 295, pp. 101–112, 2005.
2. U.S. Food & Drug Administration, n.d. Drugs@FDA:FDA Approved Drug Products (www.accessdata.fda.gov/scripts/cder/daf/).
3. U.S. Food & Drug Administration, n.d. Approved Drug Products with Therapeutic Equivalence Evaluations – OrangeBook (www.fda.gov/Drugs/InformationOnDrugs/ucm129662.htm).
4. *Chapter <3> Topical and Transdermal Drug Products – Product Quality Tests (USP 41–NF 36; *PF 44 (5)).*
5. *USP 41 Chapter <724> Drug Release for transdermal systems (TDS) and other dosage forms (USP 41 – NF36).*
6. *USP 41 Chapter <1724> Topical Drug Products – Performance Tests (USP 41 – NF36).*
7. SUPAC-SS, 1997. US Department of Health and Human Services, Food and Drug Administration. Guidance for Industry. SUPAC-SS. Nonsterile semisolid dosage forms. Scale-up and post approval changes. Chemistry, manufacturing and controls. In vitro release testing and in vivo bioequivalence documentation (www.fda.gov/downloads/drugs/guidances/ucm070930.pdf).
8. T. Higuchi, Rate of release of medicaments from ointment bases containing drugs in suspension, *J. Pharm. Sci.*, vol. 50, pp. 874–875, 1961.
9. U.S. Food & Drug Administration, Office of Generic Drugs. Draft guidance on acyclovir ointment. 2012 (www.fda.gov/ downloads/Drugs/GuidanceComplianceRegulatory Information/Guidances/ucm296733.pdf).
10. U.S. Food & Drug Administration, Office of Generic Drugs. Draft Guidance on Cyclosporine ophthalmic emulsion. 2016 (www.fda.gov/downloads/drugs/guidancecompliance regulatoryinformation/guidances/ucm358114.pdf).

11. U.S. Food & Drug Administration, Office of Generic Drugs. Draft Guidance on Benzyl Alcohol topical lotion. 2014 (www.fda.gov/downloads/Drugs/GuidanceComplianceRegulatoryInformation/Guidances/UCM428198.pdf).

12. EMA, 2014, Guideline on quality of transdermal patches (23 October, EMA/CHMP/QWP/608924/2014).

13. TJ Franz, PA Lehman, SG Raney, Use of excised human skin to assess the bioequivalence of topical products, *Skin Pharmacol Physiol*, vol. 22, pp. 276–286, 2009.

14. PA Lehman, T Franz. Assessing topical bioavailability and bioequivalence: a comparison of the in vitro permeation test and vasoconstrictor assay, *Pharm Res*, vol. 31, pp. 3529–3537, 2014.

15. U.S. Food & Drug Administration, 1998, Guidance for Industry. Topical Dermatological Drug Product NDAs and ANDAs — In Vivo Bioavailability, Bioequivalence, In Vitro Release, and Associated Studies Rockville: Food and Drug Administration, Center for Drug Evaluation and Research (CDER) (www.fda.gov/ohrms/dockets/ac/00/backgrd/3661b1c.pdf).

16. R. Holmgaard, J.B. Nielsen, E. Benfeldt, Microdialysis sampling for investigations of bioavailability and bioequivalence of topically administered drugs: current state and future perspectives, *Skin Pharmacol Physiol*, vol. 23, pp. 225–243, 2010.

17. U.S. Food & Drug Administration, 2006, Office of Generic Drugs. Draft guidance on lidocaine (www.fda.gov/downloads/Drugs/GuidanceComplianceRegulatoryInformation/Guidances/ucm086293.pdf).

18. J Medendorp, J Yedluri, DC Hammell, et al. Near-infrared spectrometry for the quantification of dermal absorption of econazole nitrate and 4-cyanophenol, *Pharm Res*, vol. 23, pp. 835–843, 2006.

19. R Mateus, H Abdalghafor, G Oliveira, et al. A new paradigm in dermatopharmacokinetics – confocal Raman spectroscopy, *Int. J. Pharm*, vol. 444, pp. 106–108, 2013.

20. KW Kim, KS Kim, H Kim, et al. *Terahertz dynamic imaging of skin drug absorption*, *Opt Express*, vol. 20, pp. 9476–9484, 2012.

21. U.S. Food & Drug Administration, 1997, US Department of Health and Human Services, Food and Drug Administration. Guidance for industry: Topical Dermatological Corticosteroids. In Vivo Bioequivalence. (www.fda.gov/downloads/Drugs/GuidanceComplianceRegulatoryInformation/Guidances/ucm070234.pdf).

22. C Herkenne, et al. In vivo methods for the assessment of topical drug bioavailability, *Pharm Res*, Jan; vol. 25(1), pp. 87–103, 2008.

23. CR Behl et al., *Book Chapter: In Vivo and In Vitro Skin Uptake and Permeation Studies: Critical Considerations and Factors Which Affect Them* – Chapter 13 (pp. 225–259), published in the book entitled *Topical Drug Bioavailabilty, Bioequivalence, and Penetration* (V. P. Shah and H. I. Maibach eds), Plenum Press (1993).

24. U Jacobi, M Kaiser, R Toll, S Mangelsdorf, H Audring, N Otberg, W Sterry, J Lademann, Porcine ear skin: an in vitro model for human skin, *Skin Res and Technol*, vol. 13, p. 19, 2007.

25. S Venkateshwaran, *In vitro-in vivo correlation for transdermal delivery. IBC International Conference on Transdermal Drug Delivery*, Coronado, 1997, pp 15–16.

26. PA Lehman, SG Raney, TJ Franz, Percutaneous absorption in man: in vitro-in vivo correlation, Skin Pharmacol Physiol, vol. 24, pp. 224–230, 2011.

27. U.S. Food & Drug Administration, 2014, Draft Guidance for Industry: Bioavailability and Bioequivalence Studies Submitted in NDAs and INDs – General Considerations (www.fda.gov/downloads/drugs/guidancecomplianceregulatoryinformation/guidances/ucm389370.pdf).

28. C Strasinger et al., Navigating sticky areas in transdermal product development, *Journal of Controlled Release*, vol. 233, pp. 1–9, 2016.

29. VP Shah, A Yacobi, FS Radulescu, et al. A science based approach to topical drug classification system (TCS), *Int J Pharm*, vol. 491, pp. 21–25, 2015.
30. U.S. Food & Drug Administration, 2000, US Department of Health and Human Services, Food and Drug Administration. Guidance for Industry. Waiver of In Vivo Bioavailability and Bioequivalence Studies for Immediate-Release Solid Oral Dosage Forms Based on a Biopharmaceutics Classification System (www.fda.gov/downloads/ Drugs/Guidances/ucm070246.pdf).
31. Concept paper on the development of a guideline on quality and equivalence of topical products EMA/CHMP/QWP/245108/2015
32. EMA/CHMP/QWP/558185/2014, 2 December 2014.
33. U.S. Food & Drug Administration, 2016, US Department of Health and Human Services, Food and Drug Administration. Guidance for Industry. Assessing Adhesion with Transdermal Delivery Systems and Topical Patches for ANDAs (www.fda.gov/downloads/Drugs/GuidanceComplianceRegulatoryInformation/Guidances/UCM504157.pdf).
34. EMA, 2014, Guideline on the Pharmacokinetic and Clinical Evaluation of Modified Release Dosage Forms (www.ema.europa.eu/docs/en_GB/document_library/Scientific_guideline/2014/11/WC500177884.pdf).
35. U.S. Food & Drug Administration, 2011, Guidance for Industry Residual Drug in Transdermal and Related Drug Delivery Systems (www.fda.gov/downloads/Drugs/GuidanceComplianceRegulatoryInformation/Guidances/UCM220796.pdf).
36. U.S. Food & Drug Administration, 2009, Draft Guidance on Ethinyl Estradiol; Norelgestromin (www.fda.gov/downloads/Drugs/ GuidanceComplianceRegulatoryInformation/Guidances/UCM162407.pdf).
37. U.S. Food & Drug Administration, 2010, Draft Guidance on Fentanyl (www.fda.gov/downloads/Drugs/GuidanceComplianceRegulatoryInformation/Guidances/UCM162427.pdf).
38. GA Van Buskirk et al., *Passive Transdermal Systems Whitepaper Incorporating Current Chemistry, Manufacturing and Controls (CMC) Development Principles*, AAPS PharmSciTech (# 2011) DOI: 10.1208/s12249-011-9740-9

# 8 Quality and Performance Tests for Dermal Drug Delivery Systems

*Margareth R.C. Marques, Tony Bennett and Gregory Fieldson*

## CONTENTS

## PART 1 – QUALITY TESTS FOR SEMISOLID PHARMACEUTICAL DOSAGE FORMS AND TRANSDERMAL DELIVERY SYSTEMS (TDS)

### 8.1 INTRODUCTION

Defined test procedures and specifications for testing topically applied drug products are required to ensure that products are manufactured to an appropriate quality so that they are safe and efficacious when they are released to the market and remain so through their shelf life. Testing is performed on all components of the drug product (active pharmaceutical ingredient, excipients and packaging) but this chapter will focus on the testing performed on the topical products themselves and any in-process tests that are particularly relevant to their manufacture.

For pharmaceutical products, authoritative guidance on which tests to include in the drug product manufacturer's specifications are given in:

- Guidance ICH Q6A – Specifications: Test Procedures and Acceptance Criteria For New Drug Substances and New Drug Products: Chemical Substances (ICH Q6A 1999).
- Pharmacopoeias, e.g., USP general chapter <3> Topical and Transdermal Drug Products – Product Quality Tests (USP 2019a).

For products packaged in containers with non-metered pumps, for some tests (e.g., viscosity, assay, etc.), with the exception of uniformity in the container test, samples needed to be collected from the pumped-out product (USP 2019a).

### 8.2 UNIVERSAL TESTS

ICH Q6A (ICH 1999) lists several universal tests for all new drug products. These tests are discussed on pp. 257–261 with respect to their application to topically applied drug products. Regulatory agencies expect all of these tests to be submitted for the registration of a new drug product and often for major post-approval changes. However, for older topical products, some tests and specifications may not have been developed when the product was first registered.

#### 8.2.1 DESCRIPTION

It is a qualitative description of the drug product. This test is a simple visual evaluation to confirm that the product is not grossly unsuitable. Failures to meet description testing signify problems with the physical or chemical integrity of the product. Description testing should be performed on all routine quality control (QC) testing (batch release and stability) and as part of testing for process validation for post-approval changes.

The test should be performed under diffuse, uniform illumination (natural or artificial daylight) under conditions that reduce shadows and non-spectral reflectance to a minimum. For topical semisolids it is performed either by examination of the material in a clear, colorless vial held against a white background, or by examination of a small portion of the sample removed from its container and placed on a clean white sheet of paper. If more contrast is needed, a black background may be used. Liquids should be examined in a clear, colorless vial held against a white or black background. In each case, lighting conditions should be carefully controlled. Suitable apparatus is described in the section 2.9.20 of the European Pharmacopoeia (EP 2019a).

If the product is prone to change in color during storage, it is advisable to include the color test in the product release and stability specifications. The acceptance criteria for the color of the product should include a numerical specification and a validated quantitative color test method (Chang et al. 2013).

- Notable aspects for semisolid products:
  - Examine the external condition of the primary pack for damage or leaks in aluminum tube crimps or other seals.
  - Internal condition of the packaging for signs of product–pack interaction including:
    - Condition of internal lacquer or coating (discoloration, pitting).
    - Condition of product contact components such as latex bands or valves which may swell or become discolored or show other damage.
  - Condition of product within the primary pack including:
    - Color.
    - Uniformity of the product.
    - Signs of separation.
    - Flow of content.
    - Signs of crystallization or coalescing of particles.
    - Foreign matter (unknown particles or lacquer).
- Notable aspects for TDS:
  - Examine the external condition of the primary packaging for damage or absence of seal.
  - Internal condition of the packaging for presence of overlay, underlay or any other additional internal packaging components.
  - Internal condition of the packaging for signs of product–package interaction including:
    - Correct quantity of transdermal systems, when multiple systems are contained in a single primary package.
    - Adhesion of the drug product to the packaging.
    - Transfer of drug product to the interior of the package.
    - Leaking of drug product from the transdermal system.
  - Condition of product within the primary pack including:
    - Color and visual uniformity of the drug product.
    - Correct and legible printing on the backing of the transdermal system.
    - Shape and size, including the dimensions of the transdermal system, and the dimensions and slit of the release liner.
    - Attachment and position of the release liner.
    - Signs of crystallization or coalescing of particles.
    - Foreign matter (unknown particles).

    ○ Organoleptic properties:
- Organoleptic tests such as odor of the product may be important, particularly for products marketed more at consumers rather than patients. Often these tests are done alongside the Description test.

### 8.2.2 IDENTIFICATION OF ACTIVE PHARMACEUTICAL INGREDIENTS (APIs)

This test confirms that the correct active ingredient is present in the drug product. It should be performed for batch release but once confirmed there is no scientific need for ongoing identity confirmation, e.g., during stability studies. There are no unique aspects to identity testing for topical products other than noting that these products often contain many excipients which may interfere with the analytical technique and the test should discriminate between compounds of closely related structures that are likely to be present. Therefore, the specificity of the tests is an important part of the test method validation.

### 8.2.3 ASSAY (STRENGTH)

This test confirms that the correct amount of the active ingredient is present in the drug product. Assay tests should be performed on all routine QC testing (batch release and stability) and as part of testing for process validation for post-approval changes. Separation of the API from all the excipients in the product usually involves a chromatography technique (e.g., high-performance liquid chromatography [HPLC]) but titration methods and other techniques are used if they can be shown to be appropriately selective. The choice of detection technique for the active content is dictated by the chemical properties of the API with UV-Vis detection being most prevalent but fluorescence detection and others are used as well. For antibiotic products, microbiological assays are sometimes used as well.

- Notable aspects for semisolid products:

    Sample preparation is the key step for semisolid products. The most common sample preparation problem is extraction of the analyte from the sample matrix. Ideally, test methods should be developed to completely solubilize the entire product and then the prepared solution is chromatographed to remove interference from the excipients. This is not always possible and often sample preparation can involve liquid–liquid extractions or solid phase extraction.

    When developing assay methods, the robustness of the sample extraction should be evaluated by varying the conditions, e.g., solvent concentrations, extraction times for shaking or sonicating solutions. Methods should be developed to avoid ambiguous situations where solutions are cloudy or frothy so that it is unclear whether the active is completely dissolved or volumetric accuracy is impaired. If partitioning between aqueous and organic phases is used, factors which affect this partitioning should be understood such as pH and temperature. Particular care should be taken with the sample preparation of microbiological assay methods where sometimes a non-robust sample preparation is hidden by the normal expectation that microbiological assays produce more variable results than chemical assays.

The test method should define how the sample is removed from the primary packaging, e.g., squeezed out through the tube nozzle or the tube is cut open with a longitudinal cut and an aliquot taken after the contents are mixed together.

Due to the use of oils and other poorly water-soluble excipients, the analysis of topical products can degrade HPLC columns, so filtration steps may be used either prior to chromatography or using guard columns just before the analytical column. If filtration is used, recovery experiments should be done as part of the method validation.

- Notable aspects for TDS:

In additional to the same concerns related to the sample preparation as for semisolid products, the test method should define whether any additional sample preparation steps are required for the TDS; for example, it may be necessary to attach the TDS to an additional substrate in order to prevent curling during extraction. Typically assay is performed on a single unit.

Due to the use of polymers, oils and other poorly soluble excipients, the analysis of TDS can degrade HPLC columns, so filtration steps may be used either prior to chromatography or using guard columns just before the analytical column. If filtration is used, recovery experiments should be done as part of the method validation.

### 8.2.4 IMPURITIES (RELATED SUBSTANCES)

Impurities arising solely from the drug substance synthesis are not usually controlled in the finished product. Instead, they are controlled by the API specification used to test and release API prior to use in the drug product. Impurities that arise in the drug product either through the manufacturing process or from degradation during the life of the product or from interaction with the primary packaging are monitored (ICH Q3B (R2) 2006).

In terms of routine QC testing, impurity testing should be performed as a minimum during stability studies. If suitable process understanding has been gained which shows that the manufacturing process does not produce new impurities, it is sometimes possible to avoid registering impurity tests in the drug product release specification for use at batch release. Instead, confirmation that the impurity content is under control is demonstrated through the stability program. Skip testing may also be considered – this is where specified tests are performed on preselected batches and/or at pre-determined intervals rather than on every batch.

Thin layer chromatography has been used in the past for impurity testing as limit tests but modern expectations are for more quantitative testing so HPLC in particular is the most prevalent technique although gas chromatography (GC) is appropriate for volatile compounds. Titrations, UV-Vis spectroscopy and other non-chromatographic techniques are not usually selective enough to determine API related impurities.

Usually the chromatographic and detection instruments are the same as for the assay and very often the assay and impurity test is a combined method for topical products.

- Notable aspects for semisolid products and TDS:
  As with the assay, sample preparation is the key step in impurity determinations for topical products. The same considerations and precautions apply.
  In addition, for impurity testing in particular, suitable blanks are useful during chromatography to determine which peaks are related to the API and which arise from other sources (excipients or their impurities or artifacts from the analysis – mobile phase contaminants, sample solvents, filtration, etc.). Although the use of blanks is not unique to topical products, the high number of excipients in topical products, the use of internal standards and the vigorous sample extractions make them especially prone to interference from non-API related peaks from other sources of contamination.

### 8.2.5 Impurities (Residual Solvents)

This test confirms that any residual solvents that are known to be present as a consequence of production or purification processes are present at levels considered to be toxicologically acceptable (ICH Q3C (R6) 2016, USP 2019b).

An assessment should be done to consider the residual solvents present in the API and excipients as well as solvents introduced during drug product manufacture. The outcome of the assessment could be that residual solvent testing may be waived on a routine basis or be tested as part of a skip testing program (as described for impurity testing on p. 260) or must be measured for each drug product batch. Providing the residual solvents do not increase through life then there is no need to perform this test upon stability.

- Notable aspects for semisolid products and TDS:
  The same considerations apply to the testing of semisolid products and TDS as for other dosage forms. In addition, the precautions noted for related impurities and assays for topical products may be relevant.

### 8.2.6 Impurities (Elemental Impurities)

This test confirms that any elemental impurities are present at levels considered to be toxicologically acceptable. The major documents relevant to elemental impurities determination are the USP general chapters <232> Elemental Impurities – Limits (USP 2019c) and <233> Elemental Impurities – Procedures (USP 2019d) and the ICH Q3D(R1): Guideline for Elemental Impurities.

Metals are most likely to arise where metal catalysis is used in the synthesis of the APIs or excipients or where the excipients are mined.

## 8.3 SPECIFIC TESTS

In addition to the universal tests, the following specific tests should be considered on a case-by-case basis.

### 8.3.1 UNIFORMITY OF DOSAGE UNITS

According to the USP <905> Uniformity of Dosage Units (USP 2019e) this test is performed to ensure the consistency of dosage units; each unit in a batch should have an API content within a narrow range around the label claim. This test is applied to TDS USP <905> which now says "not intended to apply to suspensions, emulsions, or gels in unit-dose containers intended for external, cutaneous administration".

### 8.3.2 MINIMUM FILL

According to the USP <755> Minimum Fill (USP 2019f), this test is performed to ensure that products contain the labeled quantity of product. The average fill for a batch should have not less than the labeled amount.

### 8.3.3 WATER CONTENT

The need to test water content is generally formulation dependent. Many APIs are present in drug products as either hydrates or contain water in adsorbed form. Some APIs are sensitive to water content. The presence of more than the allowable limit of water may alter the microbial, physical and chemical stability of the product (Chang et al. 2013). Water ingress or egress may occur through semipermeable packaging but not through impermeable containers such as sealed aluminum tubes.

Gross changes in water content may be determined using gravimetric methods sometimes referred to as weight loss studies performed on packaged products. Direct testing on the formulation can be done using Karl Fischer methods.

- Notable aspects for semisolid products:
  For direct water content measurement, take care to ensure complete dissolution of the sample or, at the least, complete dispersion.

### 8.3.4 MICROBIAL LIMITS (MLT)

Microorganisms may affect the efficacy and safety of the product when used by the patient. This evaluation verifies the microbiological quality of the drug product by assessing the number of viable aerobic microorganisms and to demonstrate the absence of named microorganisms (screen for specified organisms) in non-sterile finished products. The microbial limits test is applicable to non-sterile products.

The MLT test may not be necessary for formulations that have both antimicrobial and antifungal properties. Note that the presence of an antibiotic in the formulation does not necessarily allow a waiver of the MLT test since it may be possible for the product to support mold growth. Waiver of the MLT test should be based upon accepted scientific justification, e.g., contains 30% or higher amounts of alcohol (ICH Q3C 2018) or experimental evidence, e.g., the formulation passes the requirements of USP general chapter <51> Antimicrobial Effectiveness Testing (USP 2019g).

The test methods and acceptance criteria are stated in the USP general chapters <61> Microbiological Examination of Nonsterile Products: Microbial Enumeration

Tests (USP 2019h), <62> Microbiological Examination of Nonsterile Products: Tests for Specified Organisms (USP 2019i) and <1111> Microbiological Examination of Nonsterile Products: Acceptance Criteria for Pharmaceutical Preparations and Substances for Pharmaceutical Use (USP 2019j).

### 8.3.5 ANTIMICROBIAL PRESERVATIVE CONTENT

Testing for preservatives applies to non-sterile, preserved multi-dose products. All preservatives used in the formulation must be assayed on release and stability. Acceptance criteria for preservative content must be based on the levels of preservative(s) sufficient to maintain the product's microbiological quality as challenged in the USP general chapter <51> Antimicrobial Effectiveness Testing (USP 2019g). Compliance with the compendial preservative efficacy requirements throughout shelf life should be demonstrated during product development and so would not normally be considered as a routine product quality test during commercial supply. In some cases, other analytical techniques such as HPLC or titrimetry may be used to assist in the detection of certain types of preservatives, e.g., formaldehyde donor preservatives.

- Notable aspects for semisolid products:
  The methods should be specific for the preservative and together with the specifications should consider what is the analyte being detected to avoid confusion if the preservative breaks down as part of its antimicrobial action. For example, the formaldehyde donor preservatives such as imidurea can be assayed for free formaldehyde or total formaldehyde depending on whether the method uses a forced hydrolysis step.

### 8.3.6 ANTIOXIDANT CONTENT

If antioxidants are present in the drug product, tests of their content should be established unless oxidative degradation can be detected by another test method such as impurity testing. All antioxidants used in the formulation should be assayed on release. It is possible to justify not assaying for antioxidants during stability studies if lower levels than at release are shown to maintain product stability by monitoring oxidized degradants in the related impurities test. Acceptance criteria for antioxidant content should be established. They should be based on the levels of antioxidant necessary to maintain the product's stability at all stages throughout its proposed usage and shelf life (USP 2019a).

### 8.3.7 STERILITY

Semisolid dosage forms for ophthalmic application and those used in open wounds or burned areas must be sterile. The sterility is demonstrated as appropriate using the test conditions described in the USP general chapter <71> Sterility Tests (USP 2019k).

However, take note that the USP states that a satisfactory result only indicates that no contaminating microorganism has been found in the sample examined in the conditions of the test. This is because microbial contamination is rarely uniform whereas the sterility test is only performed on a limited number of samples. For pharmaceutical manufacturing the sterility test forms just one part of an overall sterility assurance program incorporating sterilization and/or aseptic manufacturing. If the specific ingredients used in the formulation do not lend themselves to routine sterilization techniques, ingredients that meet the sterility requirements described under the USP general chapter <71> Sterility Tests, along with aseptic manufacture, may be used (USP 2019k).

### 8.3.8 pH

pH may affect many physical and chemical attributes of the formulation such as chemical stability of the API, efficacy of a preservative, viscosity and emulsion stability.

Testing for pH is applicable to buffered formulations, aqueous-based formulations and formulations where the API is sensitive to pH.

This test may be waived for non-aqueous formulations and for formulations with a low water content where the pH of the formulation has been determined not to be important. pH testing is performed on release and during stability testing.

- Notable aspects of note for semisolid products:
    When developing a method, consider diluting the sample in water. If it is necessary to test neat samples, there are specialized probes available that are geared towards the food industry but work well with topical formulations. Differences in pH probe model can affect results and can be problematic for comparison of results between laboratories.

### 8.3.9 Particle Size

This test is employed to monitor the size and shape of particles, in the formulation, and to check for agglomeration. Although it is normally API particles that are monitored, often the droplet size in emulsions is measured too.

Testing for particle size applies to formulations where the API is dispersed rather than dissolved. The particle size of individual API crystals/particles or agglomerates should be measured where there is the potential for them to alter size. The potential for change to the particles should be assessed during product development during processing and stability storage. For products where there is the potential for change, testing should be done at release and on stability.

In a suspension, particle size changes can affect the release rate of the API from the formulation. More simply, larger particles can feel gritty to the patient.

For products where the API is dissolved during manufacturing, it is important during product development stability studies to understand if the API precipitates to form crystals in the formulation. This should be avoided for new products or for existing products at least understood.

For emulsion products whether the API is dissolved or not, it may be useful to try to qualitatively assess the state of the emulsion to see if that changes through life.

Droplets may flocculate, coalesce or undergo Ostwald ripening thus changing their size or shape or bunching.

True API particle sizing may be done using laser diffraction techniques where the particles are dispersed. Most commonly, API particle size and/or droplet size testing is done using optical microscopy. Dimensions can be measured either manually using a microscope fitted with a calibrated reticule or using instrumentation with imaging and analysis software. Sometimes polarized light is used to help distinguish between API crystals and other particles or droplets.

- Notable aspects for semisolid products:
  - For laser diffraction techniques, sample preparation can influence the final particle size distribution. It is good practice to ensure that the sample preparation procedure is understood, well defined and robust to avoid atypical results. For example, over-sonication to disperse particles may in contrast impart extra energy to the particles causing them to aggregate.
  - Monitoring the microscopic appearance of the formulation after processing or through stability testing is a very good visual indicator that the manufacturing has gone as designed and of the physical stability of the product during storage. However, microscopy, although visual, takes skill and experience to identify adverse trends in the API crystal habit, e.g., dispersed particles or agglomerates, or the difference between typical droplets and "lakes and pools" of emulsions beginning to separate or the uniformity of the particles or emulsion. Figure 8.1 shows a typical topical

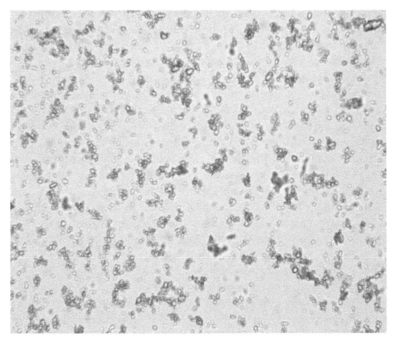

**FIGURE 8.1** Example of a microscope view for assessing particle size.

product microscope image. The challenge is to understand what the normal microscopic appearance is and then define that in a product specification in textual form referring to particle size measurements and crystal appearance for example.

## 8.4 SPECIFIC TESTS FOR TOPICALLY APPLIED SEMISOLID DRUG PRODUCTS

The following tests should be considered on a case-by-case basis for topically applied semisolid drug products.

### 8.4.1 APPARENT VISCOSITY

Viscosity is a measure of a formulation's resistance to flow and is an assessment of the rheological (flow) properties of the topical product. Only Newtonian fluids possess a measurable viscosity that is independent of shear rate, semisolid pharmaceutical dosage forms, which are non-Newtonian products, exhibit an *apparent* viscosity (USP 2019a).

For semisolid materials, the apparent viscosity is a useful holistic measurement to monitor the properties of a topical product. Changes in the manufacturing processing or the composition can affect emulsion properties such as droplet size or formation of three-dimensional cross-linked networks in gels. These physicochemical properties may in turn affect the rate of release of the active from the formulation and so affect its efficacy. On the other hand, and more obviously to a patient, the feel and ease of spreading of the product on the skin can also be affected. The apparent viscosity is a good QC tool for assessing changes to these physicochemical properties from batch to batch and through its shelf life.

The test method conditions should be well defined and adhered to for the measurement to be precise.

Apparent viscosity should be measured on release and stability. For manufacturing control, apparent viscosity may also be measured as an in-process test. However, it is important not to define viscosity specifications too tightly based on only a few batches worth of data until the commercial manufacturing and sampling process is well understood and embedded. It is useful to build specifications from a statistical assessment of the typical apparent viscosity values after 30 or so batches involving multiple manufacturing campaigns and input material batches.

It is also important to define the samples that are to be tested, as apparent viscosity can be different for samples from bulk manufacturing vessels to filled finished product which experience more shear through the filling process. Furthermore, the structures within the formulation may take days or weeks to form and can therefore produce changing apparent viscosity values so it is wise to define a window for the measurement from the date of manufacture.

Whereas the viscosity of Newtonian fluids can be measured with simple capillary glassware viscometers, apparent viscosity is measured using instrumental viscometers. There are several basic designs based on the rotation of spindles or concentric cylinders or cone-and-plates.

Spindles in particular come in a variety of sizes and shapes (discs, cylinders and T-bars). T-bar spindles can be rotated with a motorized accessory, which lowers the rotating spindle down through fresh product to describe a helical path (USP 2019l, USP 2019m, USP 2019n, USP 2019o).

- Notable aspects for semisolid products:
  The specification of apparent viscosity of non-Newtonian fluids such as semisolid topical products is tied to the measurement conditions. Aside from measurement temperature, the apparent viscosity changes with the shearing that has been applied either in the viscometer but also less obviously, but still importantly, during sampling or sample preparation.

  The apparent viscosity will change as the shear rate is varied. Thus, instrumental parameters of viscometer model, spindle type and speed and timing of the measurement have an effect on the measured viscosity and so must be defined. Although measurements can vary from measurement to measurement, it is often the stages between manufacturing and the instrument readings that are the sources of variation.

  Care must be taken to ensure that samples are taken the same way each time at the same sampling point and supplied to QC laboratories in the same type of container.

  The analyst must follow a defined sample preparation process based upon controlling each step of the preparation (e.g., is the formulation squeezed out through a nozzle or does the analyst slice open the packaging?). One common test error is the failure to remove entrapped air pockets where the spindle meets less resistance.

  If a product is to be tested by another laboratory (e.g., as a consequence of a site-to-site product transfer), it is important to transfer the knowledge of the entire chain from sampling to testing. One key consideration is that the instrument model and the spindle dimensions must all be the same to be able to apply the specification and test method successfully.

### 8.4.2 Uniformity in Containers

Poorly formulated or processed semisolid products may show physical separation during manufacturing processes and during their shelf life. This test is performed to ensure the uniformity of the formulation within the finished product container, e.g., within a tube or jar.

A visual test for homogeneity of the product may be useful, at least for an exhibit batch, to ensure no separation of phases, no synersis (extrusion of water from a gel [Chang et al. 2013]), and no changes in the appearance of the product. Figure 8.2 shows examples of phase separation and changes in the appearance of the formulation (presence of lumps).

Although uniformity is typically measured with respect to API content, uniformity of the preservative or antioxidant may also be pertinent, depending on the manufacturing process and nature of the formulation. Uniformity testing for preservatives or

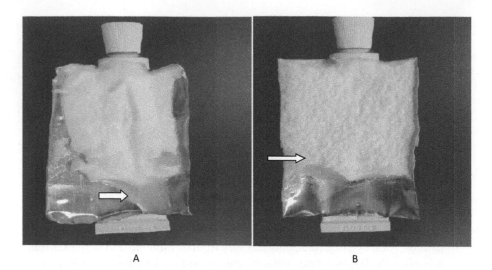

A                                    B

**FIGURE 8.2** Examples of deviation in the uniformity in the container. (A) Presence of phase separation. (B) Presence of lumps and phase separation. (© Avraham Yacobi & Satish Asotra. Used by Permission.)

antioxidants may be more common for product development and process validation rather than routine QC testing.

Non-uniformity typically arises due to physical separation of phases after storage or inadequate mixing during manufacture.

While it is important to be assured of the uniformity of the finished product at the time of batch release, it may not be necessary for it to become a product release test. Many topical products do not have a risk of physical separation at the time of manufacture, but may only start to separate during shelf life, particularly at higher temperatures such as ICH climatic zone IV and accelerated stability studies. Therefore, the requirement for uniformity in containers at time of release may be waived where initial product uniformity has been verified through process validation, continuous verification or historical data for product release.

Uniformity of content should be performed during stability testing although even then it may be waived if the formulation is a one-phase system that has no potential to separate through shelf life, such as a gel where the API is completely dissolved and is effectively in solution.

Within-tube content can be assessed by carefully removing or cutting the bottom tube seal and making a vertical cut from the bottom to the top of the tube. Carefully cut the tube around the upper rim, open the two flaps and lay the flaps open to expose the product. The exposed product is inspected for the presence of phase separation, change in physical appearance and texture, and other properties described in the product test for *Description*. Remove an appropriate amount of product from the top and bottom portions of the tube and perform a quantitative determination of the API in each portion of the product and evaluate the test results according to properly defined acceptance criteria. For semisolid products packaged in a container other than a tube, other sampling methods should be developed (USP 2019a, Yacobi 2010).

### 8.4.3 DELIVERED-DOSE UNIFORMITY IN METERED DOSE CONTAINERS

The test for delivered-dose uniformity is required for drug products contained either in metered-dose containers or in premetered unit presentations. The test for delivered-dose uniformity includes dose uniformity over the entire unit shelf life. The sampling should represent the initial, middle and final dose from the container (USP 2019a).

### 8.4.4 SPECIFIC TESTS FOR FOAMS

Foam formulations may require some additional quality tests such as foam density, foam stability, rate of collapse, delivery rate, pressure test and appearance of foam and collapsed foam (Buchta et al. 2017).

## 8.5 SPECIFIC TESTS FOR TRANSDERMAL DELIVERY SYSTEMS (TDS)

Transdermal delivery systems are formulated with an adhesive in order to maintain intimate contact with the skin and allow delivery of the desired dose of drug. Adhesion is a critical quality attribute of TDS, and they need to be designed to meet the following performance requirements:

- Easy removal of the protective release liner before use.
- Rapid adhesion to the skin upon application.
- Maintenance of adhesion through the duration of use.
- Easy removal at the end of use, without leaving residue, causing damage to the skin or any other undesirable effects.

In addition to these requirements, the adhesives must be able to maintain their performance over the shelf life of the drug product (Tan and Pfister 1999, Wokovich et al. 2006).

Testing of TDS can generally be categorized into tests of the adhesive properties, tests of the cohesive properties and other physical tests.

### 8.5.1 PEEL ADHESION TEST

TDS need to have a consistent and reliable adhesion, in order to maintain consistent clinical performance. This test measures the force required to remove TDS from a standard substrate surface. The transdermal delivery system is applied to the substrate in a controlled manner and is conditioned for specified time and temperature. It is peeled away from the substrate with an instrument that allows control of the peel angle and peel rate, and the peel force is recorded (Figure 8.3) (ASTM D6862-11, 2011). The peel adhesion test is repeated using a minimum of five independent samples.

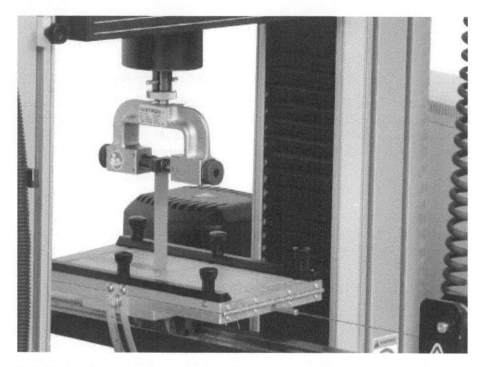

**FIGURE 8.3** Example of experimental configuration for a 90° peel adhesion test. (© Instron Corp. Used by permission.)

The product fails the test if the mean peel force is outside of the established acceptance criteria. The performance of different adhesive materials is highly varied, and there is no absolute relationship between the adhesion to standard substrates and adhesion to skin, and therefore the acceptance criteria is uniquely established for each product (USP 2019a).

### 8.5.2 RELEASE LINER PEEL TEST

TDS are most commonly provided with a protective release liner that covers the adhesive, and which must be removed by the patient prior to application. This test measures the force required to remove the protective release liner from the adhesive layer of TDS. The test sample may be conditioned using specified temperature and time. When possible, the transdermal delivery system is die cut to a uniform width for peel testing, but reservoir or form-fill-seal systems are typical run as-is. The release liner is pulled away from TDS with an instrument that allows for control of the peel angle and peel rate, and a peel force is recorded. This procedure is repeated using a minimum of five independent samples (ASTM D6862-11, 2011; Wokovich et al. 2010).

The product fails the test if the mean peel force is outside the established criteria. There are no absolute criteria for the release liner peel test; the acceptance criteria are uniquely established for each product. Generally speaking, the acceptance criteria are established based upon the usability of the drug product or peel forces at which deformation of the drug product occurs (USP 2019a).

### 8.5.3 Tack Test

Tack testing is used to evaluate the initial formation of an adhesive bond. This attribute may be correlated to the ease with which TDS are initially applied to the skin. There are several methods of tack testing that have been developed. Examples include the probe tack test and the rolling ball method. It is up to the manufacturer to decide which tack test method is appropriate for a drug product (USP 2019a).

#### 8.5.3.1 Probe Tack Method

This method measures the force required to separate the tip of the test probe from the adhesive layer of TDS. The test sample may be conditioned for a specified time and temperature prior to testing. This method uses an instrument designed to create a bond between the tip of a test probe of defined geometry and surface and TDS using a defined combination of force, time, temperature and probe velocities (application and removal). The test measures the time profile of the force required to separate the probe tip from the TDS adhesive. The integrated force and maximum force required for removal of the probe tip are recorded (Figure 8.4). The procedure is repeated for a minimum of five independent samples (ASTM D2979-01, 2009).

The product fails the test if the mean test results, either integrated force or maximum force, are outside the established acceptance criteria. The performance

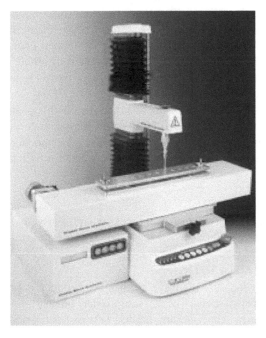

**FIGURE 8.4** Example of experimental configuration for a probe tack test. (© Texture Technologies Corp. Used by permission.)

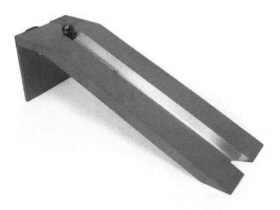

**FIGURE 8.5** Example of rolling ball equipment. (© Chemsultants Int. Used by permission.)

of different adhesive materials is highly varied, and there is no absolute relationship between the tack and clinical performance, therefore the acceptance criteria is uniquely established for each probe tack reference (USP 2019a).

### 8.5.3.2 Rolling Ball Method

This test measures the distance travelled by a defined ball on the adhesive layer of the TDS under defined conditions. The test sample may be conditioned using specific times and temperatures. The test uses a geometry designed to roll a ball of defined material, weight, size and surface, from a ramp of defined geometry and onto the adhesive layer of the TDS (Figure 8.5). The distance travelled by the ball on the adhesive layer is measured and reported. This procedure is repeated using a minimum of five independent samples (ASTM D3121-06, 2006).

The product fails the test if the mean distance travelled is outside the established acceptance criteria. The performance of different adhesive materials is highly varied, and there is no absolute relationship between the tack and clinical performance, therefore the acceptance criteria is uniquely established for each product.

### 8.5.4 Shear Test

This test measures the cohesive strength of TDS. It can be measured under either dynamic or static conditions

### 8.5.4.1 Dynamic Shear Test

Dynamic shear tests measure the force required to produce cohesive failure under the conditions of constant speed. The test sample may be conditioned using specified times and temperatures. The TDS are applied to a test panel and then pulled from the test panel at a constant speed (Figure 8.6). Dwell time, speed, type of test panel and sample size are controlled during the test. The maximum force per unit width

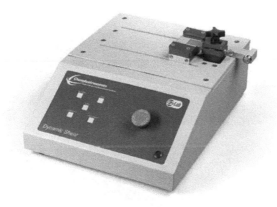

**FIGURE 8.6** Example of dynamic shear test instrumentation. (© ChemInstruments Inc. Used by permission.)

required to produce cohesive failure of the TDS from a specified area is reported. The mode of failure is evaluated to confirm that cohesive failure occurred. If another mode of failure occurs, the test result is not valid.

Dynamic shear testing may not be feasible for all TDS; the presence of multiple layers of adhesive in the system, the presence of a membrane or scrim, or the use of an emulsion adhesive system may result in the inability to achieve cohesive failure. TDS that are constructed with a peripheral adhesive ring or form-fill-seal TDS may not be suitable for this test (ASTM D1002-10, 2010; ASTM D3163-01, 2008; ASTM D3164-03, 2011; FINAT Technical Handbook, 2009).

The product fails the test if the mean test result, typically the maximum force per unit width, is outside the established acceptance criteria. The performance of different adhesive materials is highly varied, and there is no absolute relationship between the shear test and clinical performance, therefore the acceptance criteria is uniquely established for each product.

### 8.5.4.2 Static Shear Test

This test measures the time for cohesive failure to occur under conditions of constant shear force. The test sample may be conditioned using specified times and temperatures. The TDS are applied to a test pane at an angle of $2°$ from the vertical, and the sample is subjected to a shearing force by suspending weight from the TDS (Figure 8.7). The weight used, type of test panel and sample size should be controlled. The time taken for the TDS sample to detach from the test panel is reported. The mode of failure is also evaluated to confirm that cohesive failure occurred. If another mode of failure occurred, the test result is not valid (PSTC 107, 2007, ASTM D3654/D3654 M-06, 2011).

Dynamic shear testing may not be feasible for all TDS; the presence of multiple layers of adhesive in the system, the presence of a membrane or scrim, or the use of an emulsion adhesive system may result in the inability to achieve cohesive failure. TDS that are constructed with a peripheral adhesive ring or form-fill-seal TDS may not be suitable for this test.

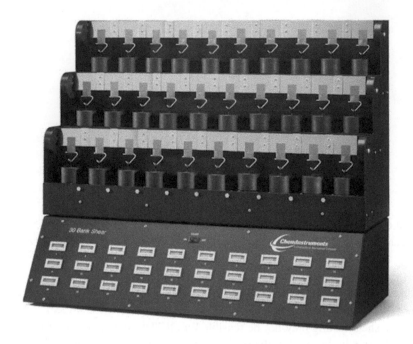

**FIGURE 8.7**   Example of static shear test equipment. (© ChemInstruments Inc. Used by permission.)

The product fails the test if the mean time required for cohesive shear failure to occur is outside the established acceptance criteria. The performance of different adhesive materials is highly varied, and there is no absolute relationship between the shear test and clinical performance, therefore the acceptance criteria is uniquely established for each product.

### 8.5.5  COLD FLOW TEST

Cold flow is the migration of adhesive beyond the boundaries of the TDS that occurs during product processing and storage. All TDS have the potential to exhibit cold flow due to the nature of pressure sensitive adhesives. A small amount of cold flow beyond the boundary of TDS is typical and does not affect the ability to remove TDS from the packaging material. When substantial cold flow occurs, it can lead to an inability to remove TDS from the packaging material and, in extreme cases, the loss of adhesive matrix and drug substance to the packaging components.

Cold flow is formulation or process dependent. Assessment of cold flow may be a combination of quantitative and qualitative methods. No single quantitative method has been identified to work universally for all TDS.

Qualitatively, appearance criteria can assess potential use issues caused by cold flow if systems are difficult to remove from pouches. Cold flow may be deemed unacceptable if release liners detach from the adhesive matrix during attempted removal from the pouch or if adhesive residue is transferred to the pouch after removal of the system.

A quantitative cold flow method captures the distance to which cold flow extends beyond the perimeter of the backing membrane. The product fails the test if the average or maximum cold flow is greater than the established acceptance criteria. A quantitative cold flow test of packaged systems does not predict any aspects of patient wear, as the test conditions are not related to wear conditions.

Several different cold flow tests have been developed. Examples include:

- Linear measurement of the radial cold flow using microscopy.
- Measuring the distance of migrated adhesive matrix at predefined and evenly spaced positions of TDS.
- Measuring cold flow by applying a reference plate in the size of the TDS plus the acceptable cold flow.
- Swabbing and stripping the migrated part of the matrix and determining it gravimetrically or by assay of the drug substance.
- Die cutting and punching out the original size of the TDS and determining the amount of migrated matrix on the outside.
- Overall area determining methods of cold flow using image analysis tools (USP 2019a).

### 8.5.6 Crystal Formation Test

Crystal formation or crystal growth of the drug substance or other excipients in the drug product during storage is a potential concern. Assessment of crystal formation potential should be evaluated using stability challenging studies such as temperature excursions, freeze/thaw, photo stability or crystal seeding during development of the product (Ma, Taw and Chiang 1996).

The relationship between crystal formation or crystal growth and drug product performance is dependent upon the drug product. Clinical and in vitro performance of some products may be insensitive to either crystal formation or growth, while other products may experience a change in performance following similar changes. The applicability of this test should be evaluated for each product.

Evaluation of crystal formation or crystal growth should be performed at release and upon stability. Crystal formation is evaluated by visual or microscopic examination of the product. The product fails if the number or size of crystals are outside the established acceptance criteria (USP 2019a).

### 8.5.7 Leak Test

This test is applicable only to form-fill-seal, liquid or semisolid reservoir TDS. Form-fill-seal TDS must be manufactured with zero tolerance for leaks because of their potential for dose dumping if a leak occurs.

In-process control methods to examine TDS for leakers or potential leakers are expected, in order to prevent incorrectly sealed products. In addition, testing of the packaged finished product is necessary to ensure the TDS do not leak over the shelf life of the product (USP 2019a).

### 8.5.7.1  In-Process Testing

The presence of leakage, or potential leakage, because of TDS manufacturing defects which may be the result of air bubbles, gel splashing or misalignment of films must be examined. Alternative methods of in-process testing exist. One such method is described on p. XX. The use of a process analytical technology to perform 100% inspection is desirable where feasible. It is up to the TDS manufacturer to decide the appropriate in-process test procedures to control for leakage.

- Visual Inspection.
  - ○ A specified number of TDS, defined based upon the batch size, should be randomly examined.
  - ○ Each sampled transdermal delivery system should be thoroughly examined for leakage.
  - ○ The product fails if any of the TDS examined have detectable leakage.
- Seal Integrity.
- TDS seals should be stress-tested to ensure that the application of pressure does not force seals to open, thereby leading to leakage.
  - ○ A specified number of TDS, defined based upon the batch size, should be randomly examined.
  - ○ Each sampled transdermal delivery system should be thoroughly examined for leakage.
  - ○ Each sampled transdermal delivery system is placed on a hard, flat surface and overlaid with a weight so that it is subjected to 13.6kg. The weight should be left in place for two minutes. Upon removal of the weight, the TDS should be visually inspected for leakage.
  - ○ The product fails if the number of TDS with a leakage after being subjected to compression by an external weight is outside the established acceptance criteria (USP 2019a).

### 8.5.7.2  Finished Product Testing

TDS may leak after they been sealed in the primary packaging material, as a result of the packaging operation itself or by user opening of the packaging. Therefore, TDS should be tested for leakage after they have been manufactured and packaged in their primary packaging material.

- A specified number of TDS, defined based upon the batch size, should be randomly tested after they have been sealed in their primary packaging material.
- Each sampled transdermal delivery system should be removed from the packaging and thoroughly examined for leakage.
- Each sampled transdermal delivery system should then be uniformly wiped with a solvent-moistened swab. Both the backing side and the release liner side of the transdermal delivery system should be wiped. The inside surface of the packaging material, including any packaging aids such as underlay or overlay films contained within the primary packaging, should also be wiped. The drug content of the swab is than assayed.

- The product fails if the total amount of drug recovered from the swab test is outside the established acceptance criteria (USP 2019a).

### 8.5.8 IN VIVO SKIN ADHESION TEST

Skin adhesion is a critical quality attribute of TDS for which there is no direct in vitro test that can be used as a quality control test. Clinical adhesion tests are commonly expected as part of the demonstration of therapeutically equivalence for generic transdermal products, in particular.

#### 8.5.8.1 FDA Requirements for In Vivo Adhesion Evaluation

FDA has included a clinical demonstration of non-inferior adhesion as part of the bioequivalence recommendation for specific transdermal products (FDA 2018). Within the guidance, the FDA recommendations are:

1. Adhesion performance of the intact test and reference listed drug (RLD) TDS must be formally evaluated and compared in the bioequivalence with pharmacokinetics endpoints and adhesion study or in a separate parallel or crossover adhesion study of single application of the active test product versus the RLD. No TDS reinforcement is allowed when the study is being used to establish adequate adhesion performance to support product approval. Adhesion scoring is to be performed at least daily, and at least just prior to removal at the end of application. For TDS that completely detach, a score of 4 should be carried forward in the adhesion analysis for all remaining observations in the application period.
2. The recommended scoring system for adhesion of TDS is indicated as follows:

   $0 = \geq 90\%$ adhered (essentially no lift off the skin)
   $1 = \geq 75\%$ to $< 90\%$ adhered (some edges only lifting off the skin)
   $2 = \geq 50\%$ to $< 75\%$ adhered (less than half of the TDS lifting off the skin)
   $3 = > 0\%$ to $< 50\%$ adhered but not detached (more than half of the TDS lifting off the skin without falling off)
   $4 = 0\%$ adhered – TDS detached (TDS completely off the skin)

3. The Per-Protocol (PP) Population evaluation of the adhesion parameter should be defined per TDS instead of per subject as follows: Adhesion Analysis – should include all TDS except those removed early for unacceptable irritation or those that dropped out of the study before the end of the application period.
4. The adhesion score and the time from application until TDS detachment (i.e., duration of TDS wear) should be evaluated for the test product and RLD, and a statistical analysis of the comparative results should be performed. In addition, the following adhesion data should be provided for the test product and RLD: (a) frequency table showing the number of TDS with each adhesion score at each evaluation time point; (b) number of TDS that are completely detached at each evaluation time point.

The adhesion evaluation of the test product and RLD must demonstrate that the upper bound of the one-sided 95% CI (Confidence Interval) of the mean adhesion score for the test product minus 1.25 times the mean adhesion score for the RLD must be less than or equal to 0. For the adhesion evaluation, the Office of Generic Drugs (OGD) also considers the number of subjects that experience detachment or unacceptable adhesion scores and how early in the application period those unacceptable scores are observed.

The same mean score could be reached with a small number of high scores (e.g., $>/= 3$) as with a larger number of low scores (e.g., 1, which are of little clinical significance). Thus, it is difficult to determine the clinical meaningfulness of a given mean score or a given difference between products with regard to mean scores. Therefore, in addition to mean scores, it is necessary to also evaluate the proportion of subjects with a meaningful degree of detachment for each product. The proportion of subjects with a meaningful degree of detachment should be no higher for the test product than for the RLD, and detachment should not occur earlier in the application period for the test than for the RLD. To be approved, the test product must be non-inferior with regard to mean adhesion scores and also show no meaningful difference with regard to degree of detachment.

In addition to the scoring methodology proposed by the FDA, an alternative scoring system has also been used to report clinical adhesion results. In the alternative system the percentage of the TDS adhered is reported directly and used for calculating the mean adhesion score.

### 8.5.8.2 EMA Guidelines for In Vivo Adhesion Studies
The European Medicines Agency (EMA) guideline on quality of TDS includes information on in vivo adhesion studies (EMA 2014). According to this guideline:

- Studies to investigate and establish the satisfactory in vivo adhesive performance of the drug product should be undertaken.
- A feasibility or pilot study should be considered to establish that the study methods and assessments can be carried out satisfactorily.
- The assessment should be undertaken throughout the proposed period of use. This is because satisfactory adhesion performance of the clinical batches used would be a requirement for any clinical conclusions to be valid and to achieve a representative number of subjects (both volunteers and patients).
- The clinical batches should be representative of the product to be marketed.

The methodology for in vivo skin adhesion testing is provided in the section 4.2.6.3.2 of this Guideline (EMA 2014):

- The investigation of in vivo adhesive performance may be included as a component part of human clinical pharmacokinetic and efficacy studies (both single dose and multi dose), or may be an independent study with either patients or volunteers.

- For TDS covering a range of different dosage strengths, as a minimum, the smallest and the largest TDS sizes should be tested in vivo. For TDS covering a range of different dosage strengths the smallest and the biggest TDS sizes should be tested in vivo.
- The elements of assessment should include:
  - The sites of application.
  - TDS application.
  - Residue formation on release 1 liner removal and on TDS removal.
  - The percentage TDS area adherence to the skin.
  - Cold flow, such as the formation of a dark ring about the TDS during use, TDS movement or displacement, wrinkling.
  - The robustness of the product to normal human behaviors, e.g., moisture resistance to washing, showering, saunas, use of moisturizers, risk of removal during exercise and/or sleeping, possible transfer to partners or family.
- The results of the study should inform the summary of product characteristics (SmPC) and product information. See also section 4.2.9 in the Guideline (EMA 2014).
- The TDS to be used as proposed. TDS reinforcement such as over-taping is not allowed.
- A satisfactory protocol, with justified visual or other scales of measurement, should be provided.
- The frequency of assessment should be stated and justified, and should include TDS administration and removal time points.
- Satisfactory and unsatisfactory performance should also be supported by photographs.
- For the determination of the percentage TDS area adherence, the following is recommended:
  - The frequency of assessment should be more than daily.
  - May be supported by analysis of photographs, to show validity of the method.
- The scores for adhesion of transdermal patches should be scaled in 5% increments as indicated:
  - More than 95% of the TDS area adheres.
  - More than 90% of the TDS area adheres.
  - More than 85% of the TDS area adheres.
  - More than 80% of the TDS area adheres.
  - More than 75% of the TDS area adheres.
  - More than 70% of the TDS area adheres.
  - Less than 70% adheres or TDS detachment is regarded as significant TDS adhesion failure.
- For TDS that completely detach during the study the score should be carried forward in the adhesion analysis for all remaining observations in the application period.
- In general, a mean adherence of greater than 90% should be expected and no instances of detachment should be seen. Poor adherence events should be investigated and possible causes and risk factors determined.

- The results should be reported in explanatory tabular and graphical formats, including:
  - ○ Frequency table showing the number of TDS with each adhesion score at each evaluation time point.
  - ○ Number of TDS that are completely detached at each evaluation time.
    A critical assessment and statistical analysis should be provided.
    For the other in vivo assessment elements as indicated earlier, similar reports, critical assessment and statistical analysis should be provided, as appropriate.

## PART 2 – PERFORMANCE TESTS FOR SEMISOLID PHARMACEUTICAL DOSAGE FORMS AND TRANSDERMAL DELIVERY SYSTEMS

### 8.6  INTRODUCTION

Dissolution/drug release testing has been employed as a fundamental tool in the formulation design and quality control of pharmaceutical dosage forms. Although initially used for solid oral dosage forms it has recently been employed for other dosage forms such as semisolid dosage forms, where it is commonly referred as in vitro release testing (IVRT), and for transdermal systems.

In vitro drug release is an important and useful tool because:

- It provides a scientific rationale for the selection of appropriate clinical candidate formulation and characterization of the dosage form.
- It ensures consistency in quality and manufacturing of a dosage form.
- It provides a uniform standard for comparing dosage forms across the industry.
- It provides a measurable index to anticipate performance of the dosage form in clinic.
- It can be used to demonstrate "sameness" in post-approval changes (changes in manufacturing site, composition, manufacturing process, etc.).
- It helps in the identification and evaluation of critical manufacturing variables.

IVRT consists of apparatus to prepare multiple solutions of the active pharmaceutical ingredient from a single aliquot of test product, typically over several hours. The set of solutions are then assayed by a separate detection method, usually HPLC. This chapter focuses primarily on the preparative aspects of IVRT, but it should be noted that an assay method for the IVRT solutions has to be developed in conjunction. Usually, this is a variation on the drug product assay method.

### 8.7  SEMISOLID DOSAGE FORMS

This section covers in vitro drug release testing only with the purpose of quality control, formulation evaluation/optimization, and post-approval changes using synthetic membranes. It does not address in vitro testing using human or animal skin. Semisolid dosage forms include, but are not restricted to, gels, lotions, creams, ointments and foams.

In vitro release testing for semisolid dosage forms is recommended as a measure of "product sameness" during scale-up and post-approval changes (FDA 1997; Chang et al. 2013; Flynn et al. 1999; Walters and Brain 2007). This method is routinely used during product development to fine-tune a formulation. However, the suggested uses of the tests to establish batch-to-batch, product certification and possible bioequivalence are fairly new and have been the subject of much debate (Olejnik, Goscianska and Nowak 2012; Shah 2005; Narkar 2010). This scenario may change in the future due to the U.S. FDA draft guidance on acyclovir ointment, issued in March 2012, recommending that bioequivalence can be demonstrated via an in vitro option if the test and reference product acyclovir ointment formulations meet all of the following criteria:

1. The test and the Reference Listed Drug (RLD) formulations are qualitatively and quantitatively the same (Q1/Q2).
2. Acceptable comparative physicochemical characterization of the test and RLD formulations.
3. Acceptable comparative *in vitro* drug release rate tests of acyclovir from the test and RLD formulations (FDA 2012).

For semisolid dosage forms, the onset of skin penetration of a drug upon contact of the semisolid formulation to the skin may be analogous to the disintegration of the drug from a solid dosage form. The rate of skin absorption will be slower than the release rate of the drug from the vehicle due to the barrier posed by the skin (stratum corneum). Therefore, the release rate of drug from semisolid dosage forms does not usually reflect absorption rate. If the effectiveness is dependent on the release of drug from the vehicle, then monitoring release rate is important for controlling the quality of the semisolid dosage product (Markovich 2001).

Although the in vitro release testing is not a measure of bioavailability, the test must be capable of detecting changes in drug release characteristics from the finished product. Changes in drug release characteristics have the potential to alter the biological performance of the drug in the dosage form. Such changes may be related to active or inactive ingredients in the formulation, physical or chemical attributes of the finished formulation, manufacturing variables, shipping and storage effects, aging effects, and other formulation factors that are critical to the quality characteristics of the finished drug product (Olejnik, Goscianska and Nowak 2012; Shah 2005).

### 8.7.1 DEVELOPMENT OF THE IN VITRO RELEASE TEST

#### 8.7.1.1 Membrane Selection

Almost all the equipment described here will require the use of a membrane to prevent mechanical disturbance of the sample by agitation of the receiving (also called receptor or dissolution) medium. The membrane must not offer significant resistance to the passage from the sample to the receiving medium. It should be an inert holding surface for the test formulation, but not a barrier. The membrane of choice should allow the drug substance to readily diffuse into the receiving medium. High porosity and minimal thickness are desirable membrane characteristics. The composition of the receptor medium should not affect the physical integrity of the membrane. Also, it should be evaluated if possible leachables and extractables from the membrane will not interfere with the quantitative procedure. It is important to confirm that there is no interaction, physical or chemical, between the membrane and the formulation. The excipients present in the formulation may affect the physical integrity of the membrane, or, in many cases, the drug substance may bind to the membrane. It is recommended that standard solutions of the drug under analysis in the receiving medium be prepared, at least, at the upper and lower concentration levels expected in the experiment, to verify the extent of drug binding to the membrane. Commonly used membranes are made of polysolfone (Tuffryn™, Supor™), cellulose acetate, nylon, Teflon™ and polycarbonate. Depending on the characteristics of the drug substance and of the dosage form, mainly in the case of lipophilic matrix, it may be necessary to pre-soak the membrane in an appropriate solvent, e.g., isopropyl miristate, to impart lipophilic character to the membrane to facilitate the diffusion of the drug substance out of the lipophilic matrix. This evaluation must be done for each product being evaluated (Zatz, Varsano and Shah 1996; Shah and Elkins 1995; Markovich 2001; Thakker and Chern 2003; Olejnik, Goscianska and Nowak 2012; Shah 2005). Realdon et al. (2005) employed a "bubble point" test to evaluate the integrity of the soaking film as well as of the membrane, during and after an in vitro release test with different types of ointments. This test can also help in the decision of using either a dry or hydrate membrane. The use of a previously hydrated membrane in testing lipophilic base ointments can guarantee constant conditions in the in vitro test.

One example of the impact of the selection of the membrane is the study done with gels containing some botanicals such as Indian penny wort, walnut and turmeric using the vertical diffusion cell. The nylon membrane showed a faster release when compared to the cellulose membrane. However, the cellulose membrane showed more discriminative power to differentiate among the three tested herbs and their formulations (Khiljee et al. 2010).

### 8.7.1.2 Quantitative Analytical Procedure

Typically the quantitative assay method is based upon the assay method for the finished product adapted to determine the amount of drug substance released from the semisolid dosage form with the appropriate sensitivity to quantify low levels of the drug in the receiving medium. Also, the specificity of the method should be carefully evaluated because there is a possibility that the receiving medium may extract components from the formulation and/or the membrane that may interfere with the quantification of the amount of drug released (Thakker and Chern 2003).

### 8.7.1.3 Selection of the Receiving Medium

Although it is desirable to have a receiving medium that is similar to the physiological condition of the skin, it is also imperative to ensure that the release of the drug can be measured appropriately. The most important factor for the selection of the receiving medium is the solubility of the drug substance in the medium. The receiving medium should provide a "diffusional sink" for the drug substance released from the semisolid formulation. The relationship of the cumulative amount of drug released versus the square root of time is derived from the Higuchi model with the assumption that there is a reservoir of the drug always available to diffuse through. As a rule of thumb, there should be no more than 30% of the total amount of the dose applied released into the medium at the end of the experiment (Thakker and Chern 2003). Typically the receiving medium will consist of an aqueous buffer that has been modified either as a hydroalcoholic medium and/or a surfactant containing medium (Markovich 2001; Olejnik, Goscianska and Nowak 2012; Shah 2005).

The pH of the medium is also an important factor for consideration. Selection of the pH of the aqueous component of the medium should be based on the pH of the formulation, pH solubility profile of the drug substance and pH of the site of application of the dosage form (Thakker and Chern 2003; Olejnik, Goscianska and Nowak 2012). A pH range of 5–6 ± 0.05 reflects the average pH of the skin (Olejnik, Goscianka and Nowak 2012).

The use of deaerated medium may be necessary to avoid the presence of bubbles on the membrane.

### 8.7.1.4   Temperature

When the dosage form is applied to the skin the temperature to be used in the test is $32 \pm 1°C$. If the dosage form is applied internally, such as vaginal creams, the temperature should be $37 \pm 1°C$ (USP 2019p).

### 8.7.1.5   Sampling Intervals

Six samples are recommended to determine the release profile of an active compound. Sampling is carried out at regular intervals with the replacement of the medium. Sampling points vary depending on the solubility of the drug substance. It is suggested that samples should be collected over at least a six-hour period, taking not less than five samples. Typical sampling intervals are 0.5, 1, 2, 4 and 6 hours. In some cases a sampling at 24 and 48 hours may be appropriated (USP 2019p; Thakker and Chern 2003; Olejnik, Goscianska and Nowak 2012).

### 8.7.1.6   Sample Application

In most cases the amount of sample introduced in the apparatus is relatively small (around 200 mg) and has no relationship with the actual use of the product by the patient because it is very difficult to define a dose for most of the semisolid products (unless packaged in a metered device). Sample application technique is very critical in order to prevent air bubbles from forming between the membrane and the semisolid preparation (Thakker and Chern 2003; Markovich 2001; USP 2019p).

### 8.7.1.7   Apparatus

Some of the current apparatus for testing semisolid dosage forms originated from in vitro skin permeation studies as is the case of the vertical diffusion cells. These diffusion cells have several common elements: two chambers, one containing a certain amount of the dosage form being tested (donor chamber) and the other containing a stirred receiving medium separated by a membrane. Care should be taken to ensure that the surface of the membrane remains in contact with the receiving medium at all times. The cell chambers are arranged in a side-by-side or vertical configuration, the latter being the most preferred. The temperature of the diffusional cell assembly is controlled using water-jackets or simply submerging the entire cell assembly into a thermostated water bath. Sufficient stirring of the receptor phase is required to minimize unstirred boundary layers thereby minimizing diffusional resistance (Markovich 2001). The other equipments that can be used for the evaluation of semi-solid dosage forms are the immersion cell, USP Apparatus 4 with a special cell for this type of dosage forms, USP Apparatus 5 (paddle over disk) and the paddle over extraction cell. All these equipments are described in the following sections.

### 8.7.1.7.1  Vertical Diffusion Cell Apparatus

The vertical diffusion cell (VDC) (Figures 8.8, 8.9 and 8.10), also known as Franz cell, was introduced by T. J. Franz in 1978 (Franz 1978; Raney, Lehman and Franz 2008), and it has been modified throughout the years. Many of the VDC systems are composed of six-cell units. Each VDC cell assembly consists of two chambers (a donor chamber and a receptor chamber) separated by a membrane and held together by a clamp, screw top or other means. In the donor chamber, the semisolid dosage

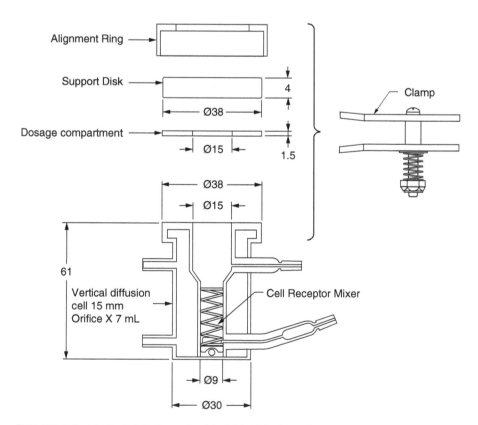

**FIGURE 8.8**   Vertical diffusion cell – Model A (All dimensions are in mm. All diameters are ± 0.5mm. All lengths are ± 2mm). (© 2019 United States Pharmacopeial Convention. Used by Permission.)

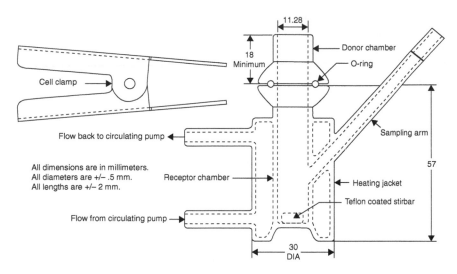

**FIGURE 8.9** Vertical diffusion cell – Model B (All dimensions are in mm. All diameters are μ0.5mm. All lengths are ± 2mm). (© 2019 United States Pharmacopeial Convention. Used by Permission.)

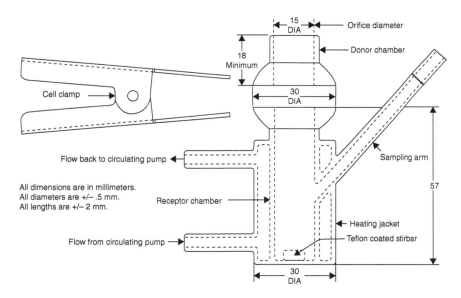

**FIGURE 8.10** Vertical diffusion cell – Model C (All dimensions are in mm. All diameters are ±0.5mm. All lengths are ± 2mm). (© 2016 United States Pharmacopeial Convention. Used by Permission.)

form sample sits on a synthetic, inert, highly permeable support membrane. A heating jacket or a suitable device should be used to maintain the temperature within the cell within the appropriate temperature range during the entire test. Usually a set of six-cell assemblies are operated together at one time (i.e., single run). For each cell, the amount of drug released ($\mu g/cm^2$) at each sampling time ($t_1$, $t_2$, etc.) is determined, and the cumulative amount release plotted versus $\sqrt{t}$ (where t = time), according to the diffusion model of Higuchi (Higuchi 1962). The slope of the resulting line is a measure of the rate of drug release. The test is often conducted with a group of six or 12 cells per run. The VDC body (i.e., donor and receptor chambers) usually is made from borosilicate glass, although other inert materials may be used. It is recommended that the cell assembly materials should not significantly react with, adsorb to or absorb the product components. The design of the VDC should facilitate proper alignment of the donor chamber and the receptor orifice. The receptor chamber should be manufactured consistently with uniform height and geometry. All the cells should have the same nominal volume, and the true volume should be measured for each individual cell. Care should be taken to minimize the inter-cell volume variability.

For the test, the VDC units are typically positioned in a stirrer rack that holds multiple VDC units (e.g., in sets of six) in the correct orientation, providing magnetic stirring at a calibrated rate and facilitating the supply of circulating heated water flow to the water jacket of the VDC. The VDC rack is typically connected to a thermostatically controlled water bath recirculator.

A magnetic nonstick stirring bar in the receptor chamber is used as the internal stirring mechanism. Aliquots of the receptor medium are drawn via the sampling arm at intervals throughout the test, and an equivalent volume of stock receptor medium is replaced.

Before initiating the test, the volume of each VDC, with the internal stirring device in place, should be determined. The rotational stirring rate is controlled within a range of ±10% (USP 2019o).

In vitro release of marketed topical corticosteroids was evaluated using the vertical diffusion cell, polysulfone membrane and 30% alcohol as a receiving medium for creams and alcohol, isopropyl myristate and water (85:10:5) as a receiving medium for ointments. The procedure showed discrimination based on the product label claim allowing rank ordering of the products related to the potency of the product (Shah 2005).

The ability of an IVRT to select the topical semisolid formulations with the most rapid release rate of ketoprofen from two closely related hydrogels was evaluated using three different receiving media: pH 7.4 phosphate buffer, isopropyl myristate and a combination of an isopropyl myristate pre-soaked membrane and pH 7.4 phosphate buffer as receiving medium. From the results obtained it was concluded that for purposes of formulation screening in the early phases of product development, an IVRT will only be useful for predicting the amount of drug available for absorption if the receptor medium has properties that closely mimic human skin. The results obtained illustrated the importance of selecting suitable receiving media (Proniuk, Dixon and Blanchard 2001). This importance was also evident in the evaluation of the IVRT of one phase systems (water- or oil-based systems) and two-phase systems (oil-in-water or water-in-oil systems) largely employed in semisolid dosage forms (Fan, Mitchnick and Loxley 2007) and for the release of ketoconazole from cream, shampoo, capillary lotion and four different formulations of gels (Mitu et al. 2011).

The influence of the composition of a semisolid formulation on the release of rutin was investigated using cellulose acetate membranes and water and ethanol (1:1) as receiving medium with VDC and a factorial design. The release followed a zero order kinetic. Urea (alone and in association with isopropanol and propylene glycol) and isopropanol (alone and in association with propylene glycol) influenced significant and negatively the rutin release form the semisolid system whereas propylene glycol 5% promote the rutin release (Baby et al. 2009).

### 8.7.1.7.2 Immersion Cell Apparatus

The immersion cell (Figures 8.11 and 8.12) (one of the trade names is Enhancer cell®) was introduced in the early 1990s (Markovich 2001). The cell consists of the following components (see Figures 8.4 and 8.5): a retaining or lock ring that secures the membrane to the cell body and ensures full contact with the sample; a washer that provides a leakproof seal between membrane, retaining ring and cell body; the membrane that should retain the sample in the sample compartment and the cell body that provides a variable depth reservoir for the sample. Model A also has an adjustment plate that allows varying the volume of the reservoir within the cell body. The plate can be completely removed to facilitate cleaning. An O-ring paired with the adjustment plate prevents leakage.

The immersion cell can be used with USP Apparatus 2 (paddle) with vessels volumes that vary from 100 mL up to 4 L, but the 150 or 200 mL vessels are the most commonly used. A flat-bottom variation of the 150 or 200 mL vessel can be used to avoid the issue of the dead space under the cell when it is used in a round-bottom vessel. If the cell is going to be used with a 150 or 200 mL vessel with USP Apparatus 2, then the appropriate modifications must be made, including holders for the small volume vessels and replacement of the standard paddle with the appropriate paddle. It also may require repositioning of any automated sampling device and/or manifold. The paddle height is adjusted to $1.0 \pm 0.2$ cm above the surface of the membrane. All the other operational parameters, such as level, vibration, wobble, etc., should be set at the same conditions defined for USP Apparatus 2 (USP 2019r, Olejnik, Goscianska and Nowak 2012). The test procedure is practically the same as for the vertical diffusion cell described on pp. 284–287.

Both vertical diffusion cell and immersion cell were used to evaluate the release of triamcinolone acetonide from hydroalcoholic gels. The study was run using ethanol and water (85.5:14:5 v/v) as receiving medium and 0.45 μm nylon as the membrane. The release rates were slightly higher and diffusion coefficients more consistent with the immersion cell when compared to the vertical diffusion cell. Notwithstanding these relatively minor differences, both equipments gave similar results (Fares and Zatz 1995).

The release of phenol from petrolatum ointments was evaluated using the immersion cell using water as receiving medium. The release rate and diffusion coefficients were reproducible and the same whether diffusion was through a synthetic membrane (nylon or cellulose acetate) or if no membrane was present.

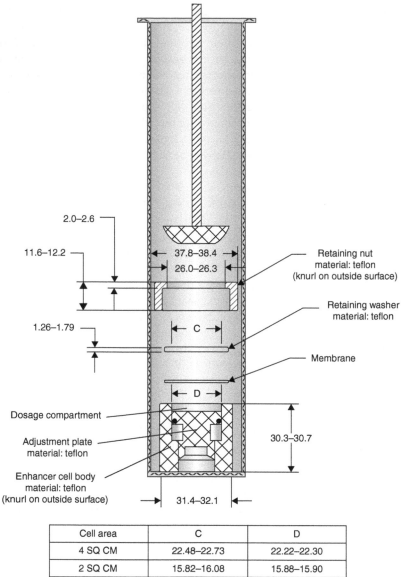

| Cell area | C | D |
|---|---|---|
| 4 SQ CM | 22.48–22.73 | 22.22–22.30 |
| 2 SQ CM | 15.82–16.08 | 15.88–15.90 |
| 0.5 SQ CM | 7.90–8.16 | 7.95–7.98 |

**FIGURE 8.11** Immersion cell – Model A assembled in a mini vessel. (© 2019 United States Pharmacopeial Convention. Used by Permission.)

However, standard deviations were greatly reduced when a membrane was used, providing improved control over the release measurement (Segers, Zatz and Shah 1997).

The discriminatory power of the vertical diffusion cell and immersion cell was compared when changing the concentration of the active ingredient in the same semisolid topical formulation. The tests were performed in conditions as nearly

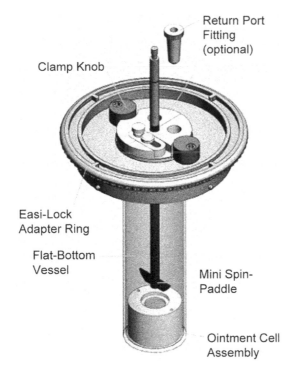

Return Port Fitting (optional)

Clamp Knob

Easi-Lock Adapter Ring

Flat-Bottom Vessel

Mini Spin-Paddle

Ointment Cell Assembly

**FIGURE 8.12** Immersion cell – Model B assembled in a vessel. (© 2019 United States Pharmacopeial Convention. Used by Permission.)

identical as possible. The receiving medium was pH 7.2 boric acid-borax buffer and 0.45 μm cellulose acetate membrane previously soaked with isopropyl myristate. Both apparatuses produced similar results for the release rate and in their response to a formulation change. The preference from one equipment over the other will depend on the laboratory decision (Rapedius and Blanchard 2001). Similar results and conclusions were obtained in evaluating the release from 1% hydrocortisone ointments (Sanghvi and Collins 1993).

Rege, Vilivalam and Collins (1998) evaluated an automated system using the immersion cell and compared the release of triamcinolone acetonide from commercial semisolid formulations. The receiving medium was ethanol and water (38:62) and membranes were regenerated cellulose, polyethylene and rat skin. The experiments were designed to determine the effect of the method variables such as the temperature of the receiving medium, receptor medium concentration, stirring speed and the choice of the membranes.

### 8.7.1.7.3 USP Apparatus 4 (Flow-Through Cell)

In flow-through cells, the receptor medium continuously flows through the acceptor compartment, and, as a result, the medium is refreshed continually. The adapter for semisolid dosage forms (see Figure 8.13) is used with the 22.6 cm cell of USP Apparatus 4. The adapter consists of a reservoir and a ring to hold the membrane.

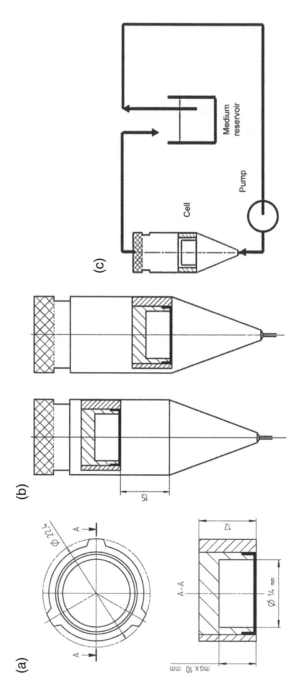

**FIGURE 8.13** (A) Adapter for topical dosage forms in USP Apparatus 4. (B) Vertical positioning of the insert using the tablet holder scoring. (C) Closed system configuration for USP Apparatus 4 (All dimensions are in mm). (© 2019 United States Pharmacopeial Convention. Used by Permission.)

The reservoir is available in different sizes that can accommodate from 400 to 1200 µL of product. The flow rate should comply with the requirements in the USP general chapter <711> Dissolution (USP 2019r) with a sinusoidal flow profile with a pulsation of $120 \pm 10$ pulses/min and a precision of $\pm 5\%$ of the nominal flow rate (USP 2019p; Olejnik, Goscianska and Nowak 2012). The other steps of the test procedure are very similar to those described for the vertical diffusion cell on pp. 284–287.

### 8.7.1.7.4 USP Apparatus 5 (Paddle over Disk)

This apparatus consists of a stainless steel disk assembly or a watchglass covered with a stainless steel screen (Figure 8.14) designed to hold the sample at the bottom of the vessel in the USP Apparatus 2 (paddle) (USP 2019s). In this case, the membrane is not required. The possibility of the formulation dissolving in the receiving medium should be evaluated (Olejnik, Goscianska and Nowak 2012).

This equipment was used to evaluate the release of tenoxicam from water-in-oil and oil-in-water ointment bases, and gels with pH 7.4 phosphate buffer as receiving medium (Makky 2002).

### 8.7.1.7.5 Paddle over Extraction Cell

The extraction cell described in the European Pharmacopoeia (2019b) is used with the USP Apparatus 2 (paddle) (see Figure 8.15).

The cell consists of a support, a cover and a membrane. The central part of the support forms a cavity where the sample is placed. The cavity has a depth of 2.6mm and a diameter that ranges from 27mm up to 52mm. The membrane is placed over the support covering the sample and the cover is held in place by nuts screwed onto bolts projecting from the support. The cell should be closed carefully to ensure that the membrane is free of wrinkles. The cell is placed on the bottom of the dissolution vessel with the cover facing up. The paddle should be at $2.5 \pm 0.2$ cm above the cell surface (European Pharmacopoeia 2019b). The other steps of the test procedure are very similar to those described for the vertical diffusion cell on pp. 284–287.

### 8.7.2 VALIDATION OF THE IN VITRO RELEASE TEST

The validation of the in vitro release testing for semisolid dosage forms can be divided in two parts:

- Validation of the sample preparation from the IVRT apparatus.
- Validation of quantitative determination of the drug release in the sample solutions removed from the IVRT apparatus.

For both aspects of the IVRT method, protocols with acceptance criteria should be prepared. The basic principles of method validation for dissolution (USP 2019q; ICH Q2 (R1) 1996) are a good basis for IVRT method validation although some modification of the experimental detail is necessary. Tables 8.1 and 8.2 contain examples of how this method validation can be done for IVRT testing.

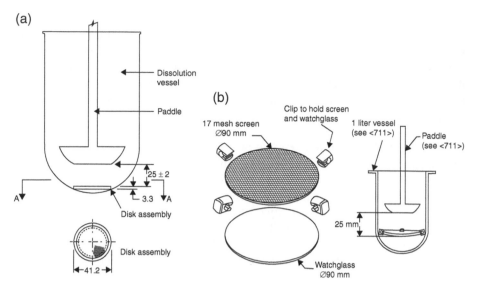

**FIGURE 8.14**  USP Apparatus 5. (A) Stainless steel disk assembly. (B) Watchglass and stainless steel screen. (© 2019 United States Pharmacopeial Convention. Used by Permission.)

## 8.8  TRANSDERMAL DELIVERY SYSTEMS

As with semisolid dosage forms, a performance test for transdermal delivery systems (TDS) also must have the ability to measure drug release from the finished dosage form, must be reproducible and reliable. Also, it must be capable of detecting changes in drug release characteristics from the finished product that may have an impact in the in vivo performance of the product.

### 8.8.1  DEVELOPMENT OF THE DRUG RELEASE TEST

#### 8.8.1.1  Quantitative Analytical Procedure

The quantitative analytical procedure employed to determine the amount of drug substance released from the TDS needs to have the appropriate sensitivity to quantify low levels of the drug in the medium. The specificity should be carefully evaluated because the medium may extract components from the TDS that can interfere with the determination of the API. Also, the interference of any accessory (double face adhesive tape, glue, etc.) used to fix the TDS on the apparatus should be investigated.

#### 8.8.1.2  Selection of the Medium

Ideally the medium should have a pH within the physiological range of the skin, pH 5–6 (Olejnik, Goscianska and Nowak 2012). Also, the solubility of the drug substance in the medium should be determined to provide the appropriate sink condition. As the drug release test for TDS has a long duration, it is important to evaluate the stability of the API in the medium in the conditions of the test.

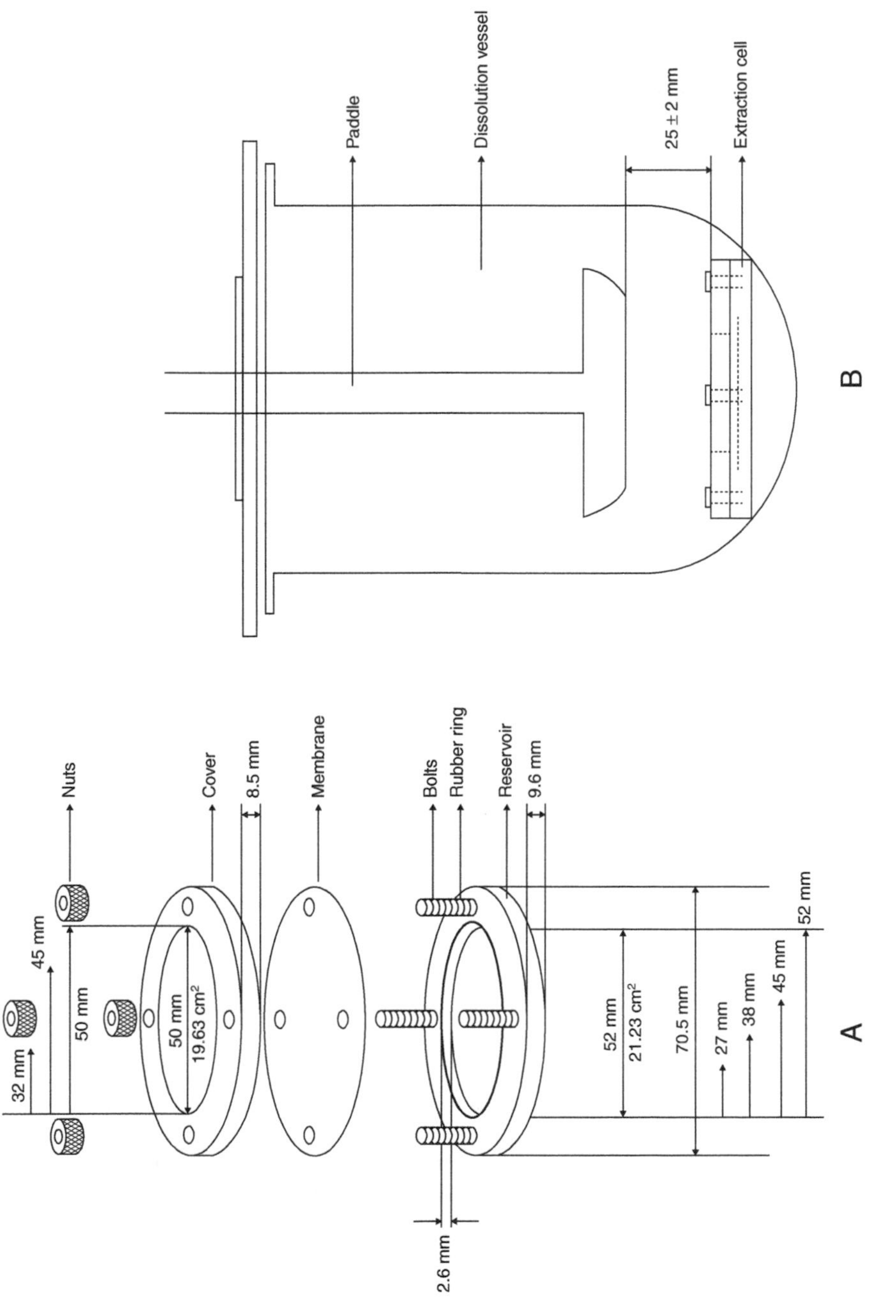


**FIGURE 8.15** (A) Extraction cell. (B) Extraction cell assembled in USP Apparatus 2.

**TABLE 8.1**

**Example of Validation Parameters for the Quantitative Determination in the IVRT Method**

| ICH Q2 Validation Characteristics | Quantitative Determination | Experimental Plan |
|---|---|---|
| Accuracy | Required | Prepare simulated IVRT solution made from placebo product. Spike the placebo solution in triplicate at three concentrations covering the lowest, midpoint and highest expected concentrations of API in an IVRT run (n=9). See Range |
| Precision (Repeatability) | Required | Assay the 9 accuracy solutions. |
| Precision (Intermediate Precision) | Not Required | Intermediate precision can be performed as part of the experimental plan for the IVRT sample preparation. |
| Specificity | Required | Assay placebo receiving solution and receiving medium to demonstrate that there are no significant interferences. If the method has been adapted from a chromatography assay for the finished product there is usually no further need to check for interference from major impurities and degradants. |
| Detection Limit | Not Required | None |
| Quantitation Limit | Required | Use one of the standard experiments for determination of quantification limit, e.g., signal to noise ratio, to confirm that the quantitation limit is below that of the lowest sample concentrations. |
| Linearity | Required | Prepare a minimum of five solutions of known concentration from the quantitation limit to beyond the highest expected sample concentration, e.g., +20%. See Range |
| Range | Required but addressed by linearity experiment | See linearity for experimental plan. Ensure that the range accommodates all strengths of the product included in the IVRT study. |
| Robustness | Required | Robustness experimentation should focus on method parameters that might reasonably vary during the IVRT assessment, e.g., test the stability of IVRT sample solutions and working standard solutions. |

*Note*: Typically the assay method from the finished product is adapted and validated for the analysis of the low concentrations obtained from the IVRT apparatus.

**TABLE 8.2**
**Example of Validation Parameters for the IVRT Sample Preparation in the IVRT Method**

| ICH Q2 (R1) Validation Characteristics | IVRT Sample Preparation Method | Experimental Plan |
|---|---|---|
| Accuracy | Not Required | Tested in the assay method experimental plan. |
| Precision (Repeatability) | Required | Run six cells with product. |
| Precision (Intermediate Precision) | Not Required | Since IVRT assessments are typically side-by-side comparisons of test and reference product, intermediate precision is useful only as an indication of how reliable IVRT release rates are from different experiments. Examples: <br> - A second analyst working independently runs six cells with the same product as in the repeatability experiment. <br> - Run six cells again on additional days. |
| Specificity | Not Required | Tested in the assay method experimental plan. |
| Detection Limit | Not Required | None. |
| Quantitation Limit | Not Required | Tested in the assay method experimental plan. |
| Linearity (Dose discrimination) | Required | In place of true linearity, IVRT validation often uses a 50% dilution of the product with placebo to confirm that the IVRT method can distinguish the two strengths. |
| Range | Required but addressed by linearity experiment. | See linearity. |
| Robustness | Required | Best addressed during method development. Parameters to be assessed include membrane binding and variation in the receptor medium composition. |

### 8.8.1.3 Temperature

As the TDS are applied to the skin, the temperature of the test should be $32.0 \pm 0.5°C$ (USP 2019s).

### 8.8.1.4 Sampling Intervals

A minimum of three time points are recommended to set the specifications. These time points should cover the early, middle and late stages of the drug release profile. The last time point should be the time point where at least 80% of the drug has been released or it should be the time when the plateau of the drug release profile has been reached. Also, it is important to measure the amount of drug release at a very early time (e.g., about one hour) to check for possible dosing dumping. Therefore, the drug release profile for TDS should be obtained at the appropriate intervals for the duration of the prescribed product treatment. In the USP monographs for Estradiol

Transdermal System, one drug release test is run for 96 hours and the other two for 24 hours each; for Clonidine Transdermal Systems, all three drug release tests are run for 168 hours; for Nicotine Transdermal Systems, the drug release tests are run from four up to 24 hours.

### 8.8.1.5 Sample Application

The release surface of the TDS, the one that contains the adhesive, should be in contact with the drug release medium during the entire test. The TDS can be fixed in the apparatus by any appropriate and validated means such as the use of double-faced adhesive tape, adhesive, membrane, nylon net, special holder (Figure 8.16), or with the aid of inert metal or polymer ring.

The TDS is applied to the holder, disk or cylinder, assuring that the release surface is as flat as possible. Care must be taken to avoid the presence of air bubbles between the membrane and the system and on the surface of the system, or wrinkles on the surface of the system (USP 2019s).

The size of holder or cylinder should be compatible with the size of the transdermal delivery system to avoid overlap of the transdermal delivery system over itself. TDS can only be cut to be fitted in the holder or cylinder if the instructions to the patient recommend cutting it in an appropriate size. In the absence of those instructions, the entire transdermal delivery system should be used.

### 8.8.1.6 Apparatus

*8.8.1.6.1 USP Apparatus 5 (Paddle over Disk)*

This equipment consists of the USP Apparatus 2 (paddle) with an accessory where the transdermal delivery system is placed. This accessory can be a disk assembly (Figure 8.14A) or a watchglass and screen (Figure 8.14B). The transdermal delivery system is applied to the disk assembly or to the watchglass, with the release surface facing the medium. Other types of holders can be used (Figure 8.16). The bottom edge of the paddle is 25 ± 2mm from the surface of the holder. The vessel may be covered during the test to minimize evaporation. The paddle is operated at the appropriate rotation speed (USP 2019s; European Pharmacopoeia 2019b).

*8.8.1.6.2 USP Apparatus 6 (Rotating Cylinder)*

This apparatus uses a stainless steel cylinder stirring element (Figure 8.17) with the vessel assembly from USP Apparatus 1. This cylinder stirring element is composed of two parts, one comprising the shaft and the upper cylinder and the other being the extension cylinder. They should be acquired all together. Both parts are serially numbered and they should be kept paired because the friction fitting is done individually for each cylinder, allowing a very tight fit. The distance between the inside bottom of the vessel and the cylinder is maintained at 25 ± 2mm during the test. The vessel may be covered during the test to minimize evaporation. The paddle is operated at the appropriate rotation speed (USP 2019s; European Pharmacopoeia 2019b).

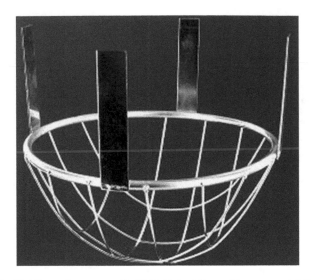

**FIGURE 8.16** Holding wire screen. (© 2019 United States Pharmacopeial Convention. Used by Permission.)

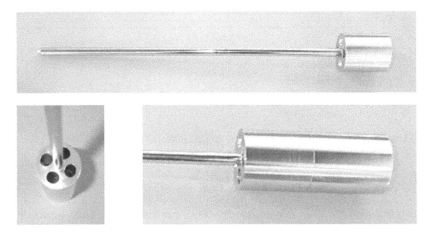

**FIGURE 8.17** USP Apparatus 6 (rotating cylinder). (© 2019 QLA-LLC. Used by Permission.)

### 8.8.1.6.3 USP Apparatus 7 (Reciprocating Holder)

This equipment consists of a set of volumetrically calibrated or tared solution containers made of glass or other suitable inert material, a motor and drive assembly to reciprocate the system vertically and to index the system horizontally to a different row of vessels automatically, and a set of suitable sample holders (Figures 8.18, 8.19 and 8.20) (USP 2019s).

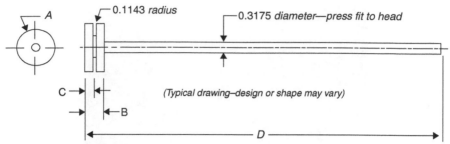

Dimensions are in centimeters.

**FIGURE 8.18** Reciprocating disk sample holder. (© 2019 United States Pharmacopeial Convention. Used by Permission.)

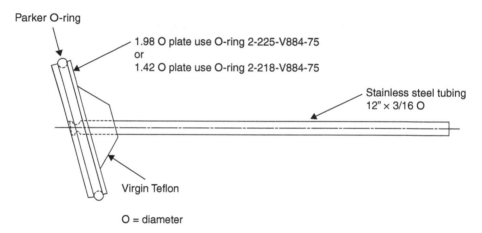

**FIGURE 8.19** Transdermal system holder – angled disk. (© 2019 United States Pharmacopeial Convention. Used by Permission.)

### 8.8.2 Validation of the Drug Release Test

The validation of the drug release test for TDS can follow the same principles as outlined in section 8.7.2 for the topical products. The method should be validated for all the TDS sizes and strengths.

## 8.9 CONCLUSION

For commercial production, dermal drug delivery systems are tested for batch-to-batch variability using routine "universal" quality control tests common to many dosage forms (tablets, respiratory products, etc.). Despite the apparently routine nature of many of these tests, the unique properties of dermal products have to be considered when developing the methods. In addition, there are some tests that are particular to the dermal drug delivery systems (semisolids and transdermal systems) which also must be well controlled to ensure reproducible

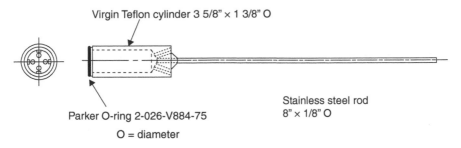

Virgin Teflon cylinder 3 5/8" × 1 3/8" O

Parker O-ring 2-026-V884-75

Stainless steel rod
8" × 1/8" O

O = diameter

**FIGURE 8.20** Transdermal system holder – Teflon cylinder. (© 2019 United States Pharmacopeial Convention. Used by Permission.)

results to minimize variation in results as a consequence of analytical error. Robust QC test methodologies produce reliable data and become the eyes of the scientists developing, transferring or improving formulations and their manufacturing processes. Quality Assurance personnel and regulators require data from QC tests as assurance that the manufacturing process has produced a quality product consistent with that approved in the product registration. Product that meets all registered specifications (and manufactured according to the current Good Manufacturing Practice regulations) would then be considered fit for use by patients and consumers.

The performance tests for semisolid dosage forms applied to the skin are usually not QC tests performed at batch release but are instead used to get a deeper understanding of the product with these holistic assessments of the product's physical and chemical properties. This knowledge provides an extra level of assurance of a consistent product after potentially significant changes during the product's life cycle, e.g., when it is transferred between manufacturing sites or improvements are made to the method of production.

Testing dermal drug delivery systems does not in itself assure quality but it is the vital endpoint in the chain of controls from medicine development into manufacturing prior to shipping out to use by patients and consumers. Knowledge of properties of the delivery system and the critical parameters of the tests themselves ensures that the results are reliable. From those results, decisions can be made regarding the quality of the finished product before it is used by the person at the end of the supply chain.

## REFERENCES

ASTM Standard D3121-06 "Standard Test Method for Tack of Pressure-Sensitive Adhesives by Rolling Ball," ASTM International, West Conshohocken, PA, 2006, DOI: 10.1520/D3121-06, www.astm.org

ASTM Standard D3163-01 "Standard Test Method for Determining Strength of Adhesively Bonded Rigid Plastic Lap-Shear Joints in Shear by Tension Loading," ASTM International, West Conshohocken, PA, 2008, DOI: 10.1520/D3163-01R08, www.astm.org

ASTM D2979-01 "Standard Test Method for Pressure-Sensitive Tack of Adhesives Using an Inverted Probe Machine," ASTM International, West Conshohocken, PA, 2009, DOI: 10.1520/D2979-01R09, www.astm.org

ASTM Standard D1002-10 "Standard Test Method for Apparent Shear Strength of Single-Lap-Joint Adhesively Bonded Metal Specimens by Tension Loading (Metal-to-Metal)," ASTM International, West Conshohocken, PA, 2010, DOI: 10.1520/D1002-10, www.astm.org

ASTM D6862-11 "Standard Test Method for 90 Degree Peel Resistance of Adhesives," ASTM International, West Conshohocken, PA, 2011, DOI: 10.1520/D6862-11, www.astm.org

ASTM Standard D3164-03 "Standard Test Method for Strength Properties of Adhesively Bonded Plastic Lap-Shear Sandwich Joints in Shear by Tension Loading," ASTM International, West Conshohocken, PA, 2011, DOI: 10.1520/D3164-03R11, www.astm.org

ASTM Standard D3654/D3654M-06 "Standard Test Methods for Shear Adhesion of Pressure-Sensitive Tapes," ASTM International, West Conshohocken, PA, 2011, DOI: 10.1520/D3654_D3654M-06R11, www.astm.org

Baby, A. R., Haroutiounian Filho, C. A., Sarruf, F. D., Pinto, C. A. S. O., Kaneko, T. M., Velasco, M. V. R. 2009. Influence of urea, isopropanol, and propylene glycol on rutin *in vitro* release from cosmetic semisolid systems estimated by factorial design. *Drug Dev. Ind. Pharm.* 35:272–282.

Buchta, R., Ding, S., Hickey, A., Houghton, M., Noland, P., Tice, T., Warner, K., Brown, W. 2017. Pharmaceutical foams. *Pharmacopeial Forum.* 43(1). www.usppf.com.

Chang, R. K., Raw, A., Lionberger, R., Yu, L. 2013. Generic development of topical dermatologic products: formulation development, process development, and testing of topical dermatologic products. *AAPS Journal.* 15(1):41–52.

EMA. October 2014. European Medicines Agency Guideline on Quality of Transdermal Patches, www.ema.europa.eu/en/documents/scientific-guideline/guideline-quality-transdermal-patches_en.pdf (accessed on May 1, 2019).

European Pharmacopoeia. 2019a. EP 9.8, Section 2.9.20 *Particulate contamination: visible particles*, Strasbourg, EDQM.

European Pharmacopoeia. 2019b. EP 9.8, Section 2.9.4 *Dissolution test for transdermal patches*, Strasbourg, EDQM.

Fan, Q., Mitchnick, M., Loxley, A. 2007. The issues and challenges involved in *in vitro* release testing for semi-solid formulations. *Drug Del. Technol.* 7(9):62–66.

Fares, H. M., Zatz, J. L. 1995. Measurement of drug release from topical gels using two types of apparatus. *Pharm. Technol.* 19(1):52–58.

FDA. May 1997. Guidance for Industry. Nonsterile Semisolid Dosage Forms. Scale-up and Postapproval Changes: chemistry, manufacturing, and controls; in vitro release testing and in vivo bioequivalence documentation, www.fda.gov/media/71141/download (accessed on May 1, 2019).

FDA. March 2012. Draft Guidance Acyclovir, www.accessdata.fda.gov/drugsatfda_docs/psg/Acyclovir_oint_18604_RC03-12.pdf (accessed on May 1, 2019).

FDA. October 2018. Bioequivalence Recommendation for Specific Products, Draft Guidance for Rivastigmine, www.accessdata.fda.gov/drugsatfda_docs/psg/Rivastigmine_transdermal%20extended%20release%20film_NDA%20022083_RV10-18.pdf (accessed on May 1, 2019).

FINAT. 2009. Technical Handbook – Test Methods, 8th Ed., FTM 18 "Dynamic shear," FINAT (Féderation INternationale des fabricants et transformateurs d'Adhésifs et Thermocollants sur papiers et autres supports), The Hague.

Flynn, G. L., Shah, V. P., Tenjarla, S. N., Corbo, M., DeMagistris, D., Feldman, T. G., Franz, T.J., Miran, D. R., Pearce, D. M., Sequeira, J. A., Swarbrick, J., Wang, J. C. T., Yacobi, A., Zatz, J. L. 1999. Assessment of value and applications of *in vitro* testing of topical dermatological drug products. *Pharm. Res.* 16(9):1325–1330.

Franz, T. J. 1978. The finite dose technique as a valid *in vitro* model for the study of percutaneous absorption in man. *Curr. Probl. Dermatol.* 7:58–68.

Higuchi, W. I. 1962. Analysis of data on medicament release from ointments. *J. Pharm. Sci.*, 51:802–804.

ICH Q2(R1). Nov 1996. Validation of Analytical Procedures: Text and Methodology, www. ich.org/fileadmin/Public_Web_Site/ICH_Products/Guidelines/Quality/Q2_R1/Step4/ Q2_R1__Guideline.pdf (accessed on May 1, 2019).

ICH Q3B (R2). June 2006. Impurities in New Drug Products, www.ich.org/fileadmin/Public_ Web_Site/ICH_Products/Guidelines/Quality/Q3B_R2/Step4/Q3B_R2__Guideline.pdf (accessed on May 1, 2019).

ICH Q3C (R7). October 2018. Residual Solvents, www.ich.org/fileadmin/Public_Web_Site/ ICH_Products/Guidelines/Quality/Q3C/Q3C-R7_Document_Guideline_2018_1015. pdf (accessed on April 30, 2019).

ICH Q3D(R1). March 2019. Guideline for Elemental Impurities, www.ich.org/fileadmin/ Public_Web_Site/ICH_Products/Guidelines/Quality/Q3D/Q3D-R1EWG_Document_ Step4_Guideline_2019_0322.pdf (accessed on April 30, 2019).

ICH Q6A. Oct 1999. Specifications: Test Procedures and Acceptance Criteria for New Drug Substances and New Drug Products: Chemical Substances, www.ich.org/fileadmin/ Public_Web_Site/ICH_Products/Guidelines/Quality/Q6A/Step4/Q6Astep4.pdf (accessed on April 30, 2019).

Khiljee, S., Rehman, N. U., Sarfraz, M. K., Montazeri, H., Khiljee, T., Lobenberg, R. 2010. *In vitro* release of Indian penny wort, walnut, and turmeric from topical preparations using two different types of membranes. *Dissol. Technol.* 17(4):27–32.

Ma, X. J., Taw, J., Chiang, C. M. 1996. Control of drug crystallization in transdermal matrix system. *Int. J. Pharm.* 142(1): 115–119.

Makky, A. M. A. 2002. Formulation and *in-vitro* release evaluation of topical tenoxicam preparations. *Egypt. J. Pharm. Sci.* 43:1–17.

Markovich, R. J. 2001. Dissolution testing of semisolid dosage forms. *Am. Pharm Rev.* 4(2):71–79.

Mitu, M. A., Lupuliasa, D., Pirvu, C. E. D., Radulescu, F. E., Miron, D. S., Vlaia, L. 2011. Ketoconazole in topical pharmaceutical formulations. The influence of the receptor media on the *in vitro* diffusion kinetics. *Farmacia*, 59(3):358–366.

Narkar, Y. 2010. Bioequivalence for topical products – an update. *Pharm Res. 6* 27:2590–2601.

Olejnik, A., Goscianska, J., Nowak, I. 2012. Active compounds release from semisolid dosage forms. *J. Pharm. Sci.* 101(11):4032–4045.

Proniuk, S., Dixon, S. E., Blanchard, J. 2001. Investigation of the utility of an *in vitro* release test for optimizing semisolid dosage forms. *Pharm. Dev. Technol.* 6(3):469–476.

PSTC 107. May 2007. Shear Adhesion of Pressure Sensitive Tape, Pressure Sensitive Tape Council, http://psatape.com.tw/pstc/pstc107.pdf (accessed on May 1, 2019).

Raney, S., Lehman, P., Franz, T. 2008. 30th Anniversary of the Franz cell finite dose model: the crystal ball of topical drug development. *Drug Del. Technol.* 8(7):32–37.

Rapedius, M., Blanchard, J. 2001. Comparison of the Hanson Microette ® and the Van Kel apparatus for *in vitro* release testing of topical semisolid formulations. *Pharm. Res.* 18(10):1440–1447.

Realdon, N., Tagliaboschi, A., Perin, F., Ragazzi, E. 2005. The "bubble point" for validation of drug release or simulated absorption for ointments. *Pharmazie* 60:910–916.

Rege, P. R., Vilivalam, V. D., Collins, C. C. 1998. Development in release testing of topical dosage forms: use of the Enhancer cell™ with automated sampling. *J. Pharm. Biom. Anal.* 17:1225–1233.

Sanghvi, P. P., Collins, C. C. 1993. Comparison of diffusion studies of hydrocortisone between the Franz cell and the Enhancer cell. *Drug Dev. Ind. Pharm.* 19(13):1573–1585.

Segers, J. D., Zatz, J. L., Shah, V. P. 1997. *In vitro* release of phenol from ointment formulations. *Pharm. Technol.* 22(1):70–81.

Shah, V. P. 2005. *In vitro* release from semisolid dosage forms – What is its value? In *Percutaneous Absorption – Drugs, Cosmetics, Mechanisms, Methods*, ed. R. J. Bronaugh and H. I. Maibach, 473–480. New York: CRC Press.

Shah, V. P., Elkins, J. S. 1995. *In-vitro* release from corticosteroid ointments. *J. Pharm. Sci.* 84(9):1139–1140.

Tan, H. S., Pfister, W. R. 1999. Pressure-sensitive adhesives for transdermal drug delivery systems. *Pharm Sci Technolo Today.* 2(2):60–69.

Thakker, K. D., Chern, W. H. 2003. Development and validation of *in vitro* release tests for semisolid dosage forms – Case study. *Dissol. Technol.* 10(2):10–15.

USP. 2019a. *USP 42 – NF 37, Second Supplement, Topical and Transdermal Drug Products — Product Quality Tests <3>.* Rockville, MD: USP.

USP. 2019b. *USP 42 – NF 37, Residual Solvents <467>.* Rockville, MD: USP.

USP. 2019c. *USP 42 – NF 37, Elemental Impurities - Limits <232>.* Rockville, MD; USP.

USP. 2019d. *USP 42 – NF 37, Elemental Impurities – Procedures <233>.* Rockville, MD; USP.

USP. 2019e. *USP 42 – NF 37, Uniformity of Dosage Units <905>.* Rockville, MD: USP.

USP. 2019f. *USP 42 – NF 37, Minimum Fill <755>.* Rockville,MD: USP.

USP. 2019g. *USP 42 – NF 37, Antimicrobial Effectiveness Testing <51>.* Rockville, MD: USP.

USP. 2019h. *USP 42 – NF 37, Microbiological Examination of Nonsterile Products: Microbial Enumeration Tests <61>.* Rockville, MD: USP.

USP. 2019i. *USP 42 – NF 37, Microbiological Examination of Nonsterile Products: Tests for Specified Organisms <62>.* Rockville, MD: USP.

USP. 2019j. *USP 42 – NF 37, Microbiological Examination of Nonsterile Products: Acceptance Criteria for Pharmaceutical Preparations and Substances for Pharmaceutical Use <1111>.* Rockville, MD: USP.

USP. 2019k. *USP 42 – NF 37, Sterility Tests <71>.* Rockville, MD: USP.

USP. 2019l. *USP 42 – NF 37, Viscosity – Capillary Methods <911>.* Rockville, MD: USP.

USP. 2019m. *USP 42 – NF 37, Rotational Methods <912>.* Rockville, MD: USP.

USP. 2019n. *USP 42 – NF 37, Rolling Ball Method <913>.* Rockville, MD: USP.

USP. 2019o. *USP 42 – NF 37, Viscosity – Pressure Driven Methods <914>.* Rockville, MD: USP.

USP. 2019p. *USP 42 – NF 37, Semisolid Drug Products – Performance Tests <1724>.* Rockville, MD: USP.

USP. 2019q. *USP 42 – NF 37, The Dissolution Procedure: Development and Validation <1092>.* Rockville, MD: USP.

USP. 2019r. *USP 42 – NF 37, Dissolution <711>.* Rockville, MD: USP.

USP. 2019s. *USP 42 – NF 37, Drug Release <724>.* Rockville, MD: USP.

Walters, K. A., Brain, K.R. 2007. Topical and Transdermal Delivery. In *Pharmaceutical preformulation and formulation*, ed. M. Gibson, 515–579. New York: Informa.

Wokovich, A. M., Prodduturi, S., Doub, W. H., Hussain, A. S., Buhse, L. 2006. Transdermal drug delivery system (TDDS) adhesion as a critical safety, efficacy and quality attribute. *Eur J Pharm Biopharm.* 64(1):1–8.

Wokovich, A. M., Shen, M., Doub, W. H., Machado, S. G., Buhse, L. F. 2010. Release liner removal method for transdermal drug delivery systems (TDDS). *J Pharm Sci.* 99(7):3177–3187.

Yacobi A. 2010. Topical Semisolid Dosage Forms. Product Quality Tests and Product Performance Testing, presentation at the PQRI – USP Workshop Topical Dosage Forms.

Zatz, J. L., Varsano, J., Shah, V. P. 1996. In vitro release of betamethansone dipropionate from petrolatum-base ointments. *Pharm. Dev. Technol.* 1(3):293–298.

# 9 Perspective on Clinical Trials for Dermal Drug Delivery Systems

*John T. Farrar and Shamir N. Kalaria*

## CONTENTS

## 9.1   INTRODUCTION

The Food and Drug Administration (FDA) began its modern regulatory functions with the passage of the 1906 Pure Food and Drugs Act focused primarily on the safety and appropriate labeling of food and drugs. With the amendment to the Federal Food, Drug, and Cosmetic Act in 1962, the U.S. Congress added the requirement that to obtain marketing approval, manufactures must conduct adequate and well-controlled trials to demonstrate the efficacy of their products in addition to the safety requirement stipulated in the original 1938 Act. Based on careful consideration of the intentions of Congress and on the science of what constituted the appropriate quantity and quality of evidence necessary to establish efficacy, the FDA has generally required at least two adequate and well-controlled studies. Over time, our understanding of the science of clinical evaluation has improved, leading to more rigorously designed and conducted clinical trials. In addition, the regulations for what the FDA requires as convincing evidence needed to conduct an adequate risk/benefit assessment have been updated to reflect this new understanding.

Recognizing that demonstrating effectiveness represented the major component of drug development time and cost, the FDA has exercised some flexibility in considering what other supporting evidence is needed to substantiate the findings of the required two well-controlled and well-conducted clinical trials. Under conditions where it would be difficult or potentially unethical to require two such studies or when the new use of an approved medication is similar enough, a single clinical trial may be all that is required. The specifics of these circumstances were outlined in the "Guidance for Industry: Providing Clinical Evidence of Effectiveness for Human Drugs and Biological Products" document published in 1998. (1) That same document outlines the Agency's growing understanding of the potential scientific limitations of a single study. Issues related to the known limitations of clinical trials serve as a loose outline for the presentation of the science of clinical trials in the rest of this chapter.

From the beginning, the process of developing any therapy for use in humans requires a series of steps including basic science, test in animals, test in small groups of humans for safety, and test in groups of patients for proof of concept followed by randomized and usually blinded human trials (1). Following initial FDA approval there is a growing expectation that there will be careful long-term follow-up to assess the longevity of the response, long-term side effects and monitoring for rare but serious side effects. Additionally useful, but rarely done, would be clinical research to determine which patient subgroups are more or less likely to respond. For the purposes of this chapter we will focus on the issues involved in the design of clinical trials either for proof of concept or the primary randomized trials necessary for approval. The contents are very general in nature which cover clinical trials required for any type of dosage forms including dermal (systemic and topical). However, if any specific design feature is required/recommended or any specific dosage forms are to be tested, the sponsor is encouraged to consult the specific clinical division of the Agency before embarking on a clinical trial.

In the first part, we present the concepts that should drive decisions about clinical trial design, including selecting the purpose or goal of the study, selecting the design features that are most likely to demonstrate efficacy if it exists, selecting the appropriate analysis for the primary outcome, and choosing the most appropriate interpretations of those results. In the second part, we present an outline of the practical implementation of those concepts as defined in the current FDA guidance.

## PART 1 – ISSUES IN CLINICAL TRIAL DESIGN

## 9.2 CHOOSING THE QUESTION AND OUTCOME

Although it may appear to be simple, the initial step to specifically define the question to be answered by a clinical trial must be carefully thought through to avoid expensive mistakes later on in the process. In the setting of trying to achieve regulatory approval, the research question is often focused on the efficacy of the treatment; however, efficacy may be defined differently depending on the treatment or disease syndrome. For the treatment of pain, the outcome is usually some change in the level of pain, but even such a seemingly simple question has an underlying complexity that is not always evident. Do we want to know the average pain, worst pain or least pain and over what time period (2)? While clearly related, these characteristics of a pain process are not identical and can provide information with very different meanings. Are we interested in reducing the pain at rest, spontaneous exacerbation of pain or the pain during activity? Specific to transdermal products, are we interested in reducing skin hypersensitivity locally (e.g., lidocaine patches), or more generalized systemic pain (e.g., fentanyl patches)? What scale should we use to measure the patient's pain response, with choices including 0–10 numeric rating scale, verbal descriptor scales, visual analogue 100mm line, faces or even color? Each of these scales have been demonstrated to be valid, but they may not all work in all populations (3). We also need to consider how to define efficacy, i.e., how much of a change would be considered clinically important. These decisions are best driven by the biology of the pain syndrome and pharmacologic properties of the treatment being considered. In addition, consideration should be given to the availability of valid and reliable measures. Deciding which measure is most appropriate for a particular study will again depend on the type of pain being studied, the presumed underlying etiology, and the anticipated activity of the therapy to be tested.

In addition to the disease entity to be studied and the symptom or sign of interest, the outcome selection will also depend heavily on the purpose of the study. Clearly if the pharmacokinetics of a drug is the primary purpose then the outcome will need to be blood or other tissue levels measured frequently at appropriate time intervals (4, 5).

If the safety of a medication is the primary focus, it will need to be reflected in the outcome(s) (6, 7). Most often the primary focus is efficacy but how it is defined will depend on the expected biological properties of the therapy (8, 9). Questions include if the treatment ever achieves a therapeutic effect, how long that effect will last and in what proportion of patients will it work satisfactorily since no therapies work in everyone. A separate question is the number of doses needed to achieve the desired effect and the safety of multiple administrations over time (10, 11).

Once the primary outcome for a study is selected, additional supportive secondary outcomes must be chosen. Frequently studies of specific therapies will also measure more global responses to ensure that benefits in one area are not offset by worsening in another. While pain is important, it is only one part of the more complex construct of quality of life. As such, global transition questions and measures of the overall effect on quality of life are a usual requirement. To improve the choice of outcomes, expert groups have been created to provide evidence-based guidance in the choice of outcomes. The oldest such group is the Outcome Measures in Rheumatology (OMERACT) which started in 1992 and in collaboration with the Osteoarthritis Research Society International (OARSI) has devised guidelines related to studies of arthritis (12). For pain, the Initiative on Methods, Measurement, and Pain Assessment in Clinical Trials (IMMPACT) group began considering these issues in 2000 and has published several papers on these topics (13, 14, 15). Choosing among the potentially relevant outcomes for clinical studies should depend primarily on the choice of the biological or clinical question to be answered.

In considering the testing of transdermal systems, they are often used to deliver drugs that have been shown to be efficacious via other delivery systems. In this case, we are generally confident that if the drug is delivered systemically in adequate amounts, it should have the desired effect. Thus issues of blood levels and the consistency of delivery over time with different skin types and/or body composition (e.g., skin changes with age, obese vs non-obese, location of the patch) become important. To study the side effects of a product, appropriate study designs will need to focus on the questions of risk rather than on efficacy. Consideration will need to be given to specific potential problems that may be inherent in transdermal systems including: direct skin toxicity from the device, drug and drug diluents; process for enhancing drug diffusion (e.g., heat, iontophoresis, etc.), or process of skin occlusion; and the potential for an allergic reaction to any of these components. Additional issues about the design of these delivery systems may influence the choice of additional outcomes including the procedure for changing of the system, exposure to unabsorbed medication and disposal of the device. The outcomes and the study designs necessary for a study of risks will need to be substantially different than those for an efficacy study.

## 9.3 DESIGN ISSUES IN CLINICAL TRIALS

Once the question has been properly formulated, the appropriate type of clinical trial must be designed. For efficacy studies a randomized clinical trial is almost always required to avoid the inherent biases and confounders present in observational studies. The advantage of an experimentally designed randomized clinical trial is that the researcher has substantial control over many of the features of the design and conduct. The primary disadvantage stems from the same issue, namely that there are many decisions to be made and it is often not obvious how to choose the best of several options. Advances in our understanding of the problems inherent in a randomized clinical trial and in the technology available to improve the conduct of such trials have provided a growing number of design types, but the gold standard remains the parallel two (or more) group comparison trial. In an increasing number of cases there is now published data to support the particular approaches but most aspects of clinical trial design reflect the preferences of the designer and the availability of the appropriate resources for the study.

In considering the design of any clinical trial, there are some key characteristics that must be considered, as outlined in Figure 9.1. While all of them are important, the underpinning of the advantage afforded by a randomized clinical trial is being able to interpret group differences found at the end of a trial on the assumption that the two (or more) groups being compared were the same at the beginning. Randomization provides the best assurance that this assumption is correct.

## 9.4 PATIENT SELECTION PROCESS

The primary consideration in the selection of a population is what aspect of a treatment is to be tested. For a study of efficacy, it is best to choose patients who are most likely to respond to the treatment to tests based on *a priori* inclusion and exclusion criteria. This is consistent with good clinical practice in which we use diagnostic criteria to help identify the most likely disease causing the patient's symptoms and then apply additional criteria at our disposal that might further refine the group to those most likely to benefit from a specific therapy. The more specific the patient group selected for a clinical trial, the higher the probability of demonstrating a true treatment effect, if a true effect exists. If the study question is to determine the potential for side effects, then an argument can be made for selecting the usually larger population of patients who are at risk of being exposed to the treatment, once it has been approved for human use. In the product development cycle, these types of trials are usually conducted only after the treatment has been shown to be efficacious in at least some more restricted groups of patients.

It is also quite common to restrict our initial testing to groups of people considered to be a lower risk, which tends to exclude children, pregnant women and the elderly. While this may make sense from the perspective of reducing the risk to these populations, it also prevents us from learning about the efficacy and potential side effects in these populations. This has important implications for the use of any therapy in these more vulnerable populations. Significant controversy still surrounds the best way to accomplish specific group testing, but there is no question that clinical trial evidence for efficacy and safety is an important and yet under achieved goal for these populations.

While from a clinical perspective the choice may seem clear, sorting out a strict definition of a clinical disease and choosing the necessary limitations to the population (age, sex, concomitant diseases and medications, etc.) can present significant problems. A primary principal of an experimental clinical trial is that the more

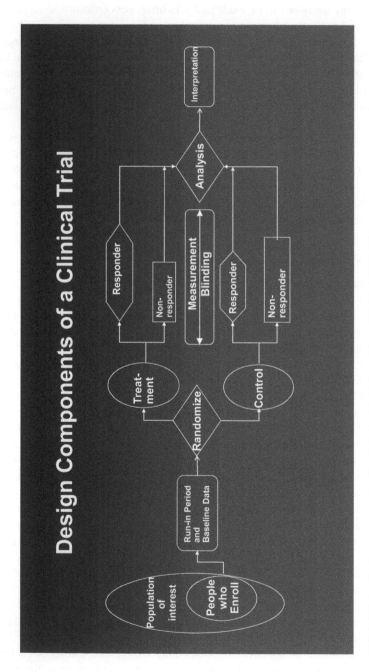

**FIGURE 9.1** Design components of a clinical trial. (Adapted from JT. Med 2010, 23.)

homogenous the test population, the less random variability will be present and the less random noise will be introduced into the study. Less random noise provides an improved efficiency in the demonstration of a true effect, if one exists. However, the difficulty with reducing variability is (1) being able to identify *a priori* the important variability stemming from a lack of understanding of the biology that leads to uninformative variability; (2) not adequately testing the new therapy in an appropriate range of people who might ultimately be administered the treatment in order to understand the potential side effect spectrum; and (3) recruiting adequate numbers of patients with the required inclusion and exclusion criteria. The decision about the appropriate population is also affected by the phase of testing, since earlier trials are often interested in knowing if any group will have a positive response, while later stage testing needs to discern what percentage of the population likely to be exposed may have a positive response. Different choices for the inclusion/exclusion criteria may lead to differing results in a clinical trial, and the design of the trial will differ as well.

Another consideration for the selection of a population is the potential usefulness of a pre-randomization testing of procedures, treatments or placebo using a run-in period. Each has its own issues and concerns. The procedure testing run-in period can be an important process to avoid protocol violations during the study, especially for complex studies. This run-in period involves having the potential subject go through the study process, including data collection, application of a dummy transdermal medications or device, and interaction with the study staff to ensure that the subjects are willing and able to carry out the necessary procedures for the study. This can often be combined with the collection of the study qualifying or baseline measurement data but may need a separate consent form, depending on the complexity of the procedures. It is much better to exclude patients who cannot appropriately complete the study requirements before their randomization than later in the study.

A placebo run-in can be very similar to the procedural run-in but it includes the use of a dummy treatment, often given in a blinded fashion, but with the intent of eliminating subjects with a large placebo response. This process is very controversial and has shown poor performance in a number of disease areas, especially depression and pain (16). The primary issue is that a single period of exposure to any treatment or placebo does not adequately define the subject as a responder (17). Rather than demonstrating a response to a placebo, the subject's responses are as likely to be due to the natural history of the disease or the regression to the mean phenomenon. Excluding such subjects appears to have no benefit for the efficiency of the subsequent clinical trial, especially of symptomatic disease (16, 17, 18). In some circumstances it can have a detrimental effect, since by keeping only those subjects who do not respond during the dummy treatment period the investigator may enhance the group of subjects who are unlikely to respond to any therapy. As such, run-in periods intended to exclude placebo subjects who appear to respond during that period are generally not recommended.

Treatment run-in periods are generally used for a different purpose and have been shown to be potentially useful in some circumstances. These run-in periods are conducted generally with open label active treatment and intended to identify patients with at least the potential to respond to the treatment. While the same issue of not being able to identify true responders in a single period of treatment also applies, this process will tend to exclude subjects with a lower than average response to the drug. This is because the patients that are likely to volunteer for a study generally have worse symptoms than average so the regression to the mean and natural history of the disease will tend towards improvement (so they remain in the study) and if the natural history of disease for a particular subject tends towards worsening, the decrement would have to be significant to overcome a true effect of the treatment. The patients excluded by this method will tend to be those who are less likely to respond to any treatment including the study treatment. Once the subjects who respond to the treatment are identified, they can either all be taken off the treatment in a washout period and then randomized to restart placebo or the study treatment (enriched enrollment), or they can be entered into a randomized withdrawal paradigm in which half are randomized to continue therapy and half are switched to placebo (randomized withdrawal). When used appropriately, these studies may have the best possibility of demonstrating an effect if a true effect exists for the treatment.

However, the use of a treatment to select the patient population to be studied remains controversial because of concerns about how the population would be identified in a clinical practice, and because it does not study the potential longer-term side effects of the treatment in the population who may subsequently be exposed to the drug once it has been approved. For approval purposes, it is unlikely that more than one of this type of study will be acceptable as a pivotal study. This issue should be carefully discussed as part of the approval process.

## 9.5   CONTROL TREATMENTS

The primary function of a control group is to isolate the effect of interest. In other words, any difference between the treated group and the control group should be attributable to the effect of the treatment we wish to study, without concerns about pretreatment difference. Often the evaluation of efficacy requires testing of a new treatment against a placebo in a randomized trial with blinding to treatment status so as to restrict the differences between groups to the specific drug effect (see the discussion of blinding in Section 9.8). Studies conducted with unblinded treatments are still valid, but the between group differences include both the actual specific physiologic effect of the treatment and the effect of being unblinded (i.e., the patient and physician's expectation of efficacy).

The primary focus of the selection of the control for a transdermal device will differ depending on whether our intention is to study the efficacy of the therapy or the efficacy of the device for the delivery of the therapy. In the first case, we would want to measure the difference between the test therapy and a placebo both being administered via the appliance. In the second case, a valid study would need to test the difference between a transdermal application and an oral or other systemic administration of the same substance. In both these cases it would be possible and important to blind the patient as to the active treatment they are receiving. But there are other situations in which it may not be possible to blind the patient for technical or ethical reasons. For example, if we were to study a surgical procedure, it would probably be considered unethical to conduct a sham operation. In that case, the difference between the study treatment and the control treatment would be both the specific results of the surgery as well as the effect of the patient's participation in the whole process of going through the surgical procedure and the expectation of benefit. The study would be a valid comparison but the implications of the results would require a careful consideration of the effect of the patient's knowledge about the type of the treatment they received.

While placebo treatments are often the control of choice, there has been a growing interest in the use of an additional positive control to test if the clinical trial design itself functioned as expected. In particular, it is possible that if a treatment effect does not differentiate from a placebo that there may be a problem with the study design or implementation of the trial such that not even a truly effective treatment would be detectable. This can be determined by the addition of an active control as an additional group using a treatment that is known to work. If the known effective treatment does not demonstrate efficacy, then the trial can be assumed to be faulty and should be repeated. This type of design helps to prevent the discarding of potentially effective treatments because of a failed trial. In situations where there exists a known effective treatment it is also not unusual for regulatory groups, especially in Europe, to demand an active comparator in order to gain information about the relative effectiveness of a new treatment compared to what already exists.

## 9.6 SELECTION OF TREATMENT AND TIMING

In the choice of a treatment design we must also consider the timing of onset of the purported treatment effect. There are different components of a patient's response, including the onset of meaningful effect, duration of the effect, multi-dose effects and any potential for the development of tolerance over time. For each component, thought must be given as to the best control group, the timing of the primary and secondary measures, and the choice of the level of the effect that will represent a clinically important or scientifically relevant response. For transdermal patches intended to provide a long period of drug availability, this will need to be tested by assessing the outcome at several appropriate time points over the intended period of administration. For short onset transdermal patches, such as some transmucosal medications, the time period will be much shorter and assessments will need to be designed to match.

## 9.7 RANDOMIZATION

The purpose of randomization is to balance both known and unknown confounding and bias at the baseline between the groups to be compared. This ensures that the initial groups are approximately equivalent prior to the introduction of the study treatment, so that any differences between the groups at the study endpoints can be attributed to the treatment. The more diverse the study population, the larger the number of patients that will be needed to ensure equivalent grouping, independent of the sample size estimated on the likelihood of response. As with all parts of a clinical trial, the implementation of the randomization needs to be carefully planned. Ideally, the randomization is done by a centralized process that is not otherwise associated with the study. This reduces the likelihood that the investigators, coordinators or patients might influence which patients get assigned to which group. A central pharmacy is often used for this process and maintains a record of the blinded assignment in case an unforeseen urgent medical situation occurs for which it is important to know the drug assignment.

The randomization is also generally assessed at the end of a trial by comparing the demographic details of the various treatment groups to show that they are not significantly different. Occasionally by chance, randomization will create groups that are uneven in some aspect. If the inequality is potentially important, the clinical trial results can be adjusted for this factor. To prevent an uneven distribution of particularly important characteristics, randomization can be produced in blocks, such that for each block of patients the important baseline characteristic is equally divided between treatment groups. This is frequently done for enrollment sites in a multi-site trial. This can be more important for smaller studies, where the potential for uneven randomization is larger.

## 9.8  BLINDING

Blinding is the process by which the study subjects, investigators, coordinators, data collectors and statisticians are kept uninformed about which subjects are in which treatment group. This is an important step in nearly all clinical trials, since this knowledge will often affect the results of the trial. For subjects, their expectation of the treatment outcome can substantially affect the reported results (19). For investigators and coordinators, knowing the subject's assignment will consciously or unconsciously affect how they treat the subject. For the data collector, this knowledge may affect the data collection such as making unconscious allowances for vague answers depending on the group assignment. Even during the statistical analysis, the process of ensuring data integrity and accuracy might be undertaken more vigorously for some entries, if the subject's group assignment is known. Since there are many people in the study who need to be blinded, it is best to describe who is blinded and how, rather than referring to a study as "double blind" or "triple blind." In situations where complete blinding of treatment is not possible, as many people as possible that are associated with the study should continue to be blinded, such as the data collectors and statisticians, for all the reasons mentioned.

## 9.9  GOOD CLINICAL PRACTICE

With any clinical study, the process of ensuring that it is conducted with the utmost care and consistency requires a careful attention to the details of all aspects of the trial. In addition, plans should be made in advance about how to deal with all known potential problems. This process is known as the development of a manual of procedures that details the specific implementation of all aspects of the trial, defining the timing of all visits, treatments and data collection instruments, as well as how to handle any possible deviations in this schedule. The responsibilities of each member of the project must be clearly spelled out and ideally the appropriate lines of communication for any issues that may arise. All staff members involved in the trial should be carefully trained on the procedures and processes to be used, and a plan for ongoing consistent monitoring, retraining and remediation designed to minimize any mistakes and detect those that do occur.

In addition it is important to carefully define the testing necessary for the inclusion/exclusion criteria and how decisions about inclusion of subjects will be made. Ideally, the decision about inclusion of subjects should be made by a group independent of the site investigators and based solely on the data collected and reported. While this may be somewhat more cumbersome than a decentralized process, it avoids the situation of site investigators viewing patients' baseline data in the most positive light because they are rewarded (monetarily or otherwise) for the enrollment of patients. For example, in a pain clinical trial the patients recruited may be encouraged, either overtly or subconsciously, to inflate their reported pain to gain participation in the study. This puts the study at greater risk of failing to show a difference when one truly exists because the artificially higher baseline pain scores reported will likely fall to the real pain level in both placebo and treated groups. Patients, as well, may want to be enrolled and overstate some of their criteria in order to be included if they know the specific requirements for inclusion either from other patients or published protocols, such as on ClinicalTrials.gov. While a central decision unit does not totally eliminate the problems with incorrect enrollment, it is likely to make it less common.

Lastly, it is important to set up systems to ensure quality control of the data. This involves several different components. Beginning with data collection, it is imperative that the data be checked for completeness, including having the study coordinator checking forms after they have been completed and before the subject leaves the study visit. All forms and/or data collected on a computer-based entry system must be monitored by the data coordinating center to ensure completeness and appropriate entries (i.e., numbers or letters or check marks in single boxes as appropriate). Any problems noted should be immediately brought to the attention of the appropriate coordinator or study staff to encourage a better review of the data collection process, to improve subject scheduling to ensure timely collections and to identify potential problem points with the data collection instruments. The amount and type of missing data, and the number of subjects who drop out, should be monitored and reported to the study steering committee on a timely and regular basis. Once the data is collected and entered, it must be kept safe, with an appropriate backup strategy and locked locations for both the online and any paper data.

While paper forms, whether computer readable or not, serve as the backup for data collected in this way, the move towards computerized data collection has created a need for new ways to ensure that there are no accidental or purposeful change of the data once entered. This requires the use of software with comprehensive and dependable tracking for changes made to the data. When data is entered from a paper form, special care must be taken that it is entered into a computer database accurately. This generally involves double data entry, or computer readable forms, as the initial entry with a subsequent careful review of the data entered by study staff. Prior to any analysis steps, any issues of data cleaning and checking must be completed. All attempts should be made to establish the actual data recorded and to have it reflected accurately in the computerized dataset.

## 9.10   THE ANALYSIS OF THE DATA

An integral part of the determination of the outcomes (both primary and secondary) is the determination of the a priori analysis plan. A primary feature must be the planned analysis of all collected data using an intention to treat (ITT) format to preserve the strength of the randomization process. Any and all drop outs must be accounted for and their data included in the analysis. Dealing with missing data is an area of some controversy as to the best approach which is beyond the scope of this chapter but is well described in a recent IOM report (20). If the primary analysis is to consider whether subjects achieve a level of response and to examine the difference in level of response between the treatment groups, then any patient who drops out of treatment can be considered a non-responder, or baseline observation carry forward (BOCF). This is considered a more conservative approach than the last observation carry forward (LOCF) process, but in using BOCF there is a loss of some degree of variability, since patients that drop out are all assigned a change in pain value of 0. Whatever method is ultimately used, it is important to remember that all methods impute the missing data in one way or another, and that the best method is to conduct the trial in such a way as to prevent as much missingness as possible. The IOM report recommends using mixed methods regression models which are less sensitive to missing data but each method has underlying assumptions about the type of missing data, namely missing-at-random (MAR), or not-missing-at-random (NMAR). A more recent method proposes using data from cumulative responder analyses (21) truncated at a specific response level that removes all missing data without consideration of the reason for missingness (22). A second key point made by the IOM report is that whatever the analysis method that is used primarily to deal with missing data, sensitivity analyses should be pre-specified to assess the robustness of the primary results to the missing data.

The statistical analysis of any data serves two primary functions. The first and most important function is to define a summary of the size of the effect. This is the primary answer to the question for which the study was originally designed and is the most important number in deciding on the clinical importance or scientific relevance of any study. The size of the effect can be represented using many units or forms, but there are only two basic constructs for this number, namely: (1) a central tendency (mean, median, mode) and a width of the distribution (standard deviation, standard error, 95% confidence interval, etc.), or (2) a proportion of the subjects who are considered responders and the range of the proportion of responders (standard deviation, standard error, 95% confidence interval, etc.). The proportion of responders is a more useful statistic from the perspective of clinical applicability, but it requires making the sometimes difficult choice of deciding what level of effect constitutes a clinically important or scientifically relevant response. For an increasing number of disease entities, the level of response that corresponds to a clinically important difference has been defined, using either anchor or distribution-based methods. The clinically important difference (CID) is applied to each individual subject to decide if he or she has achieved a response and then the proportion of responders is compared between groups. An alternate method for displaying the difference between groups at all possible levels of subject response is the use of cumulative distribution function

(CDF) curves (discussed in Section 9.11). Since both the central tendency and the responder calculations can usually be accomplished for most studies, it would seem appropriate that both be described, but this has not generally been the case in the past. It is important to understand that the CID does not apply to the level of difference between groups, which is a more difficult decision to make. Clearly the size of the difference between groups will depend on the type of disease being studied. For example, a 5% difference between groups in survival from sepsis is likely to be important, while a 5% increase in number of patients who achieve relief of their headache pain may not.

The second function of statistical analyses is to determine the probability that the result obtained could have occurred by chance. The standard cut-off is a two-sided p-value of <0.05. Most often, whether or not this level is achieved is dependent primarily on the sample size of the comparison groups. The p-value is a necessary component of any study analysis but not sufficient to provide information on the clinical importance or scientific relevance of the result. Values other than <0.05 are sometimes used depending on the type of outcome that is predefined. In particular, for clinical trials in which multiple outcomes have been defined, some process for adjusting the applicable p-value must be applied.

Whatever decision is made about how to analyze and present the data, a major component of the reporting of clinical trials is completeness and transparency about how the data were measured, collected and analyzed. This issue has become a prime concern for most journals and is being enforced by the advent of several processes that are now required for the publication of most clinical trials. The first is the requirement that such trials be registered on the ClinicalTrials.gov website prior to the initiation of data collection, so that the *a priori* hypotheses and analysis plans are public. While some trials may require changes during the conduct, these will now be available for public scrutiny and must be included in the write-up of the publication. This helps to ensure that the assumptions used to design the trial are maintained through the analysis and publication so that the reader of the publication can be confident that the authors did not cherry pick results that happened to reflect a desired outcome, rather than the original goals of the study. Second, almost all journals now require the inclusion of a Consort Statement diagram (23) in the publication to accurately account for all subjects in the trial, protecting against the presentation of results from a select subgroup of patients as the primary analysis. Subgroup analyses are often still important results as long as they are appropriately presented with all of the limitations appropriate for such analyses.

Transparency in reporting also applies to the secondary outcomes of any trial. Secondary outcomes remain substantially important in supporting (or not) the evidence derived from the primary results. They also help to provide important evidence to help us understand potential mechanisms or processes that underlie the primary outcome and contribute to our understanding of the importance of our primary findings. However, it is imperative that the study authors make clear in their publication which outcomes are primary, which are secondary and to help the reader understand how to best interpret the results based on this differentiation. As long as the authors are clear about these issues, all of the potentially important results of a study can be presented and discussed.

## 9.11   INTERPRETATION OF THE RESULTS

The potential usefulness of the results of any clinical trial to the reader will depend in large part on the understandability of the data presented and the interpretation of the potential implications that are consistent with those findings. It is the responsibility of every investigator to provide the reader with an understanding of the clinical or scientific importance of their results. In the application of clinical research data to clinical practice, the proportion of responders is more easily applied. This outcome answers the question "What is the probability that if I give a patient this treatment, they will get better enough to be considered clinically important?" This is usually the question that both physicians and patients ask about any treatment. The mean or median value of improvement in a group does not answer this question, since we will not know if everyone in the treated group from the clinical trial improved by a small amount, or how many people achieved a clinically important level of improvement. However, the selection of a cut-off point for what constitutes clinically important may seem somewhat arbitrary, and as such it is not uncommon for results to be presented for several different cut-off points.

Another method for presenting the proportion of patients who reach a specific level of response is to present the data for all possible cut-off points. This form of the data is known as a cumulative distribution function (CDF) curve (21), which has a one-to-one correlation with the normal density curve distribution of data used to graphically represent the central tendency and distribution. The CDF graphs provide data for every potential outcome value as the number or proportion of subjects who have achieved an outcome at that level or above. An example for a transmucosal form of fentanyl is presented in Figure 9.2, which has the cut-off level on the x-axis and the proportion of subjects achieving that level of effect on the y-axis (21). Based on the reader's choice of cut-off, they can read off the graph the likelihood that their patient will achieve the level of response. The probabilities of success are then used to help the clinician make a decision about using that medication, but the choice to use a treatment is dichotomous, either yes or no. Ultimately the decision about continuing the medication will also be dichotomous dependent on the level of benefit achieved, consistent with the information provided in the CDF curves shown on the graph.

## 9.12   ASSESSMENT OF SIDE EFFECTS

Studies of efficacy are not the only potential use for clinical trials. For the drug approval process and in providing data to clinicians on how to use a treatment process, the potential risks must also be assessed. Although not ideal, studies of these risks usually occur by observing all subjects exposed to the drug over time. Without a comparison group, it is impossible to distinguish between random occurrences and a true side effect of the treatment. All clinical trials also collect side-effect data but are generally not powered to detect small differences, even potentially serious ones. However, any study with a control group does provide some data on the occurrence of the side effect in the treated and non-treatment control. It is also important to consider that in a typical treatment development program it would be unusual to expose

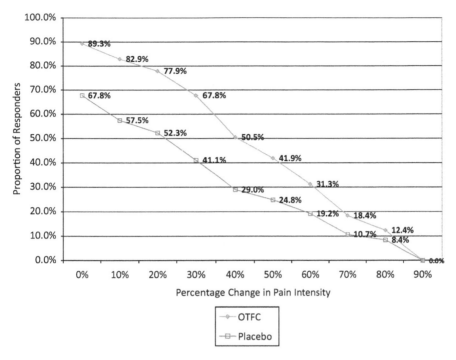

**FIGURE 9.2** Cumulative distribution function graph.

more than 10,000 subjects to a new drug before it is approved for human use. As such, we cannot know if a side effect, even death, occurs less often than 1/1,000. This fact argues for continued vigilance and active surveillance of the side effects reported in the use of any new therapy after approval.

In addition to the usual systemic side effect, dermal delivery systems must also consider other factors including the effect of a high drug concentration on local structures, the matrix material or adhesives, the occlusion of the skin, and method used to promote delivery or enhance short-term delivery. The potential consequences of accidental exposure of others to the medication must also be carefully considered, as has been seen in the use of testosterone products delivered as a cream or gel.

The process of evaluating side effects begins long before the conduct of a clinical trial with laboratory testing in cell cultures and then animals. If found safe in those groups, the product will be tested as a first time in humans, by giving increasing amounts serially to a small healthy population to evaluate pharmacokinetics, tolerability and to ensure that there are no serious side effects (phase I), followed by the use in subjects with the disease of interest striving to find the appropriate dose (phase IIA) and a proof of concept trial to learn about the potential for efficacy (phase IIB). Once the treatment has passed these hurdles without evidence of significant side-effect risks, larger phase III clinical trials are conducted to evaluate the efficacy in a population of patients. The trials must be large enough to maximize the likelihood of a significant p-value for the effect size thought to be clinically relevant, if an effect truly exists for the treatment. At least two positive phase III trials with acceptable risk profile are required for the FDA to consider a treatment for approval. This is also generally followed by an agreement on a monitoring program for the general population who will be prescribed the treatment to ensure that rarer important side effects can be detected in an appropriate time frame (phase IV). For transdermal devices, this process may be conducted separately for the device itself, followed by the drug and the device together, making the process a bit more complex.

## 9.13   CONCLUSION – PART 1

In conclusion, the most important part of designing the appropriate clinical trial for the testing of any treatment is a carefully defined question, selection of the right outcome measures, selection of the right population of patients, careful planning and monitoring of the execution of the trial, appropriate analyses of the data, and appropriate interpretation of the results. This process is well understood with a growing body of evidence on how to fit the process to a wide variety of research and clinical questions. With careful attention to detail, a clinical trial is the best method for obtaining an answer to the question of what treatments work, in whom and under what conditions. Ultimately all such trials try to answer the basic clinical question of whether the benefit of the treatment (taking into account the possible risks) is going to improve the patient's longevity or quality of life. At the end of the day, clinical trials function best when they adhere to the axiom that "A difference is a difference only if it makes a difference" (Darrell Huff).

## REFERENCES – PART 1

1. Anonymous. Guidance for Industry: Providing Clinical Evidence of Effectiveness for Human Drugs and Biological Products. In: Food and Drug Administration – Center for Drug Evaluation and Research (CDER), ed. Rockville, MD; 1998.
2. Cleeland CS, Ryan KM. Pain assessment: global use of the Brief Pain Inventory. *Annals of the Academy of Medicine, Singapore*. 1994;23(2):129–38.
3. Jensen MP, Engel JM, McKearnan KA, Hoffman AJ. Validity of pain intensity assessment in persons with cerebral palsy: a comparison of six scales. *Journal of Pain*. 2003;4(2):56–63.
4. Gschwend MH, Martin W, Arnold P, Verdun MO, Cambon N, Frentzel A, et al. Determination of the transdermal bioavailability of a newly developed diclofenac sodium patch in comparison with a reference preparation. *Arzneimittel-Forschung*. 2005;55(7):403–13.
5. Sathyan G, Zomorodi K, Gidwani S, Gupta S. The effect of dosing frequency on the pharmacokinetics of a fentanyl HCl patient-controlled transdermal system (PCTS). *Clinical Pharmacokinetics*. 2005;44 Suppl 1:17–24.
6. Katz NP. The measurement of symptoms and side effects in clinical trials of chronic pain. *Contemporary Clinical Trials*. 2012;33(5):903–11.
7. Wisniewski SR, Rush AJ, Balasubramani GK, Trivedi MH, Nierenberg AA, Investigators S. Self-rated global measure of the frequency, intensity, and burden of side effects. *Journal of Psychiatric Practice*. 2006;12(2):71–9.

8. Bolognese JA, Ehrich EW, Schnitzer TJ. Precision of composite measures of osteoarthritis efficacy in comparison to that of individual endpoints. *Journal of Rheumatology.* 2001;28(12):2700–4.

9. Gilron I, Jensen MP. Clinical trial methodology of pain treatment studies: selection and measurement of self-report primary outcomes for efficacy. *Regional Anesthesia & Pain Medicine.* 2011;36(4):374–81.

10. Gidal BE, DeCerce J, Bockbrader HN, Gonzalez J, Kruger S, Pitterle ME, et al. Gabapentin bioavailability: effect of dose and frequency of administration in adult patients with epilepsy. *Epilepsy Research.* 1998;31(2):91–9.

11. Jalali S, MacFarlane JG, Grace EM, Kassam YB. Frequency of administration of short half-life nonsteroidal anti-inflammatory analgesics (NSAID's): studies with ibuprofen. *Clinical & Experimental Rheumatology.* 1986;4(1):91–3.

12. Hawker GA, Davis AM, French MR, Cibere J, Jordan JM, March L, et al. Development and preliminary psychometric testing of a new OA pain measure—an OARSI/OMERACT initiative. *Osteoarthritis & Cartilage.* 2008;16(4):409–14.

13. Dworkin RH, Turk DC, Farrar JT, Haythornthwaite JA, Jensen MP, Katz NP, et al. Core outcome measures for chronic pain clinical trials: IMMPACT recommendations. *Pain.* 2005;113(1–2):9–19.

14. Dworkin RH, Turk DC, McDermott MP, Peirce-Sandner S, Burke LB, Cowan P, et al. Interpreting the clinical importance of group differences in chronic pain clinical trials: IMMPACT recommendations. *Pain.* 2009;146(3):238–44.

15. Turk DC, Dworkin RH, Allen RR, Bellamy N, Brandenburg N, Carr DB, et al. Core outcome domains for chronic pain clinical trials: IMMPACT recommendations. *Pain.* 2003;106(3):337–45.

16. Lee S, Walker JR, Jakul L, Sexton K. Does elimination of placebo responders in a placebo run-in increase the treatment effect in randomized clinical trials? A meta-analytic evaluation. *Depression & Anxiety.* 2004;19(1):10–9.

17. Dworkin RH, McDermott MP, Farrar JT, O'Connor AB, Senn S. Interpreting patient treatment response in analgesic clinical trials: implications for genotyping, phenotyping, and personalized pain treatment. *Pain.* 2014;155(3):457–60.

18. Dworkin RH, Katz J, Gitlin MJ, Dworkin RH, Katz J, Gitlin MJ. Placebo response in clinical trials of depression and its implications for research on chronic neuropathic pain. *Neurology.* 2005;65(12 Suppl 4):S7–19.

19. Turner JA, Jensen MP, Warms CA, Cardenas DD, Turner JA, Jensen MP, et al. Blinding effectiveness and association of pretreatment expectations with pain improvement in a double-blind randomized controlled trial. *Pain.* 2002;99(1–2):91–9.

20. Committee on National Statistics. The Prevention and Treatment of Missing Data in Clinical Trials: Panel on Handling Missing Data in Clinical Trials. Washington, DC: The National Academies Press; 2010.

21. Farrar JT, Dworkin RH, Max MB, Farrar JT, Dworkin RH, Max MB. Use of the cumulative proportion of responders analysis graph to present pain data over a range of cut-off points: making clinical trial data more understandable. *Journal of Pain & Symptom Management.* 2006;31(4):369–77.

22. Permutt T, Li F. Trimmed means for symptom trials with dropouts. *Pharm Stat.* 2017 Jan;16(1):20–28. doi: 10.1002/pst.1768. Epub 2016 Aug 15. PubMed PMID: 27523396.

23. Bian Z-x, Shang H-c. CONSORT 2010 statement: updated guidelines for reporting parallel group randomized trials. *Annals of Internal Medicine.* 2011;154(4):290–1; author reply 1–2.

24. Farrar JT. Advances in clinical research methodology for pain clinical trials. *Nature Medicine.* 2010;16(11):1284–93.

## PART 2 – SUMMARY OF AVAILABLE GUIDANCES

## 9.14   BACKGROUND

The guidances discussed in this chapter provide a general overview on the clinical trial data requirements needed to support drug effectiveness that can enable sponsors to plan sufficient and efficient drug development programs which is aligned with the FDA's current philosophy regarding "quantitative and qualitative standards" (1). In general, a dermal dosage form, be it for topical or systemic use, contains a previously approved drug substance in a different dosage form (e.g., oral or parenteral). The purpose of conducting a clinical trial with this new delivery system will be to demonstrate efficacy and safety (both local and systemic) of the drug substance in this new dosage form via the new route of administration potentially for a new indication.

For transdermal systems, in the presence of an adequate systemic concentration to establish a clinical bridge with an already approved dosage form of the same molecule via another route (e.g., parenteral or oral), a 505(b)(2) new drug application may be enough for its approval and efficacy-based clinical trials may not be needed. However, in the absence of an adequate systemic concentration, as seen in topical (local) dosage forms, generally adequate well-controlled clinical trials are needed for approval of new drug applications. For approval of generic dermal dosage forms via 505(j) applications, generally pharmacokinetic (PK) based bioequivalence (BE) trials are required for transdermal (systemic) dosage forms and clinical endpoint-based BE trials are required for topical (local) dosage forms. Again, the sponsors should consult the Agency for specific recommendation for approval either via New Drug Application (NDA) or Abbreviated New Drug Application (ANDA) routes.

### 9.14.1   LEGAL REQUIREMENTS – THE FOOD, DRUG, AND COSMETICS ACT

The laws of the USA are systematized by subject into the United States Code which contains only the currently enacted statutory language. The Federal Food, Drug, and Cosmetic Act (FDCA) and future amending statutes are codified into Title 21 Chapter 9 of the United States Code. The FDCA was initially passed by Congress in 1938 giving full authority to the U.S. FDA to oversee the safety of various food, drug and cosmetic products. The act was influenced by the death of several hundred patients due to diethylene glycol contained in elixir sulfanilamide.

The current FDCA contains ten chapters that discuss the proper steps to ensure the safety of food, drugs, devices and cosmetics. FDCA section 505 more specifically covers the regulatory approval process to help bring drugs to market. The section is separated into different subsections that describe the grounds for approval and refusal. According to section 505:

1. All new drugs must need an approved application to market.
2. Each application must contain full reports of investigations to show whether the drug is safe and effective and detailed components, composition, methods and controls.
3. The FDA will be given full authority to provide a positive or negative approval.
4. Must provide grounds for refusal or approval of a drug application.

For more information on the legal requirements pertaining to new drug approvals, please refer to Title 21 Chapter 9 USC Section 355 (2).

## 9.14.2 DEFINITION OF SUBSTANTIAL EVIDENCE

Before the 1962 Kefauver-Harris amendments to the FDCA, drug companies were only required to demonstrate that their products were safe. The amendment included a provision that required manufacturers to provide "substantial evidence" of effectiveness based on results from "adequate and well-controlled clinical studies." Study subjects would be required to give their informed consent to participate in any trial. The FDCA states that the term "substantial evidence" relates to evidence:

> consisting of adequate and well-controlled investigations, including clinical investigations, by experts qualified by scientific training and experience to evaluate the effectiveness of the drug involved, on the basis of which it could fairly and responsibly be concluded by such experts that the drug will have the effect it purports or is represented to have under the conditions of use prescribed, recommended, or suggested in the labeling or proposed labeling thereof.

Title 21 CFR 314.126 emphasizes that the only basis for approval is data from adequate and well-controlled studies. New drug applications must provide all relevant information in full details from these studies and not just summaries. Additionally, for a drug to be approved, the effect must show statistical significance on a clinically meaningful endpoint that can be replicated (3).

## 9.14.3 DEFINITION OF ADEQUATE WELL-CONTROLLED STUDIES

### 9.14.3.1 FDA Guidance: Providing Clinical Evidence of Effectiveness for Human Drugs and Biological Products

The FDA guidance on providing clinical evidence of effectiveness states that "it has been the FDA's position that Congress generally intended to require at least two adequate and well-controlled studies, each convincing on its own, to establish effectiveness of a new drug. (See e.g., Final Decision on Benylin, 44 FR 51512, 518 [August 31, 1979]; Warner-Lambert Co. V. Heckler, 787 F. 2d 147 [3d Cir. 1986])". The requirement for more than one adequate and well-controlled clinical trial demonstrates the need for independent "substantiation" of experimental results (Section 2.A). The reasons why a single clinical trial may not be sufficient enough to support effectiveness include:

1. Clinical trials may introduce "unanticipated, undetected, systematic biases."
2. Variability in human biological systems may produce certain results by "chance" alone.
3. Results obtained in a single center may be dependent on site or investigator-specific factors.
4. Scientific fraud.

There are some situations in which the efficacy of a new product or an already approved drug product for a new indication can be demonstrated without additional well-controlled clinical trials. The guidance referenced on p. 328 provides additional examples of scenarios where effectiveness can be extrapolated from data for another indication or product (Section 2.C).

When submitting clinical effectiveness data for approval of a new product or new indication, companies must also "document that the studies were adequately designed and conducted." Trial planning, protocols, trial conduct and data handling need to be submitted to the FDA in order to show that the trials were adequately designed and conducted. However, based on the types of studies conducted the FDA is able to accept "different levels of documentation of data quality, as long as the adequacy of the scientific evidence can be assured" (Section 3.B).

## 9.15   GUIDANCE DOCUMENTS

### 9.15.1 Guidance Documents Related to Good Clinical Practice

ICH E6 (R1): Good Clinical Practice – Consolidated Guidance
ICH E6 (R2): Good Clinical Practice

The ICH guidelines on good clinical practice (GCP) suggest the necessary requirements in "designing, conducting, recording and reporting" clinical trials for drug approval (4,5). By following these guidelines, compliance is assured with regards to human subject rights, safety and well-being. Credibility to the data gathered from clinical trials is also protected by adhering to this set of guidelines put forth. These guidelines help provide a uniform standard for acceptance of clinical trial data by regulatory authorities. The amended guidelines [ICH E6 (R2)] provides improved and efficient approaches with trial design due to the evolution in technology and the increased complexity and cost of clinical trials (5). Guidelines on maintaining electronic data records from clinical trials also have been added in amended guidance in the hopes of increasing quality and efficiency.

There are several principles that lay the foundation of the guidances referenced on p. 329. It is important that any "foreseeable risks and inconveniences" be weighed against the benefit for the subject before initiating a trial. Any available clinical and non-clinical information on a study product can be used to propose a clinical trial. It is important that when developing clinical trials, the trials should be in compliance with protocols that have been submitted and approved by an institutional review board (IRB) and an independent ethics committee (IEC). The guidance also discusses the qualifications of the investigators who ultimately assume the responsibility of each trial subject and is compliant with protocols approved by the IRB/IEC. Sponsors who select these investigators should heavily focus on quality management in order to "ensure human subject protection and the reliability of trial results" (Section 3.1).

The guidance also provides input on the development of clinical trial protocols and investigator brochures. An Investigator's Brochure (IB) is a:

> compilation of the clinical and nonclinical data on the investigational product(s) that are relevant to the study of the product(s) in human subjects. Its purpose is to provide the investigators and others involved in the trial with the information to facilitate their understanding of the rationale for, and their compliance with, many key features

of the protocol, such as the dose, dose frequency/interval, methods of administration, and safety monitoring procedures. The IB also provides insight to support the clinical management of the study subjects during the course of the clinical trial. If a marketed product is being studied for a new use, an IB specific to that new use should also be prepared.

(Section 7.1)

Other essential documents that are developed throughout the stages of a clinical trial should also be considered for submission to the appropriate regulatory authorities:

Essential Documents are those documents which individually and collectively permit evaluation of the conduct of a trial and the quality of the data produced. These documents serve to demonstrate the compliance of the investigator, sponsor and monitor with the standards of Good Clinical Practice and with all applicable regulatory requirements.

These documents are usually audited by sponsors and regulatory authorities in order to ensure the credibility of the trial and the reliability of data. The documents can be organized into three different sections corresponding to the stage of the trial that they were generated from: (1) before the initiation of the trial, (2) during the clinical conduct and (3) after termination of the trial (Section 8.1).

### 9.15.2 GUIDANCE DOCUMENTS RELATED TO CONTENT OF CLINICAL REPORTS

ICH E3: Structure and Content of Clinical Study Reports

This guidance provides the necessary information needed to develop a clinical study report that can be acceptable to regulatory health authorities for approval of a new product (6). The report consists of the "clinical and statistical description, presentations, and analysis" that are integrated with:

protocols, sample case report forms, investigator-related information, information related to the test drugs/investigational products including active control/comparators, technical statistical documentation, related publications, patient data listings, and technical statistical details such as derivations, computations, analyses, and computer output.

Ultimately, the report should provide a concise explanation regarding the study design, plan, methods and execution of the study. In order for the health authorities to replicate critical analyses during the review process, the clinical study report should also include individual patient data and detailed analytical methods. Safety data from the clinical study should include the detailed discussions of individual adverse events and abnormal laboratory values. Subject demographics should also be included so that potential differences in efficacy and/or safety can be characterized by subgroup. Furthermore, specific clinical guidelines for different therapeutic areas have been developed and should be used when analyzing and presenting data. The main aim of the guidance is to inform all applicants of the necessary information that should be routinely provided to regulators in the hopes of reducing future post-submission requests for additional data and clarification.

### 9.15.3 GUIDANCE DOCUMENTS RELATED TO CLINICAL STUDY DESIGN

ICH E8: General Considerations for Clinical Trials
ICH E10: Choice of Control Group and Related Issues in Clinical Trials

The ICH E8 guidance provides a general overview regarding accepted principles and practices in the conduct of clinical trials. Clinical trials should be developed and analyzed according to scientific principles in order to achieve the intended objective. The included development methodology section covers issues and considerations relating to planning a clinical program and its individual component studies (7).

The role of control groups in clinical trials is to allow "discrimination of patient outcomes caused by the test treatment from outcomes caused by other factors, such as natural progression of the disease, observer or patient expectations, or other treatments" (Section 1.2). The ICH E10 guidance discusses different types of control groups that can be potentially used to demonstrate efficacy (8). Control groups are chosen from similar patient populations as the treatment group and are treated over the same period of time. It is very important the treatment and control groups share similar baseline characteristics so that bias from other confounding factors don't play a role in determining the efficacy of a test product (8).

Issues related to the use of an active control trial to demonstrate efficacy by showing non-inferiority or equivalence are also stated in the guidance (Section 1.5). However, there are scenarios where the interpretation of the results from non-inferiority trials cannot be used as evidence to support efficacy. In order to show efficacy in a non-inferiority trial, the trial needs to have the ability to differentiate between effective, less effective and ineffective treatments.

The guidance further describes the use of each type of control group in detail and discusses the control group's ability to minimize bias, ethical and practical issues associated with its use, usefulness and quality of inference in particular situations, modifications of study design or combinations with other controls that can resolve ethical, practical or inferential concerns, and overall advantages and disadvantages (8). A flow chart is also provided in order to help guide the selection for a specific control group based on trial objectives.

### 9.15.3.1 Randomized Clinical Trials: Study Designs

Title 21 CFR 314.126 states that the whole purpose of conducting clinical trials is to determine the effect of a drug from other factors such as change in disease progression, placebo effects or biased observations. As stated before, the FDA requires at least two well-controlled trials to prove safety and efficacy before a drug can enter the market. These well-controlled trials should be double blinded, randomized and should have placebo or active treatment as controls for comparison to the studied drug. Randomized controlled trials represent the gold standard to assess the effectiveness of medications. There are three important randomized clinical trial designs that are commonly used to evaluate new drugs and indications as described in the following sections:

#### 9.15.3.1.1 Parallel Study Design

*Parallel Study Design*

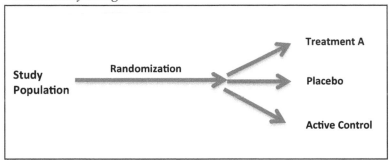

The parallel study design is a classical clinical trial approach. Subjects are randomized into different groups such as treatment, placebo or active control. Effectiveness of the drug being studied can be determined by either superiority over placebo or non-inferiority over an active control. Subjects who only complete the study are used for statistical analysis.

#### 9.15.3.1.2 Crossover Study Design

*Crossover Study Design*

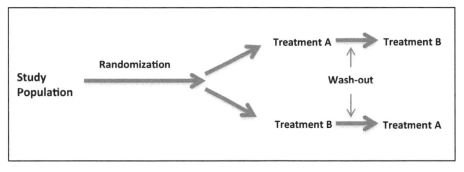

In a crossover study design, subjects are randomized to different sequences of treatments. This allows for a reduction in the source of variability and as a result there is no between-subject variability present. Each crossover subject serves as their own control. Often, crossover designs require fewer subjects to enroll. Disadvantages to this study design include a higher rate of drop-outs due to the length of the study and progression of disease. The order in which treatments are given to subjects may also influence the results of the study.

*9.15.3.1.3   Factorial Study Design*

*Factorial Study Design*

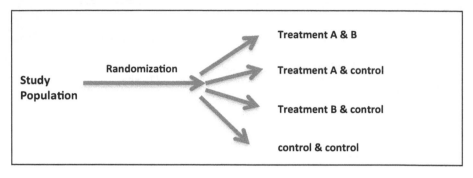

Factorial trial designs allow study investigators to look more closely at more than one treatment option in a single study. The study can be done by testing the treatments' effects independently or complementarily in order to assess if there are any treatment interactions. If the effect of treatment A differs depending on the level of treatment B, the main treatment cannot be interpreted independently due to the presence of an interaction. If there are no interactions, a single study can provide responses possible from two different studies.

## 9.15.4 Guidance Documents Related to Statistical Analysis

ICH E9: Statistical Principles for Clinical Trials

Statistics plays a key role in determining the significance of an effect due to a treatment in a clinical trial. It is important to note that the ICH E9 guidance addresses the importance of several statistical principles and not the use of specific statistical methods (9). When submitting a new application for approval, details regarding the design, conduct and proposed statistical analysis should be outlined in a well written protocol before the initiation of a trial. "The extent to which the procedures in the protocol are followed and the primary analysis is planned a priori will contribute to the degree of confidence in the final results and conclusions of the trial" (Section 1.2).

The statistical principles described in this guidance relate to minimizing bias and maximizing precision:

> The interpretation of statistical measures of uncertainty of the treatment effect and treatment comparisons should involve consideration of the potential contribution of bias to the p-value, confidence interval, or inference. Because the predominant approaches to the design and analysis of clinical trials have been based on frequentist statistical methods, the guidance largely refers to the use of frequentist methods when discussing hypothesis testing and/or confidence intervals.

(Section 1.2)

## 9.16   CONCLUSIONS – PART 2

As written in 21 CFR 315.126, the purpose of conducting adequate well-controlled studies is to confirm the effect of a drug from other factors when the drug is present in a specific dosage form and developed for a specific indication from a specific route of administration. The most important part of designing the appropriate clinical trial for the testing of any treatment is a carefully defined question, selection of the right outcome measures, selection of the right population of patients, careful planning and monitoring of the execution of the trial, appropriate analyses of the data and appropriate interpretation of the results. Although the regulatory requirements regarding the support for efficacy of a new drug product have been briefly described throughout this chapter, the sponsors are advised to consult the guidance documents listed in the following table and to the appropriate Regulatory Agencies for more specific information.

**Specific Guidance Documents Related to Clinical Trials:**

| Guidance Code | Title |
|---|---|
| E1 | The Extent of Population Exposure to Assess Clinical Safety for Drugs Intended for Long-Term Treatment of Non-Life-Threatening Conditions |
| E2A | Clinical Safety Data Management: Definitions and Standards for Expedited Reporting |
| E2B | Clinical Safety Data Management: Data Elements for Transmission of Individual Case Safety Reports |
| E2C | Clinical Safety Data Management: Periodic Safety Update Reports for Marketed Drugs |
| E3 | Structure and Content of Clinical Study Reports |
| E4 | Dose-Response Information to Support Drug Registration |
| E5 | Ethnic Factors in the Acceptability of Foreign Clinical Data |
| E6 | Good Clinical Practice: Consolidated Guideline |
| E7 | Studies in Support of Special Populations: Geriatrics |
| E8 | General Considerations for Clinical Trials |
| E9 | Statistical Considerations in the Design of Clinical Trials |
| E10 | Choice of Control Group in Clinical Trials |
| M3 | Nonclinical Safety Studies for the Conduct of Human Clinical Trials for Pharmaceuticals |
| S6 | Safety Studies for Biotechnology-Derived Products |

## REFERENCES – PART 2

1. FDA. Guidance for Industry: Providing Clinical Evidence of Effectiveness for Human Drug and Biological Products. www.fda.gov/downloads/Drugs/Guidance Compliance%20 RegulatoryInformation/Guidances/UCM078749.pdf
2. "Drugs and Devices" 21 CFR 9.355. (2011) www.gpo.gov/fdsys/pkg/USCODE-2011-title21/pdf/USCODE-2011-title21-chap9.pdf

3. "Adequate and Well Controlled Studies" 21 CFR 314.126 (2010) www.gpo.gov/fdsys/pkg/CFR-2010-title21-vol5/pdf/CFR-2010-title21-vol5-sec314-126.pdf
4. FDA. Guidance for Industry: E6 Good Clinical Practice: Consolidated Guidance. www.fda.gov/downloads/Drugs/.../Guidances/ucm073122.pdf
5. FDA. Guidance for Industry: E6 (R2) Good Clinical Practice. www.fda.gov/downloads/Drugs/GuidanceComplianceRegulatoryInformation/Guidances/UCM464506.pdf
6. FDA. Guidance for Industry: E3 Structure and Content of Clinical Study Reports. www.fda.gov/downloads/Drugs/GuidanceComplianceRegulatoryInformation/Guidances/UCM073113.pdf
7. FDA. Guidance for Industry: E8 General Considerations for Clinical Trials. www.fda.gov/downloads/Drugs/GuidanceComplianceRegulatoryInformation/Guidances/UCM073132.pdf
8. FDA. Guidance for Industry: E10 Choice of Control Group and Related Issues in Clinical Trials. www.fda.gov/downloads/Drugs/GuidanceComplianceRegulatoryInformation/Guidances/UCM073139.pdf
9. FDA. Guidance for Industry: E9 Statistical Principles for Clinical Trials. www.fda.gov/downloads/Drugs/GuidanceComplianceRegulatoryInformation/Guidances/UCM073137.pdf

# 10 Regulatory Standards for Approval of Topical Dermatological Drug Products

*April C. Braddy and Dale P. Conner*

## CONTENTS

## 10.1    INTRODUCTION

For several decades, the U.S. Food and Drug Administration (U.S. FDA) has been approving safe and effective locally acting topical dermatological drug products. These drug products are designed to deliver a topical drug to its local site of action, skin, in order to prevent or treat skin diseases and disorders. The drug product is applied to the stratum corneum which is the outermost layer of the skin. The skin disease state dictates the application site of the topical drug product. The sites on the skin can be the scalp, hand, foot, arm, leg, etc. The therapeutic drug classes consist mainly of analgesics, antibacterials, antifungals, anti-inflammatory agents (non-steroidal), antibiotics, antivirals, glucocorticoids (corticosteroids), oncologics and retinoids. The drug application site and the disease state have a direct relation to the selection of the appropriate dosage form to elicit the desired therapeutic effect.

Topical dermatological drug products are available in an array of dosage forms ranging from simple to complex. The varying dosage forms range from solutions (aqueous or oily) to semisolids, such as creams, foams, gels, lotions, ointments, pastes and sprays. These differences in dosage form can have an impact on drug absorption and thus efficacy of the drug product. The therapeutic response

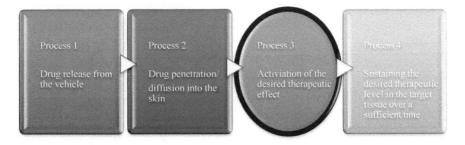

| Process 1 | Process 2 | Process 3 | Process 4 |
|---|---|---|---|
| Drug release from the vehicle | Drug penetration/diffusion into the skin | Activiation of the desired therapeutic effect | Sustaining the desired therapeutic level in the target tissue over a sufficient time |

**FIGURE 10.1** A schematic representation of the sequential process for elicitation of a therapeutic response after application of a topical dermatological drug product.

generated by application of these drug products to the skin is based on a sequential process, Figure 10.1 (Shah 2001; Weiss 2011). The site of activity (location of application on the skin), varying therapeutic drug classes and multiple dose forms are critical factors in bioequivalence (BE) assessment of topical drug products. These factors have a significant impact on the determination of the most appropriate methods that are suitable to support regulatory approval in the USA and for international regulatory authorities as well for particular drug products (Braddy et al. 2014).

There are several submission pathways to the U.S. FDA for potential approval of drug product. Three possible pathways are a new drug application (NDA) for new chemical entities, an abbreviated new drug application (ANDA) for a generic drug product or as an over-the-counter (OTC) product, Figure 10.2. The documentation that is necessary to support approval is based on the type of submission. In most instances, clinical trials are necessary for approval of NDAs. ANDAs usually contain BE studies with clinical endpoints for topical non-corticosteroid drug products. The approval can also be based on in vivo pharmacodynamic studies, pharmacokinetic studies, in vitro studies or based on a waiver from BE study requirements. This chapter will discuss the regulatory standards for approval of locally acting topical dermatological drug products based on the different types of submissions. In addition, this chapter will also discuss whether alternative approaches to comparative trials are suitable as surrogates. Particular emphasis will be on the well-established in vivo pharmacodynamic method known as McKenzie-Stoughton vasoconstrictor assay (VCA) (McKenzie and Stoughton 1962).

The Federal Food, Drug and Cosmetics Act of 1938 requires that safety be established for all new drugs that are to be marketed in the USA. The Kefauver-Harris Drug Amendments were passed in 1962 (U.S. FDA 2012b). Based on these amendments it is required that all new drug products must demonstrate not only safety but efficacy as well. In 1984, the Drug Price Competition and Patent Restoration Act (Waxman-Hatch Act) was passed. This Act currently allows for the submission of ANDAs referencing the safety and efficacy of already approved drug products (U.S. Code 1984).

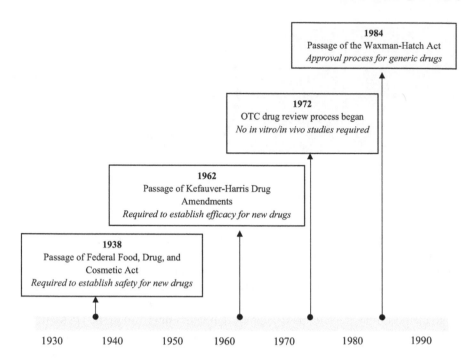

FIGURE 10.2 USFDA timeline for the regulatory basis of approval of innovator, generic and OTC products on the basis of the review of NDAs, ANDAs or OTC monograph submissions.

## 10.2 THE APPROVAL PROCESSES AND REGULATORY REQUIREMENTS FOR LOCALLY ACTING TOPICAL DERMATOLOGICAL DRUG PRODUCTS

### 10.2.1 PRE-1962

The Federal Food, Drug, and Cosmetic Act (FFD&C Act) of 1938 requires that safety be established for all drug products prior to marketing approval. It wasn't until the 1962 Kefauver-Harris Amendments that a drug product must be shown to be efficacious as well as safe (U.S. FDA 2012b). In between that 24-year time period, numerous drug products were approved. In order to address this problem of potentially ineffective drugs, in 1966 the U.S. FDA commissioned the National Academy of Sciences/National Research Council to evaluate the efficacy of all drug products approved between 1938 and 1962. Based on the results of this extensive project, many products were deemed effective and thus classified as drug efficacy study implementation (DESI) drugs (Federal Register 2012 & National Academy of Sciences 1972). This listing includes all types of topical dermatological drug products. In fact, in 1953, the first topical corticosteroid, Hydrocortisone Acetate Ointment (Cortef Acetate), was approved by the U.S. FDA based on an NDA submission. The application for this product was not approved based on comparative clinical trials. Hydrocortisone Acetate Ointment is currently listed as a DESI (Drug Efficacy

Study Implementation) drug product for the 1%, 1.5% and 2.5% dosage strengths. According to the current federal regulations, 21 Code of Federal Regulations (CFR) 320.22 (c) (U.S. Code of Federal Regulations 2013), a waiver from in vivo bioavailability and BE study requirements may be granted for a DESI drug product.

## 10.2.2 POST-1962

### 10.2.2.1 New Drug Application

Since 1938 every new drug has to be approved by the U.S. FDA based on an NDA submission. An NDA may be submitted based on section 505(b)(1) or section 505(b)(2) of the FFD&C Act. According to section 505(b) (1), extensive safety and effectiveness data are required for the drug based on its proposed uses. The quality of the product should be assured, along with proper labeling and all necessary information are to be provided in the submission. Whereas, according to section 505(b)(2), an NDA may be submitted for approval of a new drug that relies in part on studies not conducted by the applicant. The NDA submission consists of studies to establish safety and efficacy of the drug in both animal and human studies (Investigational New Drug (IND) Application 2013).

In general, for topical drug products, at least two phase-3 placebo controlled clinical endpoint trials are necessary for approval. The study has to represent the largest anticipated usage that is consistent with the clinical trials and anticipated indication and labeling. For a topical dermatological drug product, such as a corticosteroid, a phase I dermal safety study and Hypothalamic Pituitary-Adrenal axis (HPA) trials may be necessary due to systemic exposure/safety issues. The purpose of the HPA axis trial is due to the possibility of severe adrenal suppression over time due to the administration of a corticosteroid. This suppression is a major safety concern as it can lead to failure to increase cortisol levels, which results in acute adrenal insufficiency which may possibly be life-threatening. In addition, at least one phase III trial is necessary for each indication.

Applicants submitting an NDA under the provisions of Section 505(b) in the FFD&C Act are also required to document bioavailability according to 21 Code of Federal Regulations 320.21 (a) (U.S. Code of Federal Regulations 2013). Bioavailability means the rate and extent to which the active pharmaceutical ingredient (API) or active moiety is absorbed from a drug product in the systemic circulation. Bioavailability studies for topical drug products are primarily related to systemic safety. For these particular drug products, unless another validated test is available, the FDA currently recommends that a "maximal use" study be done in the patient population of interest. They provide a linkage to animal safety data, dose finding and formulation optimization in humans (Bashaw et al. 2015). In the IND (Investigational New Drug) phase, a need may arise during the pre-approval period for a topical drug product, to establish a link between the pivotal clinical trial batch(es) and the to-be-marketed formulation using alternative approaches, such as in vitro release testing or VCA approach. The alternative VCA approach is primarily utilized in an NDA submission to determine the relative potency of the corticosteroid. It is also used to compare steroid potency between different approved corticosteroid drug products. Also, the VCA approach can be used to assess bioavailability or BE in comparison of differing formulations of the same proposed drug product in comparison to other corticosteroids. The VCA approach will be discussed in greater detail in Section 10.3 of this chapter. Overall, an approved NDA drug product may become a reference listed drug (RLD) product for a proposed generic drug product.

### 10.2.2.2 Over-the-Counter Drug Products

OTC drug products can be brought to the market using the NDA process or under an OTC monograph. The OTC drug review process was established to evaluate the safety and effectiveness of OTC products marketed in the USA before May 11, 1972. In 1974, the U.S. FDA published its regulations in 21 CFR 330 for OTC human drugs which are generally recognized as safe and effective and not misbranded (U.S. FDA 2012a). The current review process is a three-phase public rulemaking process. Each phase requires Federal Register publication resulting in the establishment of drug monographs for an OTC therapeutic drug class. An OTC monograph consists of the active ingredient specific, public and a "kind of recipe" book covering acceptable ingredients, doses, formulations, labeling and, in some cases, testing parameters. The monographs for OTC products are continually updated to add additional ingredients and labeling as needed. Product conforming to a monograph may be marketed without U.S. FDA pre-approval.

In the 1950s, manufacturers applied to the U.S. FDA for approval to market topical dermatological corticosteroids as OTC products. Initially in 1957, the U.S. FDA denied this request. It wasn't until 1972 when the U.S. FDA began its OTC drug review process. Seven years later in 1979 an OTC drug monograph was approved for Hydrocortisone Acetate Ointment for external analgesic products (Joint NDAC/DODAC Advisory Committee Meeting 2005). Subsequently, in 1990, the U.S. FDA further agreed that strengths up to 1% could be sold as OTC products as well.

### 10.2.2.3 Abbreviated New Drug Applications

Since 1984, generic drug products have been approved by the U.S. FDA on the basis of an ANDA submission. The ANDA submission contains an applicant's proposal for a generic version of the RLD product. The basis of approval of generic drug products is the Drug-Price Competition and Patent Term Restoration Act of 1984, also known as the Waxman-Hatch Act (US Code, 1984). This Act modified the FFD&C Act. ANDA submissions for generic drug products generally do not require submission of costly animal and clinical studies. According to 505 (j) of the FFD&C Act, a generic drug product must be bioequivalent to the RLD product. In addition to demonstrating BE, the generic drug product must also be pharmaceutically equivalent. Pharmaceutical equivalence is based on the generic drug product containing the same amount of the API in the same dosage form as the RLD drug product and meeting compendial or other applicable standards (i.e., strength, quality, purity and identity). In vitro or in vivo BE studies serve to confirm that a generic drug product has equivalent formulation performance and safety, since efficacy has already been previously established through the NDA approval process.

According to 21 CFR 320.24, there are several approaches which are deemed acceptable for demonstrating bioavailability/bioequivalence. A listing of these approaches and their applicability to topical dermatological products are provided in Table 10.1.

## TABLE 10.1
## A Listing of the Current Bioavailability/Bioequivalence Approaches Acceptable by the U.S. FDA and their Applicability to Topical Dermatological Drug Products

| Approaches | Brief Description of Applicability for Topical Dermatological Drug Products | Examples |
|---|---|---|
| In vivo pharmacokinetic studies | Topical dermatological drug products are not generally intended for systemic absorption. In most cases, systemic absorption has more to do with safety issues than a correlation to clinical efficacy. There are some topical drug products in which the amount of systemically absorbed drug has a correlation to clinical safety and/or efficacy. | Lidocaine Patch (5%) and Diclofenac Sodium Gel, 1% (U.S. Food and Drug Administration, Bioequivalence recommendations for specific drug products 2007 & Davit 2013) Both of these drug products are systemically absorbed from the vasculature at the local site of action. The bioequivalence acceptance criteria for the 90% CIs of the PK parameters are 80.00–125.00%. |
| In vivo pharmacodynamic studies | This approach is the most commonly accepted surrogate to comparative clinical trials. In 1995, the U.S. FDA issued a Guidance for Industry Topical Dermatologic Corticosteroids: in Vivo Bioequivalence (1995). | Applicable to topical dermatological corticosteroids applied to non-scalp skin. |
| Well-controlled clinical trials | This approach is most commonly required for topical dermatological drug products. | For almost all class of topical dermatological drug products. |
| In vitro tests | This approach relies on in vitro characterization of the proposed generic and RLD products based on formulation performance. These tests can include rheological tests to assess physiochemical (Q3) properties. In vitro release testing (IVRT) using diffusion cells such as the Franz diffusion cell system is also an in vitro approach. | Example: Acyclovir Ointment (U.S. FDA, 2012d). The formulation of the test product must be Q1, Q2 and Q3 the same at the RLD product. |

**Any other approach deemed acceptable by the USDA (21 CFR 320.24 (b) (6))**
*Note*: The approaches are listed in order of accuracy, sensitivity and reproducibility (top to bottom).

### 10.2.2.3.1 In Vivo Pharmacokinetic Studies

As stated previously, in vivo pharmacokinetic studies are often not feasible or useful for topical dermatological drug products, unlike solid oral dosage forms. In most cases, topical dermatological drug products are not intended for systemic absorption. There is often no established link between the concentration in the systemic circulation and the therapeutic effect. The only link that can generally be made is to the undesired side effects that may occur due to systemic absorption. In some cases, systemic exposure may occur due to the drug being absorbed in the underlying levels of the skin, such as the epidermis, dermis or subcutaneous tissue. For this reason, other BE approaches are usually necessary.

### 10.2.2.3.2 In Vivo Pharmacodynamic Studies

The VCA approach is currently the only acceptable surrogate approach to comparative clinical trials by the U.S. FDA for topical dermatological drug products. The basis of this approach is the measurement of the pharmacodynamic effect of the drug being assessed as a function of time. The pharmacodynamic effect is temporary skin blanching (lightening of the skin). This is a result of the vasoconstriction of the skin microvasculature. On June 2, 1995, the U.S. FDA issued a Guidance for Industry: Topical Dermatologic Corticosteroids: In Vivo Bioequivalence (issued June 2, 1995), which describes the vasoconstrictor approach and how it is used to establish BE by conducting two studies: pilot dose duration-response study and a pivotal BE study, which is based on population modeling. Based on the statistical analysis of the data from the pivotal bioequivalence study, the BE criteria is 80.00–125.00%. While this approach is less expensive and requires less human subjects, it is only applicable to topical dermatological corticosteroids. All other therapeutic classes are normally required to conduct a BE study with a clinical endpoint.

#### 10.2.2.3.2.1 Bioequivalence Studies with Clinical Endpoints

BE studies with clinical endpoints are commonly required for the approval of generic topical drug products. A BE study with clinical endpoints is often designed as a randomized, blinded, parallel study using a placebo arm. The placebo arm is to confirm that there is a therapeutic response and detectable differences between the generic and RLD products. The U.S. FDA will recommend the endpoint to be used in the clinical endpoint BE study. If the RLD product is labeled for multiple indications, then the indication that is most sensitive to differences in local delivery of the drug is usually preferred. This may be due to some of the clinical endpoints not being sensitive or more sensitive to formulation differences.

These studies are usually conducted over several weeks. The assessment of the endpoint is mostly based on a dichotomous (success versus failure) or continuous (severity based on a number scale) variable. Statistical analysis on the data to establish BE varies based on the endpoint. For a dichotomous endpoint, the 90% confidence interval of the difference between the products must be within $[-0.20, +0.20]$. For a continuous endpoint, statistical analysis is performed based on the mean change from baseline. The 90% confidence interval of the generic-to-RLD ratio of means must be within $[0.80–1.25]$. Some of the major disadvantages with this approach is that the clinical endpoint may be highly variable or have a low sensitivity to detect formulation differences. In addition, these particular studies often require a large patient population (>500–600 patients). Overall, they are very costly and time consuming to perform.

*10.2.2.3.2.2 Bioequivalence Studies with In Vitro Studies* Bioequivalence studies with in vitro endpoints rely on in vitro characterization of the generic and RLD products. In certain cases (such as Acyclovir Ointment), the U.S. FDA has recently approved ANDAs based on in vitro comparisons. The studies include in vitro rheological tests (physiochemical properties (Q3) of the formulation) and in vitro drug release testing (IVRT) using diffusion cells, such as the Franz diffusion cell system. The IVRT approach is used to estimate the rate of drug release from the formulation. A difference in drug release should reflect changes in the characteristics of the drug product formulation or the thermodynamic properties of the drug product. Overall, the threshold recommendation for this approach to be considered is that the generic product must be qualitatively (Q1) and quantitatively (Q2) the same based on formulation. In addition, the generic and RLD product should not differ significantly in physicochemical properties, which includes in vitro testing. As of 2012, the U.S. FDA may accept BE studies with in vitro endpoints for Acyclovir Ointment (U.S. FDA 2012d; Davit 2013; Lionberger 2013). The regulatory acceptance of the approach is based on 21 CFR 320.24 (b) (6).

*10.2.2.3.2.2.1 Waivers from In Vivo Study Requirements* It is also possible to obtain waivers from in vivo BE study requirements for topical dermatological products. According to 21 CFR 320.22 (b) (3), waiver requests may be granted for topical solutions. Waivers are granted when BE is "self-evident." In general, BE is considered "self-evident" when the composition and components of both formulations of the generic and RLD products are Q1 and Q2 the same for both API and excipients. Some differences in excipients may be allowed as long as they do not affect safety and/or efficacy of the drug product 21 CFR 314.94(a)(9)(4). If the quantitative difference is greater than 5% or changes in the formulation impact absorption, then additional studies may be needed for approval. Also, formulation differences in processes and development may be dealt with from a chemistry, manufacturing and controls (CMC) perspective.

All topical dermatological drug products and DESI drug products that have been approved on the basis of a waiver have a therapeutic code of "AT" in the U.S. FDA Electronic Orange Book (FDA Orange Book 2014). This means the topical dermatological drug product in which chemistry and manufacturing processes are adequate and demonstrate BE. Pharmaceutically equivalent topical dermatological drug products that raise questions of BE, including those approved post-1962 and are non-solution products, are coded "AB" when adequate BE data is provided. In the absence of adequate BE data, they are coded as "BT."

### 10.2.3 Post-Approval Changes for New Drug Applications and Abbreviated New Drug Applications

In vitro studies may be acceptable for some post-approval changes for topical dermatological drug products with a semisolid dosage form. The U.S. FDA Guidance for Industry: Nonsterile Semisolid Doseage Forms Scale-Up and Postapproval Changes: Chemistry, Manufacturing, and Controls; In Vitro Release Testing and In Vivo Bioequivalence Documentation (1997), often referred to as the SUPAC-SS guidance, outlines this in vitro approach. SUPAC-SS guidance provides recommendations for post-approval changes for not only ANDA submissions, but NDA submissions as well. The guidance addresses non-sterile topical dosage forms such as creams, gels, lotions and ointments. The guidance provides the recommendations for in vitro release tests and in vivo bioequivalence tests to support changes to (1) the components or composition of formulations, (2) the manufacturing (process and/or equipment), (3) scale-up or scale-down of manufacture, and (4) site of manufacture change of its drug product. Based on the level, change will determine the data that will be necessary in order to support the acceptability of the change. As of now, the in vitro release method outlined in the SUPAC-SS guidance is based on an open chamber diffusion cell system such as a Franz cell system, usually fitted with a synthetic membrane. In most cases, in vitro release tests are useful to assess product (formulation) sameness between pre-change and post-change products. In vitro release specifications are requested for most of the submissions for routine batch-to-batch quality control as well as to avoid costly clinical-trials for post-approval changes.

## 10.3 SURROGATE FOR CLINICAL TRIALS: IN VIVO PHARMACODYNAMIC APPROACH – MCKENZIE-STOUGHTON VASOCONSTRICTOR ASSAY

### 10.3.1 BRIEF HISTORY

The preliminary work conducted by Hollander in 1951 (Hollander et al. 1951) discovered that intra-articular steroids produced blanching (whitening) of the engorged synovial membrane in rheumatoid arthritis. It was postulated that vasoconstriction produced in normal skin may be an indicator of percutaneous absorption. From the 1950s to 1960s, research began in the area of topical therapy and skin blanching. It was in 1962 that McKenzie and Stoughton published an article on assaying the potency of steroids by using vasoconstriction as an index of percutaneous absorption (McKenzie and Stoughton 1962). Three corticosteroids – Dexamethasone alcohol, Triamcinolone Acetonide and Fluocinolone Acetonide – were studied. The different corticosteroids were applied to the forearm of healthy subjects under occlusion with a perforated guard of the application sites for 16 hours after which the intensity of the skin blanching response was measured by visual assessment.

It was determined from these studies that occlusion substantially increases percutaneous absorption. The studies showed that the hydration of the skin and temperature of the skin greatly increased under these conditions. Clinical and scientific research continued in order to address the potential usefulness of this vasoconstrictor assay and its correlation to percutaneous absorption, bioavailability, potency and clinical efficacy. In 1972, Stoughton published an article on the development of the first bioassay systems to determine percutaneous absorption (Stoughton 1972). Several different research groups developed variations of the method and in two cases it was used to compare the bioavailability and activity of 31 corticosteroid ointments and 30 cream and gels (Barry and Woodford 1974, 1975). These research studies were all conducted in human subjects with occlusion and some non-occlusion of the application sites. Woodford and Barry did a comparison between the ointments and creams, and found that in most cases there were similarities in blanching profiles. Furthermore in 1984, Haigh and Kanfer conducted studies and published a report detailing the vasoconstrictor assay procedure which addressed such variables as single versus multiple time points and occlusion versus non-occlusion of the application sites (Haigh and Kanfer 1984). In addition, the results of studies performed to determine the effects of vehicle on the bioavailability and potency of the topical dermatological coritcosteroid were also reported (Stoughton 1992). The findings from these studies showed that the vehicle (i.e., change from cream to ointment for the same drug product) will impact the release rate of the cortisosteroid and may have an impact on the overall potency of the drug product with the same active ingregient, strength but different vehicle. Table 10.2 lists different corticosteroids of varying strengths on the basis of their potency.

### 10.3.2 Vasoconstrictor Assay Methodology

Five major components of the vasoconstrictor assay method are study population, site of application (on both arms), dose duration times, occlusion versus non-occlusion of the application site, and assessment of the skin blanching response. There have been several modifications based on the intended purpose of whether to determine potency, comparative evaluation of formulations or screen different topical dermatological corticosteroids. The two consistent components, no matter the purpose of the study, are only healthy human subjects are to be enrolled and the drug should be applied to the forearm (Stoughton 1972; Smith et al. 1989). This section will go into detail as it pertains to the application site, occlusion versus non-occlusion, assessment of the blanching response and selection of dose duration times based on study design.

### 10.3.3 Application Sites

The initial area of skin application as recommended by the current U.S. FDA Guidance for Industry: Topical Dermatologic Corticosteroids (U.S. FDA 1995) are as follows:

- Skin sites should be no closer than 3 to 4 cm to the antecubital fossa or wrist.
- Dose between 2–10 mg of formulation per $cm^2$ of skin surface area, and 1 cm diameter sites.
- Sites spaced as close as 2.5 cm center-to-center, either straight or staggered pattern, depending on the skin surface.

### 10.3.4 Occlusion versus Non-Occlusion of Application Sites

It is widely known that occlusion is most often used to enhance the penetration of these drug products (Zhai and Maibach 2002). This is evident by the initial studies

## TABLE 10.2
## Categorization of Approved Topical Corticosteroid Products on the Basis of Potency

| Potency | Active Ingredient | Dosage Form(s) | Strength(s) | RLD/Innovator Drug Name(s) |
|---|---|---|---|---|
| I Super High | Betamethasone Dipropionate | Cream, Augmented | 0.05% | Diprolene AF |
| | | Lotion & Ointment, Augmented | 0.05% | Diprolene |
| | Clobetasol Propionate | Cream, Ointment & Solution | 0.05% | Temovate Temovate E |
| | | Lotion & Shampoo (Solution) | 0.05% | Clobex |
| | Diflorasone Diacetate | Ointment | 0.05% | Psorcon |
| | Fluocinonide | Cream | 0.05% | Lidex |
| | Halobetasol Propionate | Cream & Ointment | 0.05% | Ultravate |
| II High | Amcinonide | Cream | 0.025% & 0.1% | Cyclocort |
| | | Ointment | 0.1% | |
| | Betamethasone Dipropionate | Ointment | 0.05% | Diprosone |
| | Desoximetaone | Ointment | 0.05% | Topicort |
| | Fluocinonide | Ointment & Solution | 0.05% | Lidex |
| III Medium-High | Desoximetasone | Cream | 0.25% | Topicort |
| | Diflorasone Diacetate | Cream | 0.05% | Psorcon |
| IV Medium | Amcinonide | Lotion | 0.1% | Cyclocort |
| | Betamethasone Dipropionate | Cream & Lotion | 0.05% | Diprosone |
| | Betamethasone Valerate | Cream & Ointment | 0.1% | Valisone |
| | Fluticasone Propionate | Cream Ointment | 0.05% 0.005% | Cutivate |
| | Hydrocortisone Valerate | Cream & Ointment | 0.2% | Westcort |
| | Hydrocortisone Butyrate | Cream | 0.1% | Locoid Lipocream |
| | Mometasone Furoate | Cream, Lotion & Ointment | 0.1% | Elocon |
| | Prednicarbate | Cream | 0.1% | Dermatop E Emollient |
| | | Ointment | 0.1% | Dermatop |
| | Triamcinolone Acetonide | Lotion | 0.025% & 0.1% | Kenalog |
| | | Ointment | 0.025%, 0.1% & 0.5% | |

*(continued)*

**TABLE 10.2**
**Categorization of Approved Topical Corticosteroid Products on the Basis of Potency (Cont.)**

| Potency | Active Ingredient | Dosage Form(s) | Strength(s) | RLD/Innovator/ Trade Names |
|---|---|---|---|---|
| **VI Low- Medium** | Alclometasone Dipropionate | Cream, Ointment | 0.05% | Aclovate |
| | Desonide | Ointment | 0.05% | -- |
| | Fluocinolone Acetonide | Cream | 0.01% & 0.025% | Synalar |
| | Fluocinolone Acetonide | Oil | 0.01% | Derma-Smoothe/ FS |
| | | Ointment | 0.025% | Synalar |
| | | Shampoo | 0.01% | Capex |
| | | Solution | 0.01% | Synalar |
| | Fluticasone Propionate | Lotion | 0.05% | Cutivate |
| | Hydrocortisone Butyrate | Cream, Lotion, Ointment & Solution | 0.1% | Locoid |
| | Triamcinolone Acetonide | Cream | 0.025%, 0.1 % & 0.5% | Kenalog, Aristostat |
| **VII Low** | Betametasone Valerate | Lotion | 0.1% | Valisone |
| | Desonide | Cream & Lotion | 0.05% | Desowen |
| | Hydrocortisone | Cream, Lotion, Ointment | 1% & 2.5% | Hytone |
| | | Solution | 1% & 2.5% | Texacort |
| | Hydrocortisone Acetate | Cream | 2% & 2.5% | Micort-HC |
| | | Ointment | 1% & 2.5% | Cortef Acetate |

performed by McKenzie and Stoughton in which occlusion of the sites for the tested drug products resulted in at least a ten- to 100-fold increase in the absorption of the low to medium potency corticosteroids: Triamcinolone Acetonide, Fluocinolone Acetonide, Hydrocortisone, and Dexamethasone when compared to non-occlusion (McKenzie and Stoughton 1962). Occlusion can also potentially alter the stratum corneum causing it to retain water and increase in temperature, along with increasing the penetration of the drug into the skin (Haigh and Kanfer 1984). Therefore, the ability to differentiate between two formulations may not be accurate or feasible under occluded conditions. However, in general, for high potency drug products occlusive covering is not needed; yet, in some cases for very low potency drug products it may be appropriate to occlude the application sites.

### 10.3.5 ASSESSMENT OF PHARMACODYNAMIC RESPONSE

#### 10.3.5.1 Visual Assessment

A visual scaling approach is used for the assessment of the blanching response which occurs after the topical dermatological corticosteroid drug product has been applied to a number of sites of the skin over a specified time period and then removed. The four-point scale (0–3) is as follows:

0 = no blanching (no change)
1 = mild blanching (visible slight change at application site)
2 = moderated blanching (visible discernible change application site)
3 = marked blanching (visibly distinct change at application site)

The degree of blanching based on visual assessment is usually accessed as the percentage of total possible score (% TPS). The % TPS is calculated based on the actual score (AS) and total possible score (TPS) (Haigh and Kanfer 1984). The AS equals the sum of the frequencies of the graded responses recorded for each preparation at each site. The TPS is the product of the maximum possible score per site (M), number of independent observers (O), number of sites per preparation arm (S) and the number of volunteers (V). The equations for the calculation of TPS and % TPS are as follows:

$$TPS = M \times O \times S \times V$$

$$\% TPS = \frac{Actual\ Score}{TPS} \times 100$$

The % TPS is then plotted versus time to yield the blanching profile (Figure 10.3).

### 10.3.5.2  Chromameter Assessment

A Chromameter® is a tristimulus instrument which is used to measure how much light is absorbed. The assessment of skin blanching using a colorimeter method was first reported by Kiraly in 1976; however, their approach was not deemed

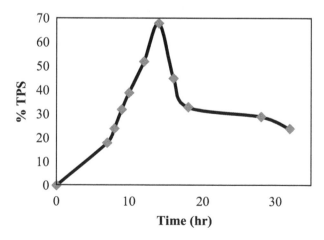

**FIGURE 10.3**  Example of a blanching profile.

beneficial at the time and therefore it was abandoned (Király and Soós 1976). It wasn't until the first initial reports in the late 1980s, in which Minolta used a colorimeter for quantification of Sodium Lauryl Sulfate irritant dermatitis and evaluation of erythema and tanning (Babulak et al. 1986; Westerhof et al. 1986; Seitz and Whitmore 1988; Wilhem et al. 1989). This led to further studies on the use of a Chromameter for measuring of blanching response in the vasoconstrictor assay study (Queille-Roussel et al. 1991). Subsequent studies have been conducted to determine using both visual and Chromameter assessment (Pershing 1995; Au et al. 2008). Based on these preliminary studies it was determined that the Chromameter can accurately measure skin color variation and produce reproducible results taking into consideration certain factors, such as the presence of hair on skin (Fullerton et al. 1996).

### 10.3.6 SELECTION OF DOSE DURATION TIME(S) BASED ON VCA STUDY DESIGN

#### 10.3.6.1 The Utilization of the VCA Approach for Evaluation of Relative Potency

For determination of relative potency, a single-point vasoconstrictor assay is utilized. The topical dermatological corticosteroid which is being studied is randomly applied to the forearm and after a specified time period, in most cases 16 hours, the site is gently washed with mild soap. After an additional specified time period, in most cases two hours, a visual assessment of the blanching response using the scale approach as described in Section 10.3.5.1 is performed. The total score is combined from all of the testing sites for the corticosteroid being evaluated and then the mean score is calculated. This value is often compared to the scores of other corticosteroids.

#### 10.3.6.2 The Utilization of the VCA Approach for Evaluation of Bioavailability/Bioequivalence

For comparative evaluation of two different formulations, a multi-point vasoconstrictor assay is utilized. Based on the current U.S. FDA Guidance for Topical Dermatologic Corticosteroids, the selection of dose duration times is vital. The recommended times may include 0.25, 0.5, 0.75, 1, 1.5, 2, 4 and 6 hours, although they can vary depending on the corticosteroid under investigation. There should be at least eight sites of application on each arm with a controlled site. After drug removal by gentle cleansing, the assessment of skin color and skin blanching response is done by one of the following ways:

- Staggered application with synchronized removal – This means the corticosteroid is applied at different dose duration times but removed from the skin at the same time. Time zero equals the time of drug removal. Chromameter readings will include 0 hours until 24 hours after drug removal, with multiple time readings at varying time points in between, along with the baseline reading prior to application of the corticosteroid to the skin.
- Synchronized application with staggered removal – This means the corticosteroid is applied at the same time for the different dose duration times and

removed from the skin at different times. Time zero equals the time of application. Chromameter readings will include six hours to 28 hours, with multiple time readings at varying time points in between, along with the baseline reading prior to application of the corticosteroid to the skin.

### 10.3.7 CORRELATION BETWEEN THE VCA APPROACH AND COMPARATIVE CLINICAL TRIALS

There has been an extensive evaluation of the correlation between the VCA approach and clinical efficacy. During the development stage of this approach from the years of 1964 to the 1980s in particular, there were numerous papers written on the correlation between the blanching response and clinical activity (Haigh and Kanfer 1984; Gibson et al. 1984). In most cases, these studies showed a correlation regardless of the design of the clinical study. For example, in 1972, in the early stages of development of the VCA approach study, a study was conducted on Fluocinonide Acetonide, 0.025% and Fluoconinolone in Base Ten at 0.02% by Burdick at Syntex Research (Burdick 1971). The study was conducted under occluded and non-occluded conditions over a specified time period of six hours, with visual assessment of the blanching response. Whereas the clinical trial was designed as a double-blind pair comparison study in steroid responsive dermatoses. The data from this study confirmed that the VCA approach can be useful in predicting clinical efficacy.

In 1985, Cornell and Stoughton (1985) reported on studies they conducted on 22 different corticosteroids of varying potency and dosage forms. The study was conducted under non-occlusive conditions and the corticosteroid drug products were applied to the skin for a specified time period of 16 hours with visual assessment of the blanching response using a four-point scale. The clinical studies were designed as randomized, double-blind, bilateral comparison evaluation carried out in outpatients with psoriasis under non-occlusive conditions. The results showed that 90% (20 out of 22) yielded comparable results between the blanching response and clinical efficacy.

In addition, the U.S. FDA commissioned Stoughton at the University of California San Diego School of Medicine to conduct studies to investigate if generic formulations were indeed equivalent to the innovator (trade name) drug products (Stoughton 1987). He investigated Triamcinolone Acetonide Cream, 0.1% (Kenalog), Triamcinolone Acetonide Ointment, 0.1% (Aristocort A), Betamethosone Cream, 0.1% (Valisone), Betamethasone Valerate Ointment, 0.1% (Valisone), Fluocinolone Acetonide Cream, 0.025% (Synalar), Triamcinolone Acetonide Cream, 0.025% & 0.5% (Kenalog). From his studies it was determined that there was a marked difference between the generic and innovator formulations containing the same cortiosteroid of the same concentration using the same vehicle. A critique of this study was written by Shah et al. discussing in depth the findings from this study (Shah et al. 1989). Based on those findings by Stoughton, the U.S. FDA also commissioned Dr. Olsen at Duke University – School of Medicine to address the issue further (Olsen 1991). His findings raised similar issues as the studies conducted by Stoughton. During this time the U.S. FDA also held numerous Advisory Committee Meetings. It was ultimately determined that the VCA approach was an acceptable approach. In addition, for the

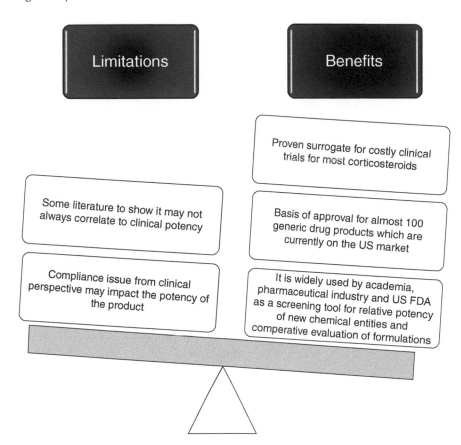

**Limitations**

**Benefits**

Proven surrogate for costly clinical trials for most corticosteroids

Some literature to show it may not always correlate to clinical potency

Basis of approval for almost 100 generic drug products which are currently on the US market

Compliance issue from clinical perspective may impact the potency of the product

It is widely used by academia, pharmaceutical industry and US FDA as a screening tool for relative potency of new chemical entities and comperative evaluation of formulations

**FIGURE 10.4** A schematic representation of the benefits and limitations of the VCA approach.

last 20 years the U.S. FDA has approved almost 100 generic topical corticosteroid drug products. There have been many discussions concerning the limitations of the VCA approach (Kirkland et al. 2006). As outlined in Figure 10.4, the benefits from a scientific, clinical and/or regulatory perspective continue to outweigh those concerns.

## 10.4 U.S. FDA HISTORY WITH THE VCA APPROACH FOR LOCALLY ACTING TOPICAL DERMATOLOGICAL CORTICOSTEROIDS

With the passage of the Hatch-Waxman for generic drug products and extensive research on the VCA approach, the U.S. FDA made the decision to recommend this assay as the basis for approval of generic drug products for topical dermatological corticosteroids. Prior to issuance of the interim guidance, Bioequivalence recommendations for specific drug products (U.S. FDA 2007, issued July 1, 1992), in order to establish bioequivalence for topical dermatological corticosteroids drug products, a single-point vasoconstrictor assay study was recommended with visual assessment of the blanching response. The following changes were made to the

(a)

**The $E_{max}$ model**

$$E = E_0 + \frac{E_{max}{}^* Dose}{Dose + ED_{50}}$$

*Where,*

E = Pharmacodynamic Effect

E0 = Baseline Effect

$E_{max}$ = Maximum fitted value "E"

$ED_{50}$ = Dose to achieve 50% of the $E_{max}$ value

(b)

**The $E_{max}$ model for Dermatological Products Data**

$$AUEC = \frac{AUEC_{max}{}^* DoseDuration}{DoseDuration + ED_{50}}$$

*Where,*

AUEC = Pharmacodynamic effect metric

$AUEC_{max}$ = Maximum fitted value of "AUEC"

$ED_{50}$ = Dose duration required to achieve 50% of the $E_{max}$ value

**FIGURE 10.5** Mathematical description of (A) the $E_{max}$ model and (B) the $E_{max}$ model for topical dermatological products.

previous recommendations: (1) a multiple dose duration study using a maximum effect ($E_{max}$) model (Figure 10.5) to describe the area under the effect curve (AUEC) (Figure 10.6). The $E_{max}$ model required the fitting of individual data. However, there were several problems identified between 1992 and 1994 upon implementation of the guidance which mainly involved the fitting of the $E_{max}$ model to the individual subject dose-response data (Singh et al. 1999). In response, the U.S. FDA held an Advisory Committee meeting and revised the recommendations. The current and revised guidance, Guidance for Industry: Topical Dermatologic Corticosteroids: In Vivo Bioequivalence (U.S. FDA 1995) currently includes two in vivo studies to establish bioequivalence between the proposed generic and RLD products. In addition, the revised guidance recommends estimation of the population $ED_{50}$ based in an $E_{max}$ model fitted to the pooled population dose-response data. Table 10.3 and Figure 10.7 provide detailed historical outlines of the VCA approach from scientific and regulatory perspectives.

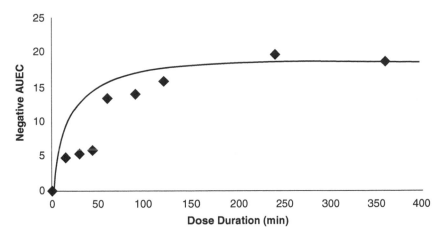

**FIGURE 10.6** Schematic representation of the relationship of AUEC to dose duration (minutes). The data is fitted to the $E_{max}$ model in order to determine the $ED_{50}$ to be used in the pivotal bioequivalence study.

**TABLE 10.3**
**Progression of USFDA Regulatory Changes to Recommendations for the VCA Approach**

| | New Drug Applications–Innovator Drug Products | Abbreviated New Drug Applications Generic Drug Products | | |
|---|---|---|---|---|
| | Present Day | Prior to July 1992 | After July 1, 1992 | 1995–Present |
| **Dose-Duration (# of time points)** | One | One | Multiple | Multiple |
| **Occlusion vs. Non-Occlusion\*\*** | Non-Occlusion | Non-occlusion | Non-occlusion | Non-occlusion |
| **Assessment** | Visual | Visual | Chromameter | Chromameter |
| **PD Modeling** | -- | -- | Individual Subject | Pooled Population |
| **Outcome** | Relative Potency | Bioequivalence | Bioequivalence | Bioequivalence |

\*\* In general, the vasoconstrictor assay is conducted under non-occlusion, unless otherwise recommended by the innovator/RLD drug product, see Section 10.3 for additional details.

## 10.5 IN VIVO VASOCONSTRICTOR ASSAY STUDY DESIGNS BASED ON THE U.S. FDA GUIDANCE FOR TOPICAL DERMATOLOGIC CORTICOSTEROIDS

### 10.5.1 PILOT DOSE DURATION-RESPONSE STUDY

The pilot study characterizes the dose duration-response relationship for drugs in terms of the $E_{max}$ model (Figure 10.5). The pilot study is conducted solely on the RLD

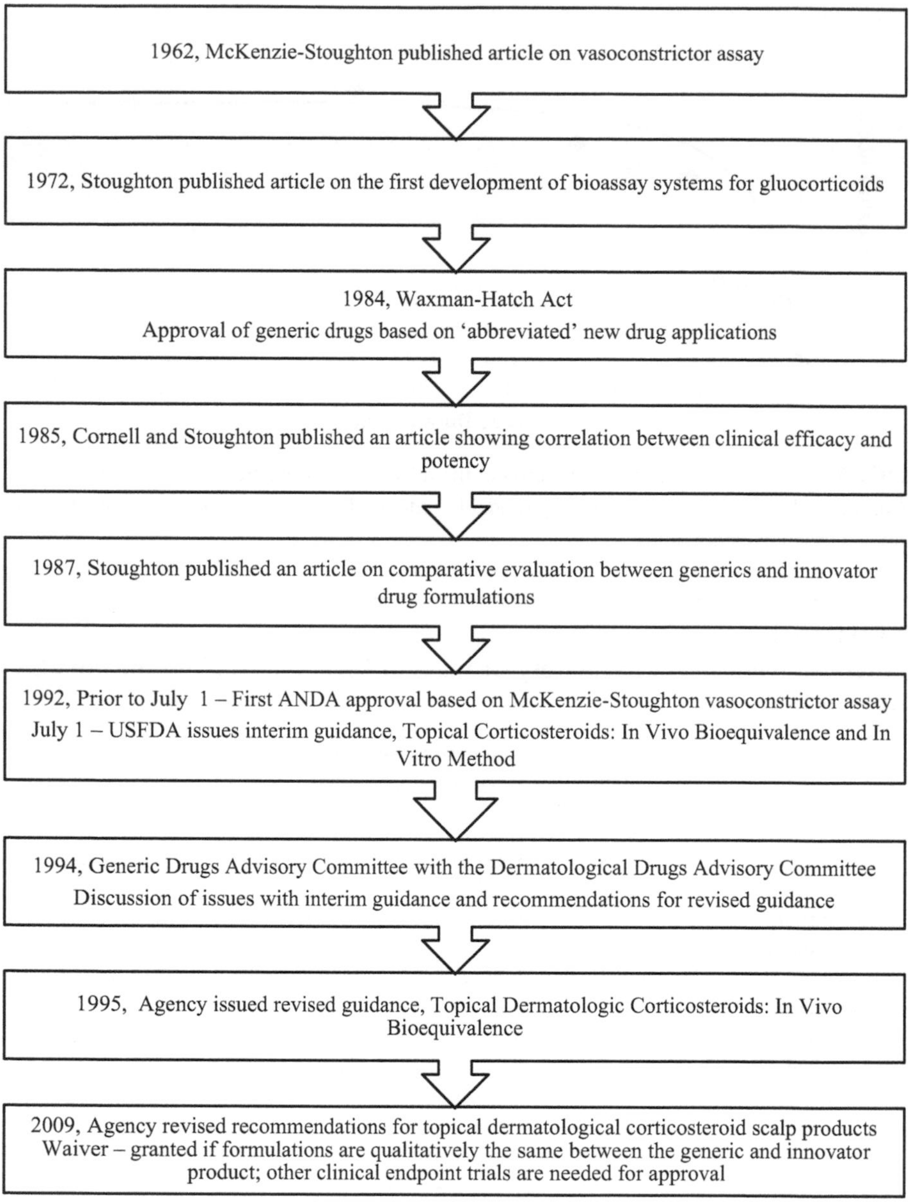

1962, McKenzie-Stoughton published article on vasoconstrictor assay

1972, Stoughton published article on the first development of bioassay systems for gluocorticoids

1984, Waxman-Hatch Act
Approval of generic drugs based on 'abbreviated' new drug applications

1985, Cornell and Stoughton published an article showing correlation between clinical efficacy and potency

1987, Stoughton published an article on comparative evaluation between generics and innovator drug formulations

1992, Prior to July 1 – First ANDA approval based on McKenzie-Stoughton vasoconstrictor assay
July 1 – USFDA issues interim guidance, Topical Corticosteroids: In Vivo Bioequivalence and In Vitro Method

1994, Generic Drugs Advisory Committee with the Dermatological Drugs Advisory Committee
Discussion of issues with interim guidance and recommendations for revised guidance

1995, Agency issued revised guidance, Topical Dermatologic Corticosteroids: In Vivo Bioequivalence

2009, Agency revised recommendations for topical dermatological corticosteroid scalp products
Waiver – granted if formulations are qualitatively the same between the generic and innovator product; other clinical endpoint trials are needed for approval

**FIGURE 10.7** Timeline for the development of the VCA approach, acceptability by the U.S. FDA and current utilization of the method of the VCA approach for topical dermatological drug products.

product. Based on the guidance, at least 12 healthy subjects are normally enrolled in the study; the RLD product is randomly applied to the skin and the dose duration is recommended to be between 0.25 to 6 hours; and Chromameter detection is used to measure the skin blanching response. In most cases, the sites are non-occluded,

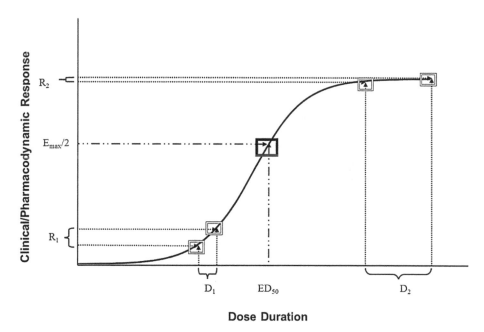

**Dose Duration**

**FIGURE 10.8** A schematic representation of the relationship between the pharmacodynamic response and dose. Depending on the given dose it will detect the pharmacological response. A low dose correlates to a low response, designated respectively as $D_1$ and $R_1$. Whereas, a high dose correlates to an oversaturation and undesirable response in which you hit a plateau and cannot achieve any more response even if you continue to increase the dose, designated as $D_2$ and $R_2$, which is also not desirable. In those two areas, one may be unable to differentiate between the two products, since the pharmacodynamic response to either product will be quite similar in those regions. However, when a dose is given which elicits 50% of the maximum response, $ED_{50}$, and correlates to 50% of the $E_{max}$ (the maximum effect), one is able to differentiate between two products based on the pharmacodynamic response.

except for in extreme cases in which the potency of the drug is extremely low and therefore detection is minimal. The data is modeled by using a non-linear fixed effect modeling method or naïve pooled data are used to determine the population $ED_{50}$ which are used in the pivotal study. The results from the study provide the necessary information to determine the $ED_{50}$, $D_1$ ($0.5*ED_{50}$, the shorter dose duration calibrator), and $D_2$ ($2*ED_{50}$ the longer dose duration calibrator) parameters to be used in the in vivo pivotal study (Figure 10.8). The appropriate selection of the dose duration sampling time points is critical in the identification of the correct $ED_{50}$ for a corticosteroid. For high potency corticosteroids, it is expected that the blanching response will be achieved at a faster rate than a lower potency corticosteroid.

## 10.5.2 Pivotal In Vivo Bioequivalence Study

The pivotal study is conducted in order to establish bioequivalence between the proposed generic drug product and the RLD product. Based on the U.S. FDA

# APPLICATION SITES

ANTECUBITAL FOSSA

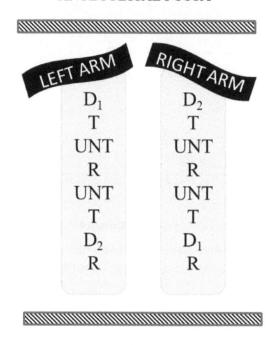

WRIST

**FIGURE 10.9** Schematic representation of application sites in the pivotal bioequivalence study. T represents the generic, R represents the RLD product and UNT represents the control. While $D_1$ and $D_2$ represent the dose durations which were determined from the $ED_{50}$ obtained in the pilot study.

Guidance for Industry: Topical Dermatologic Corticosteroids (U.S. FDA 1995), the generic (T) and RLD (R) products are applied to the skin site, along with control sites for the specified period of time (Figure 10.9). The blanching response is measured by Chromameter detection. Acceptable individual subject dose duration-response is based on an AUEC $D_2$/AUEC $D_1$ ratio of at least 1.25. The data from these subjects that meet the criteria are included in statistical analyses for determination of bioequivalence. The guidance recommends that there should be at least 40 to 60 "evaluable" subjects who meet this criteria. Locke's method is used for statistical analysis of the data (Locke 1984). In order for the generic drug product to be deemed bioequivalent to the RLD product, it must meet the 90% confidence interval of 80.00–125.00%.

## 10.6 THE DERMATOPHARMACOKINETIC APPROACH AND THE U.S. FDA EXPERIENCE

The dermatopharmacokinetic approach has been previously proposed to the U.S. FDA as a method for confirming bioavailability/bioequivalence for topical dermatological drug products (Braddy and Conner 2011). Unlike for topical corticosteroids, there is no other feasible surrogate to clinical trials for most topical dermatological products. The dermatopharmacokinetic approach evaluates the drug levels in the stratum corneum with respect to time after application and removal. Based on this, it has been proposed that it is comparable to the pharmacokinetic methods for assessment of bioavailability/bioequivalence for systemically absorbed drug products, such oral dosage form in blood, plasma or urine with respect to time. It was also claimed to provide information on drug uptake, apparent steady-state levels and drug elimination from the stratum corneum based on a stratum corneum concentration-time curve (plotted as the amount/surface area against time) (Shah et al. 1998).

This approach evaluates the rate of drug penetration from a topical dermatological drug product through the stratum corneum by application of the drug product to the area of skin; then "stripping" of the layers of the stratum corneum with tape and evaluating the kinetics of drug penetration. For establishing bioequivalence, it was proposed that if the drug concentrations from two similar formulations are the same in stratum corneum, then drug delivery to the site of activity within the skin is the same and, therefore, the safety and efficacy will also be the same. However, there were a few issues identified with this approach: healthy versus diseased skin, furrows in skin surface and hair follicles and follicular penetration on the stratum corneum. It has been postulated that if the stratum corneum is damaged or diseased, it may reduce the barrier to drug absorption allowing for a greater and more rapid delivery of the drug to the site of action and lack the ability to differentiate between different topical dermatological drug products. The skin surface is not flat and contains furrows. Therefore, the concern was that the skin-stripping method may not be a "true" measurement of the drug concentration in the skin, but instead is the drug being deposited in the furrows. Finally, as it pertains to the hair follicle and follicular penetration, some drugs could penetrate the skin more through these "holes."

The U.S. FDA had been open to the possible utlization of the dermatopharmaokinetic approach for bioavailability/bioequivalence. In an effort to devleop an appropiate guidance for dermatopharmacokinetic studies, the U.S. FDA collaborated with the University of Utah School of Medicine to conduct some studies. In two different research studies it was determined that the dermatopharmacokinetic approach was useful in the assessment of bioavaialbility/bioequivalence for topical dermatological drug products. One particular study was conducted on the retinoid, Tretinoin Gel, in order to establish possible correlation between clinical safety/efficacy and the dermatopharmacokinetic approach between different manufactures – innovator and generic (Pershing et al. 2003). The other study was conducted using the corticosteroid, Triamcinolone Acetonide cream, in which the dose responsiveness and bioequivaelnce assessment using in vitro release tests, skin stripping and vasconstrictor assay was employed to compare two different manufacturers of the drug product (Pershing et al. 2002).

Prior to and during the performance of these studies, the U.S. FDA had incorporated dermatopharmacokinetic studies into two guidances for topical dermatological products. The U.S. FDA's first experience with the dermatopharmacokinetic approach of skin stripping was in 1992 when the interim guidance for topical corticosteroids was issued. However, it was later removed from the subsequent guidance issued in 1995.

Three years later, in June 1998, the U.S. FDA issued the Draft Guidance for Industry: Topical Dermatological Corticosteroids: In Vivo Bioequivalence (U.S. FDA 1995). In this guidance, pilot and pivotal studies were proposed, along with reocmmendations for performance and validation of the skin-stripping technique. The metrics of the pivotal bieoquvalenc were time to reach the maximum concnetration ($T_{max}$), the maximum concnetration ($C_{max}$) and the area under the concerntration-time curve (AUC). The 90% confidence interval for the ratio of means (population generic means based on log-transformed data) of products were 80.00–125.00% for AUC and 70.00–143.00% for $C_{max}$. However, during years of research, along with public comments and public Advisory Committee meetings in 1998, 2001 and 2001, major issues were raised with this approach and in 2002 it was ultimately decided by the U.S. FDA to withdraw this guidance. The two major issues were regarding (1) the adequacy of the dermatopharmacokinetic method to assess bioequivalence because topical dermatological drug products are used to treat a variety of diseases and disorders in different parts of the skin, not just the stratum corneum; and (2) the lack of reproducibility of the dermatopharmacokinetic approach between laboratories. There has been some subequent research on improving this method by acedemia and the pharmaceutical industry (N'Dri-Stempfer et al. 2009; Boix-Montanes 2011); however, to date this approach is still not accepated by the US FDA.

## 10.7   CURRENT DEVELOPMENT OF ALTERNATIVE APPROACHES FOR ASSESSMENT OF CLINICAL EFFICACY AND/OR BIOAVAILABILITY/BIOEQUIVALENCE FOR LOCALLY ACTING TOPICAL DERMATOLOGICAL DRUG PRODUCTS

Overall, the U.S. FDA has continued to recognize that the assessment of bioavailability/bioequivalence of certain drug products is still hampered by the limited number of acceptable approaches. In 2003, the FFD&C Act at Section 505 (j) (8) (A) (ii) was modified to further address these limitations in the assessment of bioavailability/bioequivalence of drug products that are not intended for absorption into the bloodstream, such as of topical drug products. This modification has allowed for the assessment of bioavailability on the basis of scientifically valid measurements intended to reflect the rate and extent to which the API or therapeutic ingredient becomes available at the site of action. As we continue to progress from a regulatory and scientific perspective, the U.S. FDA continues to reiterate the importance of addressing the scientific challenges in the assessment of bioavailability/ bioequivalence. In particular, as of 2007, the U.S. FDA implemented its Critical Path Initiatives for generic drug products which includes potential method devlopment for these types of products.

The purpose of this initiative was to bring to attention, stimulate discussion and collaboration of research and development across the government agencies and the pharmaceutical industries. For topical dermatological drug products the focus is on the (1) design of BE trials with clincial endpoints; (2) in vitro characterization of topical dermatological products using rheological testing method, an in vitro release testing using diffusion cells – based on formulations that are Q1 and Q2 identical; and (3) local delivery of topical dermatological products – pharmacokinetic studies, skin stripping, microdialysis (Benfeldt et al. 2007; Chaurasia et al. 2007) and near infrared spectroscopy. Since that time additional regulatory science initiatives have been incorporated as a part of the 2012 Generic Drug User Fee Amendments (2012). This has included collaborative projects with academic groups in the area of topical bioequivalence.

## 10.8 CONCLUSION

The U.S. FDA has approved numerous new, generic and OTC products for topical dermatological products that are currently available on the market to the American public. Although the approval pathways for these drug products differ, the outcome has still been safe and effective drug products. Despite the current U.S. FDA requirements for topical dermatological drug products, there is still an effort to evaluate changes and make new progress. The U.S. FDA continues to explore the development of improved surrogate approaches which can correlate to the clinical safety and efficacy of the innovator drug product.

## BIBLIOGRAPHY

Au WA, Skinner M, Kanfer I. Bioequivalence assessment of topical clobetasol propionate products using visual chromametric assessment of skin blanching. *J Pharm Pharmaceut Sci.*, 2008; 11: 160–6.

Babulak SW, RHein LD, Scala DD, Simon A, Grove GL. Quantification of erythema in soap chamber test using the minolta chroma (reflectance) meter: comparison of instrumental results with visual assessments. *J Soc Cosmet Chem.*, 1986; 37: 475–9.

Barry BW, Fyrand O, Woodford R, Ulshagen K, Hogstad, G. Control of the bioavailability of a topical steroid; comparison of desonide creams 0.05% and 0.1% by vasoconstrictor studies and clinical trials. *Clin and Exper Dermatol.* 1987; 12: 406–9.

Barry BW, Woodford R. Comparative bio-availability of proprietary topical corticosteroid preparations; vasoconstrictor assays on thirty creams and gels. *Br J Dermatol.* 1974; 91: 323–38.

Barry BW, Woodford R. Comparative bio-availability and activity of proprietary topical corticosteroid preparations: vasoconstrictor assays on thirty-one ointments. *Brit J Dermatol.* 1975; 93: 563–71.

Bashaw ED et al. Maximal usage trial: an overview of the design of systemic bioavailability trial for topical dermatological products. *Therapeutic Innovation & Regulatory Science.* 2015; 49(1): 108–15.

Benfeldt E, Hansen SH, Volund A, Menne T, Shah VP. Bioequivalence of topical formulations in humans: evaluation by dermal microdialysis sampling and the dermatopharmacokinetic method. *J Invest Dermatol.* 2007; 127: 170–8.

Boix-Montanes A. Relevance of equivalence assessment of topical products based on the dermatopharmacokinetics approach. *Eur J Pharm Sci*. 2011; 42: 173–9.

Braddy AC, Davit BM, Stier EM, Conner DP. Survey of international regulatory bioequivalence recommendations for approval of generic topical dermatological drug products. *The AAPS J*. 2014; 17(1): 121–33.

Braddy AC, Conner DP. Regulatory perspective of dermatokinetic studies. In: Murthy SN, editor. *Dermatokinetics of therapeutic agents*. Florida: Taylor & Francis Group, LLC; 2011. pp. 193–201.

Burdick, KH. Corticosteroid bioavailability assays. Correlation with a clinical study. *Acta Derm-Venereol*, 1971; 52: 19–23.

Chaurasia CS, Muller M, Bashaw ED, Benfeldt E, Bolinder J, et al. AAPS-FDA workshop white paper: microdialysis principles, application and regulatory perspectives. *Pharm Res*. 2007; 24:1014–25.

Cornell RC, Stoughton RB. Correlation of the vasoconstriction assay and clinical activity in psoriasis. *Arch Dermatol*. 1985; 121:63–7.

Davit BM. Regulatory approaches for generic drugs: BE of topical drug products. Presented at: PQRI Workshop on the Evaluation of New and Generic Topical Drug Products – Current challenges in bioequivalence, quality and novel assessment technologies. March 11, 2013; Rockville, MD USA. www.pqri.org/workshops/Topicals2013/Davit. pdf. Accessed April 23, 2014.

FDA Orange Book. Approved drug products with therapeutic equivalence evaluations: publications. Last updated March 28, 2014. US Deparment of Health and Human Services, Food and Drug Adminsitration. www.accessdata.fda.gov/scripts/cder/ob/ eclink.cfm. Accessed April 23, 2014.

Federal Food, Drug, and Cosmetic Act. 1938 US Department of Health and Human Services, Food and Drug Administration. Last updated: December 5, 2011. www.fda.gov/ RegulatoryInformation/Legislation/FederalFoodDrugandCosmeticActFDCAct/ default.htm. Accessed April 23, 2014.

Federal Register – Docket # 98D-0388. US Department of Health and Human Services, Food and Drug Administration. www.fda.gov/ohrms/dockets/98fr/051702d.htm. Accessed April 23, 2014.

Fullerton A, Fischer T, Lahti A, Wilhelm KP, Takiwaki H., et al. Guidelines for measurement of skin colour and eryhtema: A report from the standardization group of the European society of contact dermatitis. *Contact Dermatitis*. 1996; 35:1–10.

Generic Drug User Fee Amendments. US Food and Drug Administration Safety and Innovation Act, S.3187. 3187. Congress.gov, Washington, D.C. 2012. www.congress.gov/bill/ 112th-congress/senate-bill/3187/text. Accessed October 6, 2019.

Gibson JR, Kirsch JM, Darley CR, Harvey SG, Burke CA, Hanson ME. An assessment of the relationship between vasoconstrictor assay findings, clinical efficacy and skin thinning effects of a variety of undiluted and diluted corticosteroid preparations. *Brit J Dermatol*. 1984; 111 204–12.

Haigh JM, Kanfer I. Assessment of topical corticosteroid preparations: the human skin blanching assay. *Int J Pharm*. 1984; 19: 245–62.

Hollander JL, Stoner EK, Brown EM, deMoor P. The use of intra-articular temperature measurement in the evaluation of antiarthritic agents. *J Clin Invest*, 1951: 30: 701–706.

Investigational New Drug (IND) Application. US Department of Health and Human Services, Food and Drug Administration. Last updated: October 18, 2013. www.fda. gov/Drugs/DevelopmentApprovalProcess/HowDrugsareDevelopedandApproved/ ApprovalApplications/Over-the-CounterDrugs/default.htm. Accessed April 23, 2014.

Joint NDAC/DODAC Advisory Committee Meeting. U.S. Food and Drug Adminstraion US Department of Health and Human Services. March 24, 2005. www.fda.gov/ohrms/dockets/ac/05/briefing/2005-4099B1_01_FDA-Backgrounder.pdf. Accessed April 23, 2014.

Kanfer I. Strategies for the bioequivalence assessment of topical dermatological dosage forms. *Journal of Bioequivalence & Bioavailability.* 2010; 2:102–10.

Király K, Soós G. Objective measurement of topically applied corticosteroids. *Dermatologica.* 1976; 152 Suppl.: 133–7.

Kirkland R, Pearce DJ, Balkrishnan R, Feldman SR. Critical factors determining the potency of topical corticosteroids. *J Dermatol Treat.* 2006; 17: 133–5.

Lionberger R. FDA critical path initiatives: opportunities for generic drug development. *AAPS J.* 2008 Mar; 19(1):103–9.

Lionberger R. Challenges of assessing bioequivalence of topical pharmaceutical products. Presented at: PQRI Workshop on the Evaluation of New and Generic Topical Drug Products – Current challenges in bioequivalence, quality and novel assessment technologies. March 11–13, 2013; Rockville, MD USA. www.pqri.org/workshops/Topicals2013/Lionberger.Challenges.pdf. Accessed April 23, 2014.

Locke CS. An exact confidence interval from untransformed data for the ratio of two formulation means. *J Pharmaokinetic Biopharm,* 1984; 12:649–55.

Maibach HI. In vivo percutaneous penetration of corticoids in man and unresolved problems in their efficacy. *Dermatologica;* 1976; 152 Suppl. 1: 11–25.

McKenzie AW, Stoughton RB. Method for comparing percutaneous absorption of steroids. *Arch Dermatol;* 1962; 86; 608–10.

New Drug Application. US Department of Health and Human Services, Food and Drug Adminstration. Last updated: June 10, 2019. www.fda.gov/drugs/types-applications/new-drug-application-nda. Accessed October 6, 2019.

N'Dri-Stempfer B, Navidi WC, Guy RH, Bunge AL. Improved bioequivalence assessment of topical dermatological drug products using dermatopharmacokinetics. *Pharm Res.* 2009; 26: 316–28.

Olsen, EA. A double-blind controlled comparison of generic and trade-name topical steroids using the vasoconstriction assay. *Arch Dermatol.* 1991; 127:197–201.

Pershing LK. Assessment of topical corticosteroid-induced skin blanching response using the visual mckenzie-stoughton and colorimeteric methods. *Drug Inf J.* 1995; 29: 923–34.

Pershing LK, Bakhitan S, Poncelet CE, Corlett JL, Shah VP. Comparison of skin stripping, in vitro release, and skin blanching response methods to measure dose response and similarity of triamcinolone acetonide cream strengths from two manufactured sources. *J Pharm Sci.* 2002; 91: 1312–23.

Pershing LK, Nelson JL, Corlett JL, Shrivastava SP, Hare DB, Shah VP. Assessment of dermatokinetic approach in the bioequivalence determination of topical tretinoin gel products. *J Am Acad Dermatol.* 2003; 48:740–51.

Queille-Roussel C, Poncet M, Schaefer, H. Quantification of skin-colour changes induced by topical corticosteroid preparations using the minolta chroma meter. *Br J Dermatol.* 1991; 124: 264–70.

Seitz JC, Whitmore CG. Measurement of erythema and tanning responses in human skin using tri-stimulus colorimeter. *Dermatologica.* 1988; 177:70–5.

Shah, VP. Progress in methodologies for evaluating bioequivalence of topical formulations. *Am J Clin Dermatol.* 2001; 2:275–80.

Shah VP, Flyn GL, Yacobi A, Maibach HI, Bon C, Fleischer, NM, Franz TJ, et al. AAPS/FDA workshop report. Bioequivalence of topical dermatological dosage forms – methods of evaluation of bioequivalence. *Pharm Res.* 1998; 15:167–71.

Shah, VP, Peck, CC, Skelly, JP. 'Vasoconstriction' – skin blanching – assay for glucocorticoids – a critique. *Arch Dermatol*. 1989; 125:1558–61.

Singh GJ, Adams WP, Lesko LJ, Shah VP, Molzon JA, Williams RL, Pershing LK. Development of in vivo bioequivalence methodology for dermatologic corticosteroids based on pharmacodynamic modeling. *Clin Pharmacol Ther*. 1999; 66:346–57.

Smith EW, Meyer E, Haigh JM, Maibach HI. *The human skin-blanching assay as an indicator of topical corticosteroid bioavailability and potency: an update*. In: Percutaneous absorption: mechanisms – methodology – drug delivery. New York: Marcel Dekker; 1989. pp. 443–60.

Stoughton, RB. Some bioassay methods for measuring percutaneous absorption. *Adv Bio Skin*. 1972; 12:535–46.

Stoughton, RB. Are generic formulations equivalent to trade name topical glucocorticoids. *Arch Dermatol*. 1987; 123:1312–4.

Stoughton, RB. *Vasoconstrictor assay – specific applications*. In: Topical Corticosteroids, Surber C Maibach HI, editors. Basel: Krager: 1992. pp. 42–53.

US Code. The Waxman-Hatch Act. The Drug Price Competition and Patent Term Restortation Act of 1984 (popularly known as the Waxman-Hatch or Hatch-Waxman Act) is codified at 21 U.S.C. 355 of the Food, Drug and Cosmetic Act and 35 U.S.C. 271 (e) and 35 U.S.C. 156 of the Patent Act. 1984.

U.S. Code of Federal Regulations. 2013. 21 Parts 300 to 499. US Departmetn of Health and Human Services, Food and Drug Adminstration. Last updated 01 June 2013. www.accessdata.fda.gov/scripts/cdrh/cfdocs/cfcfr/cfrsearch.cfm. Accessed April 23, 2014.

U.S. FDA. Guidance for industry: topical dermatologic corticosteroids: in vivo bioequivalence. US Department of Health and Human Services, Food and Drug Adminsitration. 1995. www.fda.gov/downloads/Drugs/GuidanceComnplianceRegulatoryInformation/Guidance/ucm070234.pdf. Accessed April 14, 2014.

U.S. FDA. Guidance for industry: nonsterile semisolid doseage forms scale-up and postapproval changes: chemistry, manufacturing, and controls; in vitro release testing and in vivo bioequivalence documentation. US Department of Health and Human Services, Food and Drug Administration. 1997. www.fda.gov/downloads/Drugs/GuidanceComplianceRegulatory Information/ Guidances/UCM070930.pdf. Accessed February 26, 2013.

U.S. FDA. Guidance, bioequivalence recommendations for specific drug products. US Department of Health and Human Services, Food and Drug Administration. 2007. www.accessdata.fda.gov/scripts/cder/psg/index.cfm?event = Home.Search#letterSearchBar. Accessed October 6, 2019.

U.S. FDA. Drug applications for Over-the-Counter (OTC) drugs. US Department of Health and Human Services, Food and Drug Administation. Last updated: October 18, 2012a. www.fda.gov/Drugs/DevelopmentApprovalProcess/HowDrugsareDevelopedandApproved/ApprovalApplications/Over-the-CounterDrugs/default.htm. Accessed April 23, 2014.

U.S. FDA. For consumers: Kefauver-Harris amendments revolutionized drug development. US Department of Health and Human Services, Food and Drug Administration. 2012b. www.fda.gov/ForConsumers/ConsumerUpdates/ucm322856.htm. Accessed April 23, 2014.

U.S. FDA. Generic Drug User Fee Act program performance goals and procedure. US Department of Health and Human Services, Food and Drug Administration. 2012c. www.fda.gov/downloads/ForIndustry/UserFees/GenericDrugUserFees/UCM282505.pdf. Accessed April 23, 2014.

U.S. FDA. Guidance, bioequivalence recommendations for Acyclovir Ointment. US Department of Health and Human Services, Food and Drug Administration. 2012d. www.fda.gov/downloads/Drgs/Guidance ComplianceRegulatory Information/ Guidances/UCM296733.pdf. Accessed April 23, 2014.

U.S. FDA Approved Drug Products. US Department of Health and Human Services, Food and Drug Adminsitration. www.accessdata.fda.gov/scripts/cder/daf/. Accesssed October 6, 2019.

Weiss SC. Conventional topical delivery systems. *Dermatol Ther.* 2011; 24(5): 471–6.

Westerhof W, Van Hasselt BA, Kammeijer A. Quantification of UV-induced erythema with a portable computer controlled chromameter. *Photodermatology.* 1986; 3:310–4.

Wilhem KP, Surber C, Maibach HI. Quantification of sodium lauryl sulfate irrant dermatits in man: comparison of four techniques: skin colour reflectance, transepidermal water loss, lass Doppler flow measurement and visual scores. *Arch Dermaol Res.* 1989; 281: 293–5.

Zhai H, Maibach HI. Occlusion vs. skin barrier function. *Skin Res Technol.* 2002; 8:1–6.

# 11 Gaps and Future Considerations for Development of Transdermal and Topical Delivery Systems

*Caroline Strasinger*

## CONTENTS

## 11.1 INTRODUCTION

Although the manufacturing of transdermal and topical delivery systems has been around for several decades, difficulties with quality control and regulation of these complex dosage forms are prevalent. Little progress has been made with respect to how transdermal and topical delivery systems (collectively TDS) are developed, manufactured and regulated in comparison to their oral or parenteral dosage form counterparts. Since the first transdermal system came to market in 1979, the number of transdermal systems and similar dosage forms recalled from the market has increased; the majority as a result of quality related issues ranging from drug crystallization, to reservoir leakage, to adhesive issues.[1] Many of these quality issues affecting the marketplace may be ascribed to outmoded ways of development, manufacture and

361

control of complex delivery systems. Common deficiencies range from scarce raw material qualification and understanding, to inadequate process development and product controls, to excessive residual drug loads, among several other identifiable deficiencies in the topical and transdermal drug delivery system realm. This chapter briefly discusses quality considerations with regard to TDS development and manufacturing and explores the regulatory challenges and common deficiencies of transdermal drug delivery system development, manufacturing and control.

## 11.2  TRANSDERMAL SYSTEMS AND QUALITY DEVELOPMENT

Although Title 21 Section 314.50 of the Code of Federal Regulations discusses the general requirements of drug applications (NDAs and ANDAs), it does not address issues specific to transdermal and topical systems thereby leading to scientific gaps in the manufacturing and regulation of TDS. Regulatory Agencies have been quite vocal in encouraging Quality by Design (QbD) principles to mitigate many quality related issues across the field of pharmaceutics.[2] While encompassing all the aspects of QbD discussed in ICH Q8, 9 and 10 may not be possible with a complex dosage form such as TDS, incorporating several of the tools or concepts of QbD throughout development and manufacturing may prove beneficial in the long term. By taking a general quality approach, critical quality attributes (CQA) that affect product purity, strength, drug release, permeability and stability may be identified early in development. By identifying CQA and building a knowledge base of raw materials early in the development process, a well-designed and systematic approach to drug development is inherent. The next step for manufacturers is then to demonstrate a mechanistic understanding of material attributes and process parameters to the drug product CQA; risk assessments may aid manufacturers in relating raw material attributes and manufacturing steps to their effects on the final drug product. Furthermore, by utilizing process analytical technology (PAT) to design, analyze and control manufacturing, sound product quality can be assured.

Because of the complexity of transdermal drug delivery, identifying CQA as well as a quality target product profile (QTPP) may be difficult. Although no final FDA guidance exists, one can conceive that CQA for a particular transdermal product may encompass everything from the traditional aspects of drug permeability, adhesion properties and in vitro release to attributes that have more recently become evident due to quality related deficiencies in the marketplace such as cold flow, residual solvents, residual drug and reservoir seal. Similarly, QTPPs may touch on in vivo and in vitro delivery rates, residual drug in the TDS, adhesion to skin, lack of irritation to the skin, and avoidance of dose dumping. PAT affords the opportunity to take a dynamic and often innovative approach to produce a product with consistent quality while also reducing wastes and overall costs.[3] Table 11.1 indicates areas in which regulators and industry representatives alike have identified possible areas to incorporate PAT tools into the manufacturing process of passive type transdermal systems.[4]

In the end, the incorporation of some of the basic concepts of ICH Q8, 9 and 10 into the transdermal development may allow manufacturers to manage some of the complexity associated with the dosage form. By defining CQA and QTPPs, and

**TABLE 11.1**
**Incorporation of PAT into Passive Transdermal Manufacturing Process**

| | | Matrix | Reservoir | |
|---|---|---|---|---|
| Manufacturing Step | Liquid Blending | Coating, Drying, Laminating | Filling, Laminating, Sealing | Die Cutting, Pouching |
| Possible PAT tools | On-line viscometry | Infrared (IR) monitoring for laminate defects | At-line leak detection | Size rejection |
| | Video microscopy* | In-Line temperature and moisture sensing | In-line fill weight monitoring | Alignment for multilaminate systems |
| | FTIR/NIR* | In-Line Coat Weight/ Thickness testing | Visualization equipment for imperfections† | Pouch seal integrity |

\* Real-time monitoring for particle size, crystal formation and polymer characteristics.
† Real-time monitoring for pinholes, tears and cuts in the backing membranes and heat seals.

incorporating PAT, whether it be multivariate analysis during development or process analyzers during production, manufacturing firms have a means to evaluate progress during development and manufacturing and subsequently prevent many quality issues post-approval.

## 11.3 COMMON DEFICIENCIES WITH TRANSDERMAL DRUG DELIVERY SYSTEMS

### 11.3.1 RAW MATERIAL QUALIFICATION

It is well recognized that transdermal systems can be as simple as a drug substance dissolved in a single adhesive or a highly complex multi-component, multi-adhesive, multi-laminate matrix. Excipients can include various adhesive systems, permeation enhancers, solubilizers, plasticizers, softeners or tackifiers, all of which intricately influence the physical and pharmacokinetic properties of the TDS. As such, characterization and control of critical excipients, namely adhesives, is critical to the safety, efficacy and quality of the drug product.[5]

Proper qualification of adhesives, as well as other key excipients during the development stages, can be highly beneficial to transdermal and topical drug product manufacturers. A sound knowledge base of the critical parameters and characteristics of adhesives and excipients, both prior to and post drug formulation, aids in defining optimum drug product quality attributes in transdermal and topical formulations, as well as assisting in a seamless post-approval change process should the manufacturer or manufacturing process of the raw materials change.

Looking specifically at the adhesive component, proper qualification would include an assessment of the adhesive at three main stages of the adhesive life cycle: as a readily available polymer, the adhesive as a lamina, as well as the adhesive in the final drug product. Testing the adhesive as the supplied raw material provides insight into subtle differences that may exist for the same adhesive but supplied by different manufacturers or an altered manufacturing process. Examining the adhesive as a lamina, or as a film without the drug substance or other drug product excipients, does much of the same as testing the adhesive as a raw material, however, as a lamina would highlight the functional parameters of adhesion as well as potential impurity differences. Additionally, assessing the adhesive in the final drug product will identify any relevant changes related to drug product compositional interactions that may exist. Proper qualification of the adhesives used to formulate the drug product may include the following when applicable:

- Readily available polymer: Molecular weight distribution, polydispersity, spectroscopic analysis (IR), thermal analysis, intrinsic viscosity, and measurement of residual monomers, dimers, solvents, heavy metals, catalysts and initiators.
- Adhesive as a laminate (without drug or other formulation-specific excipients): Residual solvents, extractable and leachables, and an evaluation for peel, tack, shear and adhesion.
- Adhesive in the final drug product: Residual monomers, dimers and solvents, viscosity, IR identification, loss on drying, impurities, and content uniformity. Functionality parameters to be assessed include but are not limited to peel, shear, adhesion, tack, in vitro drug release and in vitro drug permeation.

### 11.3.2 IN-PROCESS CONTROL

Product and process controls of any drug manufacturing platform are of significant interest for both manufacturers and regulators alike. In-process testing, manufacturing controls, product specification and stability of the drug are critical to assuring the manufacturing of a quality drug product. Unfortunately, gaps in scientific understanding of transdermal and topical dosage forms in addition to inadequate process and product controls can lead to less than desirable TDS.

For drug-in-adhesive systems, a uniform adhesive mix is desired prior to casting the laminate in order to assure consistency across and throughout the uncut laminate during the manufacturing process. Similarly, reservoir systems require that the gelled reservoir solution be well mixed and consistent in composition prior to dosing. Without a consistent adhesive matrix or gelled reservoir solution, content uniformity of the final drug product cannot be assured. For this reason, identifying critical process parameters and establishing sound in-process controls at the mixing stages are critical for the overall manufacturing of the drug product.

For many formulations the order of addition of components, mixing speed, temperature and time significantly affect the adhesive formulations. During process development, great care should be taken in determining the influence and importance of each parameter. Sampling for in-process testing of the adhesive mix should be from top, middle and bottom of the mixing vessel. Proper tests are product specific but may include a variety of identification and assay or potency methods, visual examination for color, clarity, air entrapment or undissolved particles or agglomeration of excipients or drug substances, and viscosity. Other tests may be applicable and all avenues and considerations for proper control of the mixing steps should be explored. As previously mentioned, the incorporation of PAT at this stage of the manufacturing process may prove beneficial. According to the *Guidance for Industry – PAT a Framework for Innovative Pharmaceutical Development, Manufacturing and Quality Assurance*, "a process end point is not a fixed time; rather it is the achievement of the desired material attribute."[3] During the blending process the use of infrared technology or other real-time monitoring methods may allow manufacturers to determine when solvation has been achieved or confirm when a homogenous blend of the drug/ adhesive solution is obtained; thus the blend can then be moved to the laminating or casting stage of production.

Akin to many other dosage form manufacturing processes, transfer from one stage to the next is not always immediate. Often, adhesive mixes are held for a period of time before being transferred to casting, drying and laminating for a variety of reasons. Similarly, after laminating, the matrix is often rewound and stored for a period of time before transferring to die cutting and pouching. As expected, anytime there is an interruption in the process, whether intended or not, regulators are interested in the effects such hold times may have on the finished product. To address potential regulatory questions, manufacturers may want to provide in their drug application packages a summary of, and justification for, all established hold times. Data from in-process sampling and other quality control measures may aid in supporting claims of minimal to no impact on the final drug product. Additionally, if individual products are held for a period of time prior to release to the marketplace, justification for this hold time or equilibration period would also be of interest to regulatory agencies.

### 11.3.3 DRUG PRODUCT SPECIFICATION

It is only natural that drug product specification is given substantial focus by manufacturers and regulators alike in the drug approval and post-approval settings. Despite the attention, the drug product specification for dermal drug delivery systems in the past has not provided adequate quality control of the drug product, as demonstrated by product recalls, stability issues and the sometimes need for post-marketing changes to the formulation or manufacturing process. While product specifications such as appearance, identification, assay, degradation products and in vitro release may seem obvious, methods that are not congruent across most pharmaceutical dosage forms and often overlooked, as well as deficiencies within these methods and acceptance criteria, lead to poorly controlled drug products. By having a thorough scientific understanding of the product in the development stage and by incorporating robust quality principles, a sounder product specification can be conceived and designed.

In 2008, Schwarz Pharma Manufacturing recalled its rotigotine transdermal system (Neupro) for crystal formation of the drug substance in the drug product.[6] More recently, Ortho-McNeil-Janssen Pharmaceuticals recalled lots of its fentanyl transdermal system (Duragesic) also for observed crystals in the transdermal matrix.[7] Given that the majority of drug substances used in dermal formulations are solids and must be dissolved into adhesive matrices or other delivery vehicles, the potential for drug recrystallization is highly possible. By including a method and acceptance criterion in the specification for the observation of crystals to be monitored at release and throughout stability, greater quality control can be assured. During product development stability challenging studies such as crystal seeding, temperature excursions, photostability and freeze/thaw can be conducted to possibly predict the likelihood for crystallization to occur in individual formulations during storage.

The pressure sensitive adhesives (PSA) used in transdermal systems must be able to deform under slight pressure; adhesion occurs by applying pressure which induces a liquid-like flow of the PSA and wetting of the skin surface. Although the fluidity of the adhesive is required for adhesion, it can cause a quality issue commonly known as cold flow. Cold flow is the creep or oozing of the adhesive matrix beyond the parameter of the backing membrane. The presence of cold flow may result in increased or unintentional exposure to the drug substance, make it difficult for the patient to remove the transdermal delivery system from the pouch and/or release liner, and cause a "tacky" ring around the perimeter.[8]

Although the cold flow phenomenon is inherent to transdermal and topical systems, special consideration during product development as well as adequate control in the product specification may result in better product design and greater quality control. During development, manufacturers may investigate different adhesives, excipients and their subsequent interactions with the drug substances and consider using cold flow as one of their CQA. Additionally, manufacturers may also explore a number of release liner designs, packaging configurations, as well as within matrix/non-rate controlling membranes to add structural support for the matrix and perhaps decreased cold flow.

To adequately assess cold flow at release and throughout stability may require a combination of quantitative and qualitative methods. In the product specification, appearance criteria can assess potential use issues caused by cold flow if systems are difficult to remove from pouches, if release liners detach from the adhesive matrix during attempted removal, as well as adhesive residue transferred to the pouch after removal of the system. A quantitative cold flow method can capture the degree to which cold flow extends beyond the perimeter of the backing membrane. Regardless of the method(s), cold flow around the perimeter of the system that may remain attached to the TDS when the release liner and the pouch are removed should be assessed. Due to the intrinsic properties of the release liner, the adhesive composition has greater affinity for the backing membrane and the exposed adhesive perimeter than the release liner itself. For this reason, it is common to experience adhesive "stringiness," "balling" and other similar phenomenon around the edge of the backing membrane and the perimeter of the system after removal of the release liner and pouch. With increased tackiness around the perimeter during product use (wear), the potential for the system to detach from the skin is increased.

As previously mentioned, adhesion characteristics are critical for proper product design and therapeutic use. Equally as important, having adequate specifications and acceptance criteria for release and stability is essential. Specification and acceptance criteria, if properly set, powered and justified with scientific data, can detect adhesive property changes that may be due to raw material variation that may not always be evident in raw material acceptance criteria and testing. Additionally, adhesive testing at release and stability allows for monitoring for undesirable trends throughout the life cycle of the product. Adhesion testing can be done by a variety of methods but typically consists of adhesion to steel or other suitable substrate, peel from release liner, probe tack, and shear.

Other tests that are not common to other dosage forms or require slightly different design include a test for residual monomers, content uniformity, pouch integrity and microbial examination. In more detail, residual monomers from the adhesive component of the product may be present despite drying efforts and should be tested for and adequately controlled. Although USP <905> is frequently used to assess content uniformity, much like other dosage forms, providing a sampling plan to regulators often aids in assuring that uniformity across and throughout the uncut drug laminate is maintained. Additionally, for some system designs, uniformity within a single transdermal or topical system unit may be necessary to assess at release, particularly if the system is designed to be cut such as the Lidoderm® Lidocaine Patch 5%.[9] A variety of standard methods can be used to ensure the immediate container closure, most commonly a pouch, is properly sealed at release and throughout shelf life; regardless of the method, a specification and acceptance criteria should be included in product specification or as an in-process test. Microbial examination methods may or may not be necessary as part of the regular specification, and are based on product design. Often times drug/adhesive matrices are solvent-based systems and are not growth promoting mediums; however, regulators often request to see justification for lack of microbial methods; USP methods are typically employed in such instances. Conversely, water-based reservoir systems, whether passive or part of an active system like iontophoresis, as well as newer technologies such as microneedles, may require more substantial and consistent microbial testing.

### 11.3.4 STABILITY

The previous discussion of specification and acceptance criteria segues nicely into the latter stage of product development, i.e., manufacturing; stability. Issues such as crystal growth, decrease in adhesion, increase in peel from release liner, cold flow, adhesive impurities and changes in in vitro release may not manifest until later in the shelf life. As such, adequate testing and acceptance criteria are equally important throughout the shelf life for transdermal and topical systems. Additionally, referring to the previous discussion of hold times, manufacturers should recognize that shelf life of a product begins when the drug substance is committed to the adhesive matrix for transdermal systems not when the laminate is die cut and pouched into individual units.

An area that is commonly overlooked in stability studies is the impact the identifying label on the backing membrane may have on stability. In general, transdermal and topical system backing membranes are labeled with, at a minimum, the drug product name and strength, to be visible throughout the duration of wear. Additional information may be requested to be added to the identifying label or to ensure that the label is visible during disposal depending on the individual product and its intended use. Regardless of the actual marketed wording, the labeling technique should be applied in the early phases of clinical trials in order for the impact on stability to be adequately assessed. Methods of applying the identifying label are unique to the individual product. Ink printing, embossing, debossing or laser etching are just a few of the techniques that have been explored over the history of TDS manufacturing. Similar to the backing membrane itself, any inks utilized should be assessed for leachables and extractables and should not interact with the drug product itself throughout the duration of shelf life. Embossing, debossing and laser etching are physical methods to label a backing membrane, which if applied after the drug/adhesive matrix has been laminated, introduces stress to the matrix and may lead to crystal formation or other undesirable quality issues. As such, choosing a labeling technique and applying a label of some kind is important early in development to thoroughly assess the impact on stability; the text presentation can always be finalized at a later point in time.

Taking a life-cycle approach towards TDS development may provide insight into and eventually prevent many post-marketing issues. It is common knowledge that an adhesive matrix is not a rigid structure. Just as pressure sensitive adhesives must have a degree of flow in order to adhere to the skin, the lack of rigidity may also lead to migration of drug substances and excipients within the matrix over the shelf life of the product. By obtaining a scientific understanding of the impact of raw material variation on finished product lots as well as of changes that may occur to a drug matrix on stability, a safer and more effective drug product can be manufactured and marketed throughout its intended shelf life with potentially fewer product quality related recalls. As alluded to before, in addition to sometimes having multiple drug substances, many TDS formulations include multiple non-miscible adhesives, solubilizers, permeation enhancers, softeners, internal membranes or many other possible excipients, Naturally, over time, some of these components can be expected to realign based on physical and chemical properties inherent to the components. During product development, stability studies and even in post-marketing exploration, it may be prudent for manufacturers to visually assess the surface and cross-sectional changes in drug product matrix via high-powered microscopy, elemental mapping or other scientific means. By exploring the impact of raw material variation and taking a life-cycle approach to TDS, greater product control can be assured in development, manufacturing and market.

### 11.3.5 Residual Drug

Although it is well recognized that transdermal and topical delivery systems require greater drug loads than that which is delivered into systemic circulation or utilized to provide therapeutic effect during wear, excessive drug loads have shifted into the purview of regulatory agencies very recently. In 2011, the FDA issued the *Guidance for Industry: Residual Drug in Transdermal and Related Drug Delivery Systems* which recommends "that sufficient scientific justification to support the amount of residual drug in TDS, transmucosal delivery systems, or topical patches be included in an application."[10] The level of information should be sufficient enough to demonstrate product and process understanding and assure that a science- and risk-based approach has been taken to minimize the amount of residual drug in a system after use. Discussing the impact of different adhesive systems explored, use of permeation enhancers or other excipients, as well as providing in vitro skin permeation data of development formulations may help with justification of the residual drug amount. Additionally, the guidance should be considered during clinical trial as it is important to assess the residual drug amounts in the transdermal systems after use rather than just theoretical assessment.

## REFERENCES

1. "2000–2010 Recalls by Dosage Form and Problem Area." *The Gold Sheet*. May 2011, Vol. 45, No. 5.
2. Aksu, B., De Beer, T., Folestad, S. et al. 2012. Strategic Funding Priorities in the Pharmaceutical Sciences Allied to Quality by Design (QbD) and Process Analytical Technology (PAT). *European Journal of Pharmaceutical Sciences*. 47(2): 402–405.
3. U.S. Department of Health and Human Services Food and Drug Administration. *Guidance for Industry PAT – A Framework for Innovative Pharmaceutical Development, Manufacturing, and Quality Assurance*. September 2004. www.fda.gov/downloads/ Drugs/GuidanceComplianceRegulatoryInformation/Guidances/ucm070305.pdf
4. Strasinger, Caroline. "Regulatory Challenges: Gaps and Future Consideration for Transdermal Systems." Improved Development/Regulation Transdermal Systems, DIA, Arlington, VA. 15 SEP 2011. Conference Presentation.
5. Buskirk, G.A., Arsulowicz, D., Basu, P. et al. 2012. Passive Transdermal Systems Whitepaper Incorporating Current Chemistry, Manufacturing and Controls (CMC) Development Principles. *AAPS PharmSciTech*, 13(1) (March): 218–230. www.ncbi.nlm. nih.gov/pmc/articles/PMC3279638/pdf/12249_2011_Article_9740.pdf.
6. U.S. Food and Drug Administration. Enforcement Report for May 14, 2008. U.S. Food and Drug Administration, 30 APR 2009. Web. 4 Nov. 2012. www.fda.gov/Safety/Recalls/ EnforcementReports/2008/ucm120506.htm
7. U.S. Food and Drug Administration. Enforcement Report for June 6, 2012. U.S. Food and Drug Administration, 07 JUN 2012. Web. 4 Nov. 2012. www.fda.gov/Safety/Recalls/ EnforcementReports/ucm307229.htm
8. Wokovich, A.M., Prodduturi, S., Doub, W.H. et al. Transdermal drug delivery system (TDDS) adhesion as a critical safety, efficacy and quality attribute. *European Journal of Pharmaceutics and Biopharmaceutics*. 64 (2006) 1–8.
9. Endo Pharmaceuticals Inc. *How to Apply the Lidoderm® Patch*. Endo Pharmaceuticals, September 2012. Web. 12 Nov. 2012. www.lidoderm.com/patch.aspx.
10. U.S. Department of Health and Human Services Food and Drug Administration. *Guidance for Industry: Residual Drug in Transdermal and Related Drug Delivery Systems*. August 2011. www.fda.gov/downloads/Drugs/GuidanceComplianceRegulatoryInformation/ Guidances/UCM220796.pdf

# 12 Regulatory Challenges in Chemistry, Manufacturing and Controls

## Gaps and Future Consideration for Locally Acting Topical Dermal Systems

*Shulin Ding*

## CONTENTS

## 12.1 INTRODUCTION

Locally acting topical dermal systems are those pharmaceutical preparations that are applied on the outer surface of the body and intended for local action with minimal systemic exposure. The most commonly known dosage forms are solutions, suspensions, lotions, creams, ointments and gels. Recently, foams have increasingly gained popularity, and several prescription foam products have been approved by the FDA. Topical sprays, nail lacquers, sponges, swabs (pledgets) and locally acting topical patches also exist on the market of prescription drugs but are less common.

The dosing of locally acting topical dermal systems is usually imprecise. Typically, an instruction such as "apply a thin layer over the affected area" is all that is given in the section of Package Insert for dosage and administration. Another characteristic of locally acting topical dermal systems is that there is a general lack of knowledge in local pharmacokinetics (PK) due to difficulty in measuring PK parameters (such as $C_{max}$ and AUC) in local tissues. This lack frustrates the effort to correlate clinical performance with local PK parameters. Consequently, the use of clinical endpoints has been the typical regulatory approach for bioequivalence evaluation and determination (with the exception of topical steroids which have the option of using vasoconstriction study to establish bioequivalence for generic product development).

The limitation in local PK knowledge and tools impedes the chemistry, manufacturing and controls (CMC) development of locally acting dermal systems for both new and generic drugs. For the new drugs, it is difficult to identify and confirm clinically relevant critical product attributes. Novelty through formulation or process innovations is, therefore, hard to substantiate. For the generic drugs, the difficulty in demonstrating bioequivalence without a clinical study has resulted in much fewer generic dermal products when compared with systemic products.

## 12.2 RECENT AND FUTURE TREND

### 12.2.1 INDUSTRIAL INNOVATIONS

Despite the development challenges and the lack of tools, the field of dermal products is still reasonably active. One major focus of recent activities in this field has been method development and optimization for dermal product assessment. The following methodologies have gained particular attention, and been proposed by the industry for regulatory acceptance: in vitro release testing (IVRT) and in vitro skin permeation testing (IVPT) for quality assessment, and dermatopharmacokinetics (DPK) as well as microdialysis for bioequivalence determination. Previously, a separate pharmacodynamic method, vasoconstriction, has already been accepted by the FDA for bioequivalence determination of glucocorticoids.

In addition to method development and optimization, new dermal products are regularly proposed to the FDA, and a significant number of new drug applications (NDAs) are approved every year. A review of recently approved dermal products and what are being proposed to the FDA for the near future shows that the formulation as well as container/closure system have grown more complex and diverse, and new excipients with interesting physicochemical and even biological properties are being explored to improve dermal drug delivery. Complex active ingredients such as plant extracts and proteins are also included in the prospect of dermal products.

The more complex and diverse formulations, container/closure systems and active ingredients often present significant challenges to the regulators notably in areas such as dosage form determination, control strategy over active ingredient, formulation and process, and designation of multiple active ingredients in conjunction with the combination drug policy. Following are some examples of the proposed innovations and their regulatory challenges (i.e., gaps).

### 12.2.1.1 Foams

Dermatological foam products have gained popularity in recent years. The earlier ones are all aerosols. Recently, due to advancement in technology, foam-creating mechanical pumps become available for the pharmaceutical industry to produce non-aerosol foams.

The non-aerosol foams are hazardless and cheaper to manufacture. It affords the industry an alternative to produce foam products, and at the same time posts a regulatory challenge as to whether the differences between the foams produced by these two types of technologies are distinct enough to warrant the creation of subcategories, aerosol and non-aerosol, under the dosage form of foam.

Pharmaceutically, an obvious formulation difference exists between aerosol and non-aerosol foams because the former requires the use of propellants whereas the latter does not. The physical characteristics (density, firmness, breaking time, etc.) of the produced foams appear to be somewhat different too between the two technologies. The clinical significance of these apparent physicochemical differences is, however, to be determined since typically the labeling of dermatological foams instructs patients to rub the foams into the treated area. Rubbing would presumably break all foam structures, and thus potentially eliminate or mitigate the physicochemical differences caused by propellants.

There is a general consensus that the need to make a decision on the dosage form for foams is urgent. However, a scientifically sound decision cannot be made at this time due to a lack of knowledge in physicochemical characteristics of pharmaceutical foams including drug release and penetration characteristics.

### 12.2.1.2 Film-forming Formulations

The earlier approved nail lacquers were film-forming organic solutions. The medication leaves a residual film behind on the treated area after the evaporation of the volatile components of the formulation. The film is considered to be a potential drug reservoir that can continuously supply the active ingredients to the tissues and also a protective layer to prevent the wear off the medication through rubbing. Therefore, potentially this type of dosage form may reduce dosing frequency, and thus become an extended-release dosage form.

The film-forming concept has recently been applied to other dermatological diseases beyond nail infections. Furthermore, the formulation proposed is not necessarily a solution; it can be a suspension, an emulsion, a cream, etc. Obviously, nail lacquer is no longer an appropriate dosage form nomenclature for this kind of product. An appropriate one that conforms to current nomenclature standards will need to be decided by the regulators.

One can expect that CMC information to support such a product may be more than what is typically required for a simple solution/suspension/emulsion. The resultant film and the raw material of the excipient responsible for film-formation may need to be characterized and controlled. If reduction in dosing frequency can be substantiated for certain indications, in vitro drug release (IVRT) would then likely be considered as a critical quality attribute and included in drug product specification.

### 12.2.1.3 Liposomes/Vesicles/Nanoparticles
The technologies of liposomes, vesicles and nanoparticles have been introduced to dermatological formulations in recent years with an aim to increase drug penetration and thus bioavailability in the targeted local tissue. These technologies are very complex, and their technical challenges in formulation, characterization and scale-up are well documented. For these complicated technologies, it cannot be emphasized enough the importance of conducting a comprehensive product characterization early on. Early identification of critical product attributes and important manufacturing process parameters is essential to the eventual success in the development. In vitro drug release is a potential critical product attribute for this kind of product. Therefore, it is prudent to undertake its method development and validation early. Classification of this kind of product for dosage form will also be an interesting task.

### 12.2.1.4 Pumps and Applicators
Due to technology advancement and product life cycle management, many recent proposed products involved innovations in the container/closure system design such as adding a pump head or an applicator to the approved bottle configuration, or a co-packaged pump head or applicator. The inclusion of a dropper or a brush for the patients to administer a dermal medication is not a new idea but the sophistication and diversity of the newly proposed pumps and applicators is unprecedented. Questions have been raised regarding the regulatory status of these pump heads/applicators (e.g., are they devices?), and the type of studies needed to approve such a product.

### 12.2.1.5 Organic Volatile Formulations
A non-aqueous, volatile formulation was uncommon in the past due to challenges in manufacturing and handling as well as concerns related to safety (i.e., extractables/leachables) and quality (solvent evaporation, leakage and deterioration of the container/closure). The interaction of the organic solvents with the plastics of the container/closure systems may cause discoloring, blistering, cracking and swelling of the bottles, caps, valves, gaskets, etc. Organic, volatile formulations require tight,

well fit container/closure systems to prevent loss of volatile ingredients and leakage, and clean, inert plastics as fabrication materials for the container/closure to minimize the undesirable extractables/leachables.

With the availability of cleaner medical grade plastics in recent years and more sophisticated manufacturing equipment/process, the aforementioned CMC challenges have been overcome. Multiple NDAs have been received proposing fully organic, volatile formulations for dermal indications. More products with such nature are expected to be proposed to the FDA in the future.

### 12.2.1.6 Penetration Enhancers and Transport Peptides

The use of organic solvents and surface active agents to enhance drug penetration has been a formulation strategy for topical drug delivery for many years. The FDA recognizes the potential of these solvents/surfactants for penetration enhancement, and has never regarded them as "active ingredients." The FDA may request the inclusion of a routine identity and assay test over the "penetration enhancer" in the drug product specification to assure the expected penetration enhancement but has never required the same degree of CMC control and GMP (Good Manufacturing Practice) as that is required for active ingredients.

A new class of penetration enhancers for proteins has emerged in recent years. These biological penetration enhancers, also known as transport peptides, can react with specific receptors on the barrier membrane (e.g., skin) to open the pathway for proteins to cross. Without the presence of transport peptides, the penetration of proteins would be negligible, but with their presence the penetration might be significant enough to reach the therapeutic level. The role of transport peptides has been regarded by some regulators as equivalent to an active ingredient based on their interpretation of drug laws. However, to others the transport peptides are just functional excipients because the actual moiety that exerts the pharmacological activity is the protein molecule. Those who attempt to develop a topical protein product should look out for the FDA's final position on the regulatory status of transport peptides.

### 12.2.2 USP INITIATIVES

Since the turn of the century, USP Council of Experts has actively undertaken standard-setting activities to keep the compendial standards and information up-to-date. One recognized urgent need is the establishment of a compendial taxonomy and glossary for pharmaceutical dosage forms so that pharmaceutical preparations can be categorized in a non-ambiguous, uniform way. Such a system will not only benefit prescribers and patients but also carry a significant legal and regulatory implication since dosage form has been regarded as a factor in the determination of pharmaceutical equivalence according to the Orange Book.

In 2002, a USP Ad Hoc committee composed of members with expertise in pharmaceutical dosage forms, biopharmaceutics and nomenclature was formed to work with the Pharmaceutical Dosage Forms Expert Committee in the development of a compendial taxonomy and glossary. The result of the joint effort, a Stimuli article, was published in 2003 (Reference 1). The article describes a three-tiered taxonomic scheme with an associated glossary of terms. Additionally, the taxonomy is

**TABLE 12.1**
**Three-Tiered Taxonomic Scheme Described in the Stimuli Article**

| | | |
|---|---|---|
| Tier One | Route of Administration | Oral |
| | | Parenteral |
| | | Mucosal |
| | |    Oropharyngeal |
| | |    Rectal |
| | |    Nasal |
| | |    Ophthalmic |
| | |    Otic |
| | |    Urethral |
| | |    Vaginal |
| | | Skin surface |
| | |    Transdermal |
| | |    Topical |
| | | Lungs |
| Tier Two | Physical State | Solid |
| | | Tablets |
| | | Capsules |
| | | Chewable tablets |
| | | Powders |
| | | Pellets |
| | | Suppositories |
| | | Lyophilizate |
| | | Inserts |
| | | Tapes |
| | | Gauzes |
| | | Plasters |
| | | Semisolid |
| | | Gels |
| | | Creams |
| | | Gums |
| | | Pastes |
| | | Ointments |
| | | Foams |
| | | Liquid |
| | | Solutions |
| | | Suspensions |
| | | Emulsions |
| Tier Three | Drug release pattern | Immediate release |
| | | Modified release |
| | | Extended release |
| | | Delayed release |

considered to be a basis for the General Policies and Requirements Division of USP Council of Experts to support the extension of the USP performance test to dosage forms other than oral solids (Reference 2). The Stimuli article concluded with a recommendation that USP Expert Committees could be assigned or Advisory Panels could be formed to develop and revise the needed tests and general chapters for quality standards of dosage forms under each route of administration.

Advisory Panels for each route of administration have been established since 2004. Through the panels' effort the general information chapter on pharmaceutical dosage forms, USP <1151>, has been revised, and two new general chapters on topical products, USP <3> Topical and Transdermal Drug Products – Product Quality Tests, and USP <1724> Semisolid Drug Products – Performance Tests, have been added to the USP.

The extension of the USP performance test such as in vitro release test (IVRT) to non-oral-solid dosage forms, and utilizing the performance test to link, is a new USP initiative. This concept plus the tiered taxonomy and the differentiation of quality tests from performance tests are being incorporated in every chapter/draft chapter mentioned earlier. Given in the following list are brief summaries for the revised USP <1151> and the new general chapters USP <3> and USP <1724>, and USP <603>.

- *USP <1151> Pharmaceutical Dosage Forms*
  The tier concept of the Stimuli article was incorporated into the revised General Information chapter USP <1151>. The revised chapter focuses on the second tier of the compendial taxonomy, and is organized according to the physical attributes of each particular dosage form. The revised chapter is much more comprehensive than the obsolete version because general manufacturing principles, quality control information, packaging and storage, labeling and use, etc. are included in the revised chapter for most dosage forms in addition to providing a definition. The revised chapter is divided into four sections:

  General Consideration: Serves as the introductory section, covering tier concept, dosage form definition and tests to ensure compliance with pharmacopeial standards for dosage form performance.

  Product Quality Tests, General: Provides comprehensive testing strategy to ensure safety and efficacy of the commercialized drug products. Some tests (such as description, identity, assay and impurities) are universally applied; some tests are dosage form specific.

  Dosage Form monographs: Provide general description, definition, discussion of general principles of manufacturing or compounding, and recommendations for proper use, storage and labeling.

  Glossary: Provides definitions for terms used in medicine and serves as a source of official names for official articles. The glossary clearly distinguishes preferred from not preferred terminology.
- *USP <3> Topically Applied Drug Products – Product Quality Tests*
  This chapter provides a list of product quality tests for topically applied drug products. The quality tests are divided into two categories: universal tests (such as description, identification, assay and impurities) and specific tests (such as uniformity of dosage units, preservative content, antioxidant content,

particle size, pH, sterility, microbial limits, etc.). Special sections are devoted to apparent viscosity for semisolids, uniformity test in containers, and specific tests for transdermal delivery systems. As indicated in the title of this general chapter, all of the tests described in this chapter are intended for the quality of the product. Although product quality tests are important in the overall control strategy for the finished dosage form, none of the quality tests are considered to be a performance test.

- *USP <1724> Semisolid Drug Products – Performance Tests*
  This chapter provides general information about in vitro drug release testing of topically administered semisolid drug products and lotions, the theory and applications of such testing, descriptions for three different drug release apparatus designs and application of drug release testing. USP General chapter <3> Topical and Transdermal Drug Products—Product Quality Tests provides information related to product quality tests for topical and transdermal dosage forms, USP <724> Drug Release provides procedures and details for testing drug release from transdermal systems, and this chapter (USP <1724>) is intended to provide procedures for determining drug release from topically administered semisolid dosage forms and lotions.

- *USP <603> Topical Aerosols*
  This chapter is intended for topical aerosol products. The chapter states that the product quality test for topical aerosols should follow USP <5>, USP <61>, USP <62>, USP <755> and USP <604>. Furthermore, there are special considerations and quality requirements including:
  ○ Delivery rate and delivered amount.
  ○ Pressure test which is only applicable for topical aerosols fitted with a continuous valve.
  ○ Minimum fill and is per USP <755>.
  ○ Leakage rate as directed by USP <604> Leak rate.
  ○ Number of discharges per container.
  ○ Delivered dose uniformity.

### 12.2.3  FDA QUALITY INITIATIVES

- *Dosage Form Standardization*
  Since the issue of SUPAC-SS (Guidance for Industry, Nonsterile Semisolid Dosage Forms) in 1987, FDA has not had any major quality initiative that addresses the specific needs of dermatological products until the publication of the manuscript entitled "Topical Drug Classification" by Buhse et al. in 2005 (Reference 3). The purpose of this manuscript as stated in its Abstract and Introduction was to obtain a scientifically based, systematic classification of dosage forms for topical products so that physicians can be guided by dosage form for desirable physical properties in prescribing topical products for a patient.

  The subject of topical product classification began to receive FDA's attention in the late twentieth century since the creation of a generic drug market in the USA. Because the FDA defines pharmaceutical equivalence in the Orange

Book as "same active drug ingredient, same strength, same dosage form and same route of administration," the term "dosage form" begins to carry regulatory and legal implications. Consequently, dosage form determination becomes a critical component of CMC review in the drug approval process.

Although the work of Buhse et al. covered only a few common topical dosage forms, and the characterization was not comprehensive, the classification system developed by them is scientifically sound enough for the FDA to apply its main principles to the CMC review of new drug applications. On June 21, 2006, FDA revised its CDER Data Standards Manual for the definition of lotion, cream, ointment and paste based on the classification system developed by Buhse et al. This is a major milestone in the nomenclature history of topical dosage forms. Concurrently, USP revised USP <1151> Pharmaceutical Dosage Forms to be consistent with CDER Data Standards Manual. To-date, although no official guidance had been issued for topical drug classification, CDER Data Standards Manual and the decision tree contained in Buhse's manuscript have been served as the main guiding references for CMC reviewers in dosage form determination for topical products (see Figure 12.1).

The thought process of the decision tree is not without some ambiguity, but is consistent with the tiered taxonomy published in 2003 (Pharmacopeia Forum 29[5]) by USP Ad Hoc committee. The taxonomy assigns physical state (i.e., solid, semisolid or liquid) as the first tier for consideration next to the

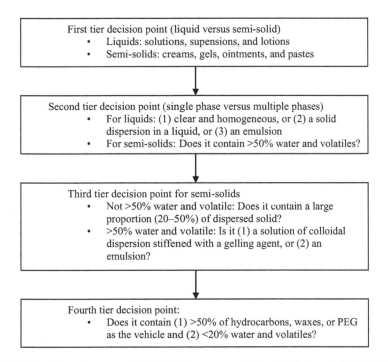

**FIGURE 12.1**   Thought process in the decision tree published by Buhse et al. in 2005.

route of administration. The pharmaceutical industry has recognized the value of the decision tree and some have expressed a desire to see a further expansion of the decision tree and better definition of the dosage form (e.g., cream versus lotion) through applying knowledge of rheological properties.

- *Quality by Design*
  Quality by design (QbD) is an essential element of the FDA's initiative "Pharmaceutical Quality for the 21st century: A Risk-Based Approach." The initiative, launched in 2002, is the Agency's effort to modernize drug quality regulation and regulatory processes, and QbD concept with its principles are adopted as a vehicle to accomplish the objectives set by the initiative as follows:
  - To encourage the early adoption of new technological advances by the pharmaceutical industry.
  - To facilitate industry application of modern quality management techniques, including implementation of quality systems approaches.
  - To encourage implementation of risk-based approaches.
  - To ensure that regulatory review and inspection policies are based on state-of-the-art pharmaceutical science.
  - To enhance the consistency and coordination of FDA's drug quality regulatory programs.

  Quality by design (QbD) as defined in ICH guideline Q8(R2) is a systematic approach to development that begins with predefined objectives and emphasizes product and process understanding and process control, based on sound science and quality risk management. The emphasis of QbD is placed on a thorough understanding of the product and process by which it is developed and manufactured along with a knowledge of the risks involved in manufacturing the product and how best to mitigate those risks.

  An illustrative example given by ICH Q8R for the QbD approach to the development of a pharmaceutical product includes the following key QbD elements:
  - Targeting the product profile.
  - Determining the **Critical Quality Attributes** (CQA).
  - Linking raw material attributes and process parameters to CQA and performing **risk assessment**.
  - Developing a **design space**.
  - Designing and implementing a **control strategy**.
  - Managing product life cycle, including continual improvement.

  Elements 1 and 2 are activities to acquire product understanding, Elements 3 and 4 are activities to acquire process understanding and Elements 5 and 6 are activities to achieve process control. Much more elaboration for each QbD element can be found in ICH Q8R and relevant publications.

  To facilitate the implementation of QbD, and to ensure international harmonization in regulatory processes, the FDA has collaborated with international health and regulatory organizations via participation in the International Conference on Harmonization (ICH) to develop ICH QbD related guidelines for the three major regulatory regions. The following three QbD related ICH guidelines have been finalized since the initiation of the Pharmaceutical Quality initiative:

○ ICH Q8(R2) Pharmaceutical Development, August 2009.
○ ICH Q9 Quality Risk Management, November 2005.
○ ICH Q10 Pharmaceutical Quality system, June 2008.

Additionally, the FDA also completed and issued many QbD-aligned CDER guidance's in the first decade after the introduction of the initiative. Some examples are:

○ Guidance for Industry: PAT – A Framework for Innovative Pharmaceutical Development, Manufacturing, and Quality Assurance, September 2004.
○ Guidance for Industry: Q10 Pharmaceutical Quality System, April 2009.
○ Guidance for Industry: Process Validation: General Principles and Practices, January 2011.
○ Guidance for Industry: Q8, Q9, & Q10 Questions and Answers – Appendix: Q&As from Training Sessions (Q8, Q9, & Q10 Points to Consider), July 2012.
○ Guidance for Industry: Q11 Development and Manufacture of Drug Substances, November 2012.

The Agency's effort in implementing QbD within the Agency's internal regulatory processes for quality review has also progressed significantly in the first decade after the introduction of the initiative. A few highlights are:

■ CDER's Office of New Drug Quality Assessment (ONDQA) has established a new risk-based pharmaceutical quality assessment system (PQAS) based on the application of product and process understanding.

■ ONDQA has initiated and completed a CMC pilot program for QbD submissions. Twelve submissions (nine NDAs and three supplements) were accepted into the program, and 11 of them have been approved. One submission was withdrawn. The learning from this pilot program has been shared with the industry.

■ CDER's Office of Generic Drugs (OGD) announced a Question-based Review (QbR) process for its CMC evaluation of Abbreviated New Drug Applications (ANDAs) in 2005, and began to implement in 2007. QbR focuses on critical pharmaceutical quality attributes. It is designed to assess a sponsor's implementation of FDA's Quality Initiative for the twenty-first century.

■ CDER's Office of Biological Products (OBP) launched a QbD pilot program in 2008. A group of ten applications and supplements have been selected for this pilot program.

■ EMA-FDA QbD pilot program started in 2011. The pilot program is a collaboration between the FDA and the European Medicines Agency (EMA) to review applications containing Quality by Design (QbD) elements in parallel. Reviewers from both agencies will separately assess the applications which are submitted to both the FDA and the EMA. The pilot program was initiated to address industrial concern that certain ICH guidelines may be interpreted differently in Europe and the United States.

The concept and principles of QbD have been well adopted by many industries for many years, but its application to pharmaceutical product development did not begin until the turn of the century. Although significant progress has been made by the FDA in the first decade after the introduction of the initiative both internally and externally, there is still much work to be done in order to have the full embracement of QbD by the pharmaceutical industry.

The experience to-date suggests that QbD may be more readily embraced by the large pharmaceutical companies for the development of oral solids, and nasal sprays. It is less appealing to the development of dermatological products such as creams and lotions. Among all QbD applications reviewed by ONDQA as of December 2012, most are for tablets and none is for a dermatological product.

The dermatological market size may be small when comparing with other therapeutic sectors, but the formulation, container/closure system and manufacturing process of dermatological products can be as complicated and technically challenging as other dosage forms. The incidences of manufacturing deviations, batch failure and product recalls are no strangers to this sector. It is imperative for the manufacturers of dermatological products as a part of the industry to be closely involved in the quality initiative in order to remain competitive.

## 12.3 DEVELOPMENT CONSIDERATIONS

The considerations described in this section are guided by recent USP and FDA initiatives, and devoted to the development of future dermatological products. The emphasis is on those elements that are unique to dermatological products and have not been regularly taken into consideration in the past. Some of the ideas have recently been adopted by USP and ICH (e.g., USP <1151>, <3> and <1724>; ICH Q8, Q9 and Q10) but some are still being discussed. Standard CMC regulatory requirements are not covered in this section; they are the content of multiple chapters throughout this book.

The development of a dermatological product should begin with the establishment of a targeted product profile. The profile should include not only the required properties for clinical, toxicology, biopharmaceutics and clinical pharmacology, but also the required properties for CMC such as dosage form, formulation, container/closure system, stability and shelf life.

Traditional dermatological product development was often empirical in CMC activities. Clinical development proceeded in hast without adequate formulation characterization. Critical quality attributes were either not identified or identified too late to be measured for the pivotal clinical batches. Without knowing the values of the critical quality attributes for the pivotal clinical batches, the link between the pivotal batches and commercial batches is unsubstantiated. Consequently, the clinical performance established through phase III trials and stated in the product labeling cannot be assured for the future commercial batches. CMC overlook is usually due to an ignorance of the clinical/regulatory implications of CMC elements (e.g., dosage form, container/closure, etc.). The overlook often leads to development set back. In certain cases, a phase III re-do and/or registration stability study re-do is the price to pay.

Following are development considerations for selective CMC topics:

### 12.3.1 DOSAGE FORM

The selection of the targeted dosage form must include a consideration of clinical indication, and treated area. Gels and lotions are usually more favorable for acne and rosacea, whereas creams and ointments are typical for psoriasis. Sprays and foams penetrate better and deeper; therefore, they are preferable for hairy areas. However, their mists can easily get into eyes and nostrils; therefore, they should be refrained from directly applying onto face and scalp.

Dosage form is one of the four factors in the determination of pharmaceutical equivalence according to the Orange Book. Consequently, it carries a regulatory implication, and can determine whether an application should be sent to Office of Generic Drugs (OGD) or Office of New Drugs, and whether it should be a new NDA or a supplement.

Dermatological dosage forms were not standardized until 2006. Before the standardization, the dermatological market was very chaotic in this matter. Products with similar formulations can be called lotion by one company and cream by another. The chaos resulted in many regulatory and legal problems.

Both FDA and USP have adopted the concept published by Buhse et al. in 2005 for the definition of the following seven dermatological dosage forms: cream, lotion, gel, ointment, solution, suspension and paste. There are many more dermatological dosage forms available on the market beyond those covered in Buhse's 2005 article. Some of the dosage form nomenclatures are dictated by container/closure systems rather than the formulations. Wipe, sponge, swab, spray and foam are just a few examples. The formulation inside a bottle/can of these products may be a solution or an emulsion, but the dosage forms granted are normally based on the final physical form presented to the patients rather than the physical form of the formulation in the container.

It is imperative to understand that the physicochemical properties of a product must match its granted dosage form throughout its shelf life for regulatory reasons. The FDA grants only one dosage from for each product. Therefore, close attention must be paid to viscoelastic properties of the formulation when developing a product with a targeted liquid or semisolid property.

### 12.3.2 FORMULATION

Much consideration should be put into the formulation development. The targeted formulation properties are influenced by factors such as clinical indication, treated area, population, dosage form, shelf life, storage condition, aesthetic appeal, etc. To achieve the targeted properties, decisions need to be made in many formulation variables such as organic content, volatile content, viscoelastic properties and choice of excipients in addition to pH value, type of buffers, preservatives, antioxidants, chelating agents, etc. The following discussion focuses only on the four factors in the first group because they are unique for dermatological formulations whereas the second group consists of common formulation ingredients that deal with stability and the microbiological attribute of the formulation.

- *Volatile Content*
  Volatile organic solvents such as ethanol, isopropyle alcohol are commonly used in dermatological formulation for two main reasons: (1) to enhance the penetration of the active ingredients, and (2) to dissolve poorly water soluble active ingredients or other formulation excipients. However, high content of volatile organic solvents may require special package design and capping/ sealing operation to prevent evaporation of volatile solvents and gross leak of formulation. A significant evaporation of volatile solvents would change the formulation composition. Leakage is a failure of the package in its protection of the formulation. Neither is acceptable from a quality perspective. High volatile content may also trigger a concern with flammability of the formulation; therefore, a flammability warning may be needed on the product label.

- *Viscoelastic Properties*
  Viscoelastic properties dictate the runniness and spreadability of the formulation. The formulation becomes runny when its viscosity is too low. The formulation may not spread readily when its viscosity is too high. Certain indications (such as head lice) do not favor a runny formulation out of a concern that the formulation may get into the eyes, but do want a good spreadability.

  Viscoelastic properties are a formulation attribute that is often overlooked by the developer. The properties can be affected by scale-up, process change, temperature and time. Because the key property that distinguishes liquids from semisolids is flowability, a significant change in viscoelastic properties can change dosage form from cream to lotion or vice versa as discussed in Section 12.3.1.

- *Organic Content and Choice of Excipient*
  Dermatological products are notorious for high organic content. Many of them are formulated with waxes, lipids, petrolatum, polyethylene glycols, silicon oils, fatty alcohols and their esters, surfactants, gums, glycerin, propylene glycol, organic solvents, etc. Many ingredients are mixtures, and many are polymeric materials. The high organic content is necessary for some semisolid products such as ointments, creams and pastes in order to produce the needed viscoelastic properties for semisolids, but it also creates an undesirable greasy skin feel and reduces spreadability.

  Some of the excipients are incorporated in the formulation for their function as "emollients," "moisturizers" or "humectants." Emolliency, moisturization and humectancy are in vivo skin effects, which cannot be substantiated solely by physicochemical data. The function of an excipient in a formulation should be based on its physicochemical properties unless its skin effect can be substantiated.

  It is advisable to formulate a dermatological product with excipients whose functions in the formulation can be demonstrated. In other words, incorporation of ingredients with unsubstantiated merits is not advisable because of the associated risks that can be brought to the product due to compatibility, stability, variations in raw materials and supply issues. Additionally, from the perspective of QbD, the more complex the formulation becomes, the more difficult it is to acquire the correct product understanding.

One more caution that formulators of dermatological products should be aware of is that an excipient can function as an unintended active ingredient. For example, titanium dioxide as an over-the-counter (OTC) sunscreen ingredient may be questioned for its function in a formulation intended for the indication of rosacea. Titanium dioxide may be added to the formulation for a purpose other than sun-protection, but because of its sun-protection ability, titanium dioxide may provide clinical benefit to rosacea patients; therefore, it may be deemed as the second active ingredient in the product. Another example is petrolatum in the approved diaper rash product Vusion ointment. Vusion was approved in 2006 with three active ingredients: miconazole nitrate, white petrolatum and zinc oxide. Petrolatum is the base of the ointment, but deemed to be an active rather than an excipient.

### 12.3.3 CONTAINER/CLOSURE SYSTEM

Container/closure systems of dermatological products did not receive adequate attention in the past. They have often been under qualified, and their implications in clinical performance are overlooked. The imprecise dosing and low safety risk of dermatological products may be the reasons responsible for a general disregard of the necessity to acquire proper knowledge of the container/closure system including clinical implications.

- *Qualification of Container/Closure System*
  The developers of demagogical products frequently rely on test results of USP <661> Containers, compliance with indirect food additive regulations, and registration stability studies data to support the proposed container/closure system for marketing authorization. The relevant tests prescribed by USP <661> for dermatological products are four physicochemical tests (nonvolatile residue, residue on ignition, heavy metals and buffering capacity). These four tests are only a qualitative crude evaluation of extractables from plastics, and they were initially designed to evaluate plastics that contact aqueous formulations.

  However, as stated in the Section 12.2.1, recent dermatological formulations tend to contain a high level of organic solvents, and container/closure systems have grown much more diverse both in design and fabrication materials. USP <661> alone is no longer adequate to assess the safety (i.e., extractables/leachables) of the container/closure system that contacts organic formulation and involve unusual plastics or rubbers. Functionality of the container/closure system is another area that requires qualification for a novel container/closure design.

A proper qualification of container/closure system for future dermatological products should address the following four general considerations by conducting additional studies other than USP <661>:

○ To address the consideration on **protection** (e.g., from light, from solvent evaporation, from leakage):

Include Package Integrity and Weight Loss tests in the registration stability studies (and/or in-use stability study if applicable and warranted). The package integrity test should examine both interior and exterior of the immediate container at batch release and stability studies. It should also include an examination for leakage. If warranted, a leakage test can employ a sophisticated method (such as pressure or current rise) other than visual examination.

Include photostability study per ICH Q1B in the stability program.

○ To address the consideration on **compatibility** (e.g., drug uptake by plastic, discoloration or texture change of plastic, etc.):

Conduct special compatibility study on the effect of the plastic on the formulation and vice versa. The study should be done on an individual, formulation-contacting packaging component.

○ To address the consideration on **safety** (e.g., extractables/leachables):

Conduct a risk assessment based on the chemical composition of formulation-contacting plastics and assuming worst case scenario.

Conduct special extractables study on high-risk plastics. The study should be done on an individual, formulation-contacting, high-risk packaging component (rather than the entire container/closure system). The major extractables should be monitored in registration stability studies if warranted.

○ To address the consideration on **performance** (functionality, drug delivery, etc.):

Include functional tests in registration stability studies or in-use stability study, whichever applicable, for container/closure systems such as pump or applicator.

- *Changes in Container/Closure Design: Clinical Implications*
One should not assume that a container design change carries no or minimal clinical concern. Recently, pump configuration has been approved and added to the product line of a few existing approved creams and gels (which were packaged in bottles, tubes or sachets originally). The addition of an applicator to the existing approved product has also been proposed to the FDA for multiple products. Pump heads and applicators have potentials to impact clinical dosing and administration. More sophisticated ones may be considered as a device and human factor studies may be required for approval. Following are examples of clinical questions that may be raised for post-approval changes in container/closure design (e.g., adding a pump head or an applicator):

○ Does the proposed change involve a device? Does this change produce a combination product?

○ Does the proposed change affect the dosage form?

○ Does the safety or functionality of the proposed new container/closure system warrant a clinical trial?

○ Does the proposed new container/closure system deliver approximately the same dose as the original one?

○ Are there concerns regarding microbiological contamination of the surface of the applicator?

- *Changes in Container/Closure Design: Dosage Form Implication*
As stated earlier in Section 12.3.1 on dosage forms, people should be aware of dosage forms dictated by container/closure systems such as wipe, sponge, swab, spray, foam, etc. The formulation inside the bottle/can of these dosage forms may be a solution or an emulsion but the dosage form granted is based on the final physical form presented to the patients rather than the physical form inside the container. Therefore, when a pump head is mounted on the top of a bottle of a solution, the dosage form may need to be changed to spray or foam depending on the physical form after being pumped out. However, cases where there is no change in dosage form also exist if the original physical form remains unchanged from the perspective of the patients. Examples are gels, creams and ointments packaged in a bottle with a mounted pump head or a cartridge mounted with an applicator head. They remain to be called gels, creams and ointments.

- *Special Consideration for Closure Design*
The design of container/closure systems for dermatological products should abstain from bearing a resemblance to oral liquid products. This is due to a concern with medical errors (e.g., accidental ingestion). A child-resistance closure may even be preferable in some cases.

Child-resistance closure is especially requested by the FDA for the liquid products developed for head lice treatment because of a fatality caused by the accidental ingestion of Lindane lotion. Incidences of mistaking a tube product as toothpaste by children have also been reported.

## 12.3.4 Manufacturing

- *QbD Approach to Process Development, Scale-Up and Commercial Manufacturing*
The manufacture of dermatological products can be complicated and technically challenging. The incidences of manufacturing deviations, batch failure and product recalls are no strangers. To improve manufacturing consistency and process reliability, a QbD approach may be useful. A QbD approach emphasizes product and process understanding and process control. It is based on sound science and quality risk management.

Figure 12.2 is a flow chart showing the QbD approach to establish the knowledge base of the manufacturing process.

- *Special Attention to Filling/Capping/Installation*
For dermatological products involving pump head or applicator, people should be aware of the impact of assembly process (e.g., fully automatic versus semi-automatic) on package integrity and the performance of pump head and

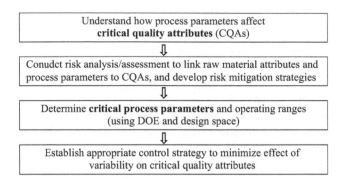

FIGURE 12.2  QbD approach flow chart to establish the knowledge base of the manufacturing process.

applicator. The semi-automatic process may produce units with poor container performance regarding functionality. Similarly, special attention needs to be paid to the impact of process on the performance of the container/closure system regarding protection from solvent evaporation and leakage, especially for highly volatile organic formulations. Pilot scale may suffer from a higher incidence of defects such as loose cap/crooked cap. Therefore, the batch release and stability data generated from pilot scale batches regarding weight loss, leakage and package integrity may not be representative for commercial batches.

### 12.3.5 STABILITY

- *Registration Stability Studies*
  The registration stability batches should be manufactured using the to-be-marketed container closure system and a process that is representative of the commercial-scale process including filling/capping/mounting process (per ICH Q1A). However, filling/capping/mounting process has often been overlooked. The batch manufacture for registration stability and phase III batches may be initiated before finalization of the design of a pump head or applicator, or the filling/capping/mounting operation may use a semi-automatic pilot process which produces many more defects than the fully automatic process.
  The stability protocol of the registration stability batches should include all critical product attributes and functionality tests when the container/closure system involves a mounted pump head or applicator. The protocol should also investigate different orientation of the container/closure system, and include package integrity (including leakage) and weight loss tests. The analytical samples should be taken from the discharged formulation from the pump or applicator head.
- *In-Use Stability Studies*
  When warranted, an in-use stability study should be conducted to support the proposed in-use period. The physicochemical integrity and the functionality of the pump head or applicator need to be demonstrated throughout the intended

use period. Additionally, the discharged formulation should be demonstrated to meet the product specification throughout the intended use period. The in-use stability study is needed regardless of whether the pump head or applicator is co-packaged or not.
- *Special Stability Studies*
Special stability studies such as photostability, freeze/thaw and cool/warm cycling studies are conducted to support shipping/handling of the product.

## 12.4  CONCLUSION

The various challenges described in Section 12.2.1 on Industrial Innovations are the potential "gaps" between the pharmaceutical industry and the regulators as seen by this author. Some are nomenclature in nature. Some are due to unprecedented technologies. To minimize the "gaps" the FDA and the USP have started initiatives to modernize regulatory and compendial standards for quality and nomenclature. The industry is encouraged to pay attention to the initiatives in order to remain competitive. In the following list are the recommendations from the author for the development of a Next Generation of Topical Product:

1. Application of QbD principles to acquire adequate product/process understanding, and identify critical quality attributes and process variables.
2. Early development of an in vitro drug release method (if applicable) as a routine quality control measure and to assist needed bridging for scale-up, site change, formulation modifications, etc.
3. Inclusion of container/closure considerations in the in-use stability and registration stability studies (e.g., samples taken from discharged formulation, functionality, leachables, etc.).
4. Adequate qualification of container/closure system including extractables/ leachables and functionality.
5. Accurate understanding of the definition for the intended dosage form.
6. Awareness of the impact of assembly process (e.g., fully automatic versus semi-automatic process) on functionality (e.g., pump) and package integrity (e.g., leakage).
7. Awareness of the need of human studies (e.g., human factor study) for some post-approval container/closure changes (e.g., adding a sophisticated applicator).

## REFERENCES

1. Keith Marshall et al. Development of a Compendial Taxonomy and Glossary for Pharmaceutical Dosage Forms, *Pharmacopeia Forum* 29(5), Sep-Oct, 2003.
2. Roger L. Williams, Standards-Setting Activities of the US Pharmacopeia During the 2000–2005 Cycle, *Drug Information Journal*, vol. 40, pp.317–329, 2006.
3. Lucinda Buhse et al., Topical Drug Classification, *International Journal of Pharmaceutics*, vol. 295, pp. 101–112, 2005

## DISCLAIMER

This book chapter reflects the views of the author and should not be construed to represent FDA's views or policies.

## ACKNOWLEDGMENT

The technical edit provided by Dr. Sarah Ibrahim is gratefully acknowledged.

# 13 Development of Topical and Transdermal Dosage Forms
## *Regulatory Perspective*

*Amit Mitra and Sarah A. Ibrahim*

## CONTENTS

The skin is one of the most extensive and readily accessible organs but serves as a barrier to the environment surrounding us. It is elastic, rugged and under normal physiological conditions, self-generating[1]. Drug development, either for topical or transdermal products, represents an added layer of both complexity and opportunity for the drug developer and clinician. Even though transdermal drug delivery takes advantage of the relative accessibility of the skin, only a small number of drug products are currently available via this route of administration. In many cases, a drug's physical properties, including molecular size and polarity, limits its capacity to be delivered across skin. Similarly, the biological properties of drug molecules including dermal irritation/sensitization and insufficient bioavailability due to limited skin permeability have posed additional constraints to this delivery technology. Irritation and sensitization can be caused by the drug, the adhesive or other excipients on the skin from the applied formulation. Still, there are a number of notable examples of successful transdermal products on the market. Approved transdermal systems include clonidine, estradiol, estrogen/progestin, fentanyl, methyl salicylate, methylphenidate, nicotine, nitroglycerin, oxybutynin, rivastigmine, rotigotine, selegiline, scopolamine and testosterone. In recent years several Investigational New Drug (IND) Applications have been received by the Food and Drug Administration.

## 13.1  ANATOMY AND PHYSIOLOGY OF THE SKIN

The skin is the largest organ in the body with a surface area in the adult male of approximately $1.73m^2$. Although the skin is often thought of as a barrier of uniform thickness, it is varying in both thickness and in the type and distribution of hair follicles and sebaceous glands which provide alternative routes of absorption (Figure 13.1). The outer layer of the epidermis, known as the stratum corneum, is approximately 10–15 cells thick and is composed of dead skin cells (corneocytes); the lower portion of the epidermis is viable and is nourished by papillary plexus that extend upward from the dermis into the epidermis. The corneocytes themselves

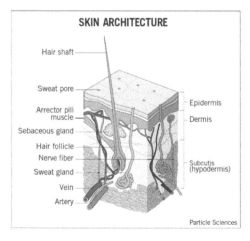
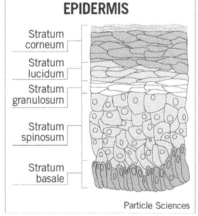

**FIGURE 13.1**   Skin structure.

are arranged in a so-called "bricks and mortar" pattern with lipids representing the mortar holding the cells in place. The organization of the stratum corneum is what makes it an effective barrier to both water loss and to the environmental challenges (including drug penetration). Thus drug delivery across skin is a balance of the degree and rate of penetration down into the proper skin layer for either local (i.e., into the epidermis) or systemic (i.e., into the dermis) drug delivery.

While seen as a continuous membrane, the skin is in a dynamic equilibrium. On an average every two weeks the stratum corneum is replaced in a process of "flaking off." In support of this remodeling process the dermis plays the key role in supporting the flexibility of the skin as it contains the elastin and collagen fibers that give skin its strength and resilience. The dermis also contains the sensory nerve fibers for pain, touch and temperature. This organization, notably the lack of nerve endings in the stratum corneum, has been utilized for drug delivery of otherwise impenetrable products by the use of microneedles which penetrate and pierce the stratum corneum and the epidermis yet remain above the sensory nerve endings. In doing so, microneedles present a viable route for the delivery of proteins, vaccines and other macromolecules or small molecule drugs that have either solubility or charge properties that hinder their penetration[2]. Microneedles also represent a flexible route of delivery as the depth of penetration is related to needle length and can be developed to only penetrate the stratum corneum or deeper to the dermis. They also come in a variety of presentations from a hand-held roller for cosmetic use[3] to transdermal systems using coated, dissolvable, hydrogel or hollow, microneedles that provide access to a reservoir of drugs[4].

In developing products for dermal delivery there is a primary bifurcation. Most "topically" applied products are intended to treat diseases that manifest themselves in the skin (e.g., acne, psoriasis, atopic dermatitis, etc.). As such, the formulations themselves are directly applied to the diseased skin. In contrast, products intended for systemic delivery, such as transdermal drug delivery systems (TDDS) (e.g., scopolamine, fentanyl, etc.) or topical gels (testosterone) are applied to intact skin. In diseased skin the normal protection (barrier function) provided by the stratum corneum is compromised resulting in less resistance to drug entry and a correspondingly higher bioavailability[5]. This loss of barrier function is assessed by measuring the transepidermal water loss (TEWL), a measure of the loss of water vapor across the skin. For products intended for transdermal delivery they are never to be applied to diseased skin. For these products, drug delivery studies are always conducted on normal skin, such that the formulation factors (adhesive, programmed delivery rate, system vs skin control) can be evaluated in a reproducible manner. Diseased skin is inherently variable from patient to patient and within an individual patient (lesion to lesion) as no two lesions are ever identical.

Thus in deciding on the formulation for development, consideration should first be given to the site of application and the physiologic state of the skin (healthy vs diseased) itself. After that has been determined then the formulation elements over which the drug developer has control can be considered.

## 13.2 PHYSIOCHEMISTRY AND DERMAL DELIVERY

Once one has decided on the site of application (for a transdermal product) or the ideally sized application area and severity of disease for a topical product, the physiochemistry of the drug substance becomes the key issue for formulation development, and the clinical pharmacology of the drug-biologic system interaction.

Whether a topical or transdermal formulation, the bioavailability of any topically applied product is the result of the complex interaction between the drug substance, formulation-dosage form and skin factors that impact the barrier function of the skin (disease, heat, sweat, adhesion, occlusion, etc.). These interactions can be optimized through proper formulation development to yield a favorable profile over time in either the target skin layer or systemic availability. As noted previously, using the "bricks and mortar" analogy, diffusion into and through the stratum corneum is the rate-limiting step for the transdermal transport of drugs. The "mortar" being composed ceramides, fatty acids, cholesterol and cholesterol esters, giving the advantage to lipophilic compounds. Taking that as a starting point, an examination of some currently marketed transdermal agents reveals some similar physiochemical properties (Table 13.1).

From Table 13.1 we can see that, in general, transdermally available drugs are of low molecular weight and generally have low melting point. A high octanol:water partition coefficient is not always necessary[6]. The key feature seen with topically applied products with systemic activity is that of a small efficacious dose, i.e., a high potency. For example, methylphenidate has a generally unfavorable octanol:water coefficient but, as the effective dose (orally) is < 20 mg, a transdermal system was feasible, delivering 1.1 mg/hr. Acetaminophen, on the other hand, has both a lower molecular weight than the other agents listed and its octanol:water partition coefficient and melting point is not that unreasonable for a transdermally delivered drug, suggesting that it *might* be a viable candidate for dermal delivery. However, as the lowest, generally effective dose of acetaminophen is 325 mg every six hours, this would yield a total daily dose of 1,300 mg of acetaminophen to be delivered transdermally. To accommodate this amount of mass transfer from a TDDS or a cream/lotion, etc. into and through the skin to the systemic circulation would require both a sophisticated

**TABLE 13.1**

**Physiochemical Properties of Selected Topical and Transdermal Agents vs Acetaminophen[c]**

|  | MW | M.P. (Celsius) | Octanol:Water | Dose (oral or IV) |
|---|---|---|---|---|
| Oxybutynin | 357 | 129 | 2.9 | 5 mg |
| Fentanyl | 336 | 87.5 | 860 | 100 mcg |
| Hydrocortisone[a] | 324 | 217 | 1.61 | n.a. |
| Scopolamine | 303 | 197 | 0.98 | 0.4-0.8 mg |
| Tretinoin[a] | 300 | 180 | 6.3 | n.a. |
| Terbinafine[a] | 291 | 195 | 3.3 | 250 mg |
| Testosterone | 288 | 155 | 3.32 | [b] |
| Methylphenidate | 233 | 42 | 0.38 | 5-20 mg |
| Nicotine | 162 | 79 | 15 | 1 mg |
| Acetaminophen | 151 | 168 | 0.46 | 325 mg |

a Topically delivered therapeutic agents.
b Testosterone is dosed to a therapeutic level and individualized to the patient.
c Physical chemical properties obtained from PubChem, http://pubchem.ncbi.nlm.nih.gov

formulation with extreme permeation enhancement and a large size patch (in the order of a sheet of notebook paper!), the antithesis of pharmaceutical elegance.

Using the same standards, it would appear that Terbinafine is an outlier, with an oral dose of 250 mg. This is, however, misleading as when the oral route is used for onychomycosis or other topical fungal infections, the normal dynamic is reversed. In this situation, there is a need to build up systemic blood levels to allow the drug to migrate from the blood out to the skin, instead of the mass transfer occurring the other way around. Generally, without resorting to heroic efforts on behalf of the formulator, most transdermal to topically available daily doses are under 20 mg and are ideally as low as possible to keep the system size/application area unobtrusive.

The physiochemistry of the drug–skin interaction is also related to how the skin responds to environmental factors during drug application. The classic example here is that of transdermally delivered fentanyl. Fentanyl, following dermal application, builds up a significant subcutaneous reservoir due to its high lipophilicity. When the skin is then exposed to heat, resulting in vasodilation, the subsequent rapid uptake of fentanyl can lead to toxic levels[7]. While the existence of these factors was always recognized in theory, it was brought home in a dramatic sense with the deaths associated with transdermal fentanyl[8]. While some of the reported deaths were due to extraction of fentanyl or improper use (use in non-opioid tolerant patients), reports continue to be published in the literature regarding the effect of heat and/or a compromised skin barrier that result in adverse outcomes[9].

While this is true of all dosage forms with specific delivery issues to a greater (inhalational) or lessor extent (direct intravenous injection), dermal products also have considerations in regards to the environment to which they are exposed to. While they should not be drivers of development, product usage questions such as "Does the patient live in a warm or cold climate? Does the patient engage in vigorous exercise or have a sedentary lifestyle?" should always be a consideration for products with a high octanol:water partition coefficient, coupled with both a high potency and a potential for life threatening adverse events.

## 13.3 TOPICAL DRUG DELIVERY

Moving from the general to specific routes of delivery, topical drug products represent a broad variety of dosage forms and presentations including creams, ointments, lotions, gels, sprays, powders and mousses. While there are broad and distinct physical differences between the products, they generally share the common element that systemic delivery is undesired and can in fact lead to systemic toxicity. However, there are exceptions such as the aforementioned case of topically applied testosterone for replacement therapy, but they are the exceptions that "prove the rule."

While there is a general belief that there is a hierarchy of absorption where one dosage form has a higher bioavailability than another, this is not abided out in practice. Ointments, for example, may demonstrate the highest bioavailability for a particular drug, but for another drug the lotion may exhibit this highest bioavailability. It is the interaction of drug, formulation and the pathophysiology/severity of diseased skin that determines in vivo bioavailability for topical products. This distinction is relevant for clinical dose selection as it is common that, in the marketplace, topical drug products will exist in multiple presentations, often as an ointment and a cream, or as a lotion and a gel. There are cases where some products, such as Terbinafine, are approved as cream, solution, gel and as a spray powder in addition to oral tablets and granules. This range of dosage forms for a single product is testament to both a variety of indications (topical and systemic) and the varied sites of application where one formulation is preferred over the other for a variety of reasons including cosmetic and convenience. These latter two elements, cosmetic and convenience, cannot be overlooked in a topical product.

### 13.3.1 TRANSFERABILITY AND WASHING

A special consideration for topically applied products is that they are "open" dosage forms. That is, once applied (or dosed) they are open to the environment vs a "closed" dosage form (such as a transdermal system) where the drug is contained within a matrix or layered system, thus minimizing (but not eliminating) inadvertent exposure. For topical products, there is a demonstrated concern that anyone who comes into contact with the site of application will likely be exposed to the drug which can result in systemic exposure. This concern has been demonstrated in practice with regards to replacement testosterone therapy where transference of drug to children has resulted in symptoms of precocious puberty, aggression and mood changes[10,11]. A post-marketing review conducted by the FDA resulted in both a box warning being added to AndroGel 1% and Testim 1% in May 2009 describing the concern and steps to minimize transfer of drug to partners or children. Although this represents the extreme case, in vivo transfer studies looking at transfer via direct skin contact and mitigation strategies need to be conducted as part of the safety assessment to develop appropriate labeling and patient instructions regarding the risk of transfer.

Related to transfer, and a recommended method to reduce the risk and degree of transfer, is the issue of washing. That is, what level of washing is effective to remove drug residue from the hands following application or from the site of action. In addition, studies to assess the timing of showering related to absorption are recommended. Patients need to be told how long they should refrain from showering/washing to allow absorption of topical products to occur. Using testosterone as an example, showering 15 or 30 minutes after application resulted in ineffective systemic levels. Additional studies were able to demonstrate that if subjects refrained from showering for 2 hours they were able to achieve a sufficient degree of systemic absorption to achieve therapeutic effect. The goal in performing transferability and showering/washing studies is to mitigate the risk of inadvertent exposure while assuring an efficacious exposure[12,13].

### 13.3.2 TOPICAL IN VIVO BIOAVAILABILITY TESTING – GENERAL DESIGN FACTORS

As noted on p. 395, minimization of systemic absorption is a goal of all topical products intended for local delivery. In general, their site of action resides not in a distant tissue target but either in the stratum corneum (as in the case of antifungals), in the sebaceous gland (for acne treatments) or at the basal cell layer (for psoriasis). In the USA, the FDA requires that all drug products include as part of their development an assessment of the bioavailability of the product. The regulations call for assessment of bioavailability "…at the site of action." For a topical product, this would be either the stratum corneum or the epidermis/dermis junction, depending on the disease in question. To date, while many methods have been proposed – tape stripping, confocal Raman, near IR and microdialysis – none of them have achieved regulatory acceptance. However, the FDA has remained a supporter of research in these areas and has participated in many public workshops to that effect.

Currently, the U.S. FDA recommends that sponsors undertake a Maximum Usage Trial (MUsT) bioavailability assessment. This trial is designed to "maximize" those factors that affect topical absorption under planned "usage" conditions. As analytical methods have improved, the ability of the MUsT paradigm to resolve entire plasma level time curves in a majority, if not all subjects, has added to the Clinical Pharmacology knowledge base. This paradigm has been presented in multiple national meetings since the mid-1990s.

### 13.3.2.1 Biopharmaceutical Considerations

Pharmacokinetic studies to assess the degree of and/or potential for systemic absorption may be needed to fulfill the requirements of 21 CFR part 320 (Bioavailability and Bioequivalence Requirements). Under this section, a new drug application (NDA) must either contain an assessment of in vivo bioavailability or sufficient information which would allow the Agency to issue a waiver of in vivo bioavailability testing. In general, waivers of in vivo biostudies are the exception and are only granted in specific cases. Because of the variable dosing nature of topical products, it is recommended that studies of the in vivo assessment of systemic exposure be done under so-called maximal use conditions. The recommended elements of such a maximal use study are as follows:

1. A formulation identical to the clinically studied/to-be-marketed formulation should be used.
2. The study should be done in an adequate number of patients with area of involvement and disease severity index/measuring toward the upper end of that in the proposed indication to include at least the face, shoulders, chest and back.
3. The topical dosing used should represent the maximal dosing anticipated in both phase III trials and in the proposed package insert for the following:
   a. Frequency of dosing.
   b. Duration of treatment.
   c. Use of highest proposed strength.
   d. Extent of involved area to be treated at one time.
   e. Amount applied per square centimeter.
   f. Method of application/site preparation.
4. The analytical method should be properly validated for both parent compound and metabolites.

The objective of this study is to maximize those elements affecting dermal penetration such that systemic absorption can be determined. We recommend, when possible, that the resulting pharmacokinetic data be analyzed using standard pharmacokinetic metrics (AUC, $C_{max}$, $T_{max}$). It is also recommended that the study protocols incorporate evaluations for cutaneous safety.

The goal, as outlined in this trial, is to assess the absorption within the upper range of planned use. Not unrealistic use, but planned use, i.e., at the highest dose and strength proposed by the sponsor for marketing. The data from such studies can be re-assuring as to the systemic safety, provided that under such conditions either no circulating drug levels are detected or that the levels fall within the demonstrated safety margin from the toxicological studies program. A more recent description of this methodology has been published that maintains the rubric presented in the FDA Guidance document, but also provides a deeper explanation of the elements and the overall goals of this trial approach[14].

This test is not one focused on the efficacy of the product, but on its safety. At the present time, in vivo Clinical Efficacy trials are necessary for demonstrating bioequivalence. While this represents a real-world test, there has been and remains interest in developing other technologies focused on measuring the drug at the actual site of action. Such a test, or more like tests optimized for different dosage forms or situations, would allow for a more rapid development program by allowing formulation optimization and formulation changes to be incorporated more readily. However, with the exception of the Hypopituitary-Adrenal Axis suppression test, to date there is no accepted in vivo methodology for assessment of bioequivalence for topical products.

## 13.4 TRANSDERMAL

In comparison to "topical" products intended for local delivery, transdermal products – be they transdermal systems, sprays or gels – are designed to penetrate and produce systemic exposure to achieve their therapeutic effect. Understandably, transdermal drug delivery offers several important advantages over more traditional dosage forms. The steady permeation of drug across the skin allows for more consistent serum drug levels, often a goal of therapy. The lack of peaks in plasma concentration can reduce the risk of side effects. In addition, if toxicity were to develop from a drug administered transdermally, the effects could potentially be reversed by removing the TDDS. However, some drugs develop a depot within the skin and continue to deliver systemically even after product removal. Another advantage is convenience, especially for systems that require only once weekly application. Such a simple dosing regimen can aid in patient adherence to drug therapy. First pass metabolism, an additional limitation to oral drug delivery, can be avoided via transdermal administration. Furthermore, drugs that are degraded by stomach enzymes, extreme GI pH, surfactants in the gastrointestinal system may also be candidates for transdermal delivery. However, various extrinsic factors result in variability to the transdermal absorption. Those include temperature, humidity, race, age, gender, anatomical site, general health of the subject, disease and trauma, bathing/cosmetic habits, occlusion and hydration of the skin. The system adhesion, physical state of the drug, presence of skin penetration enhancers, solubility of the drug in the TDDS components (concentration gradient), irritation of the skin caused by TDDS composition are common factors that can change the skin permeability intrinsic to the TDDS properties.

The most common TDDS are either skin controlled or system controlled (i.e., the system incorporates a rate controlling membrane). These systems are "closed" delivery systems, in that they contain uniform quantities of drug and are discrete systems. Although they are considered closed systems, transferability is possible through loss of product adhesion and reattachment to another subject. Compared to direct topical transfer, the risk of transferability is less with the "transdermal"-based systems.

In general, when discussing transdermal drug delivery, one is primarily concerned with the chest, upper arm and back. These are not the only sites available but they do represent large surface areas that are easily accessible and allow for rotation. The non-exclusivity of these sites is shown by the use of the post-auricular area for transdermal scopolamine and the thighs for some topical testosterone replacement products.

### 13.4.1 TRANSDERMAL DRUG DELIVERY SYSTEMS (TDDS)

Passive transdermal drug delivery systems (TDDS) are drug delivery systems designed to deliver systemic levels of a drug substance across the skin to achieve a therapeutic effect. Passive TDDS, for the purpose of this document, are systems that do not use heat, electrophoresis, iontophoresis, sonophoresis, microneedles or other mechanical approaches to induce or control transdermal drug delivery. In order to maintain consistent release rates, transdermal systems contain a surplus of active molecule. A stable concentration gradient is the mechanism used to maintain consistent release rates and constant serum drug levels. Most transdermal systems contain nearly 10–20 times the amount of drug that will be absorbed during the time of application. Thus, after removal, most TDDS may contain as much as 95% of the total amount of initial drug loading in the drug product. Therefore, patients and health care providers are expected to exercise care when disposing of used TDDS. This becomes even more critical for DEA (Drug Enforcement Administration)-scheduled drugs such as narcotics, which are amenable to abuse, and diversion. Common instructions for disposal of used systems typically include folding them in half with the adhesive sides stuck together and flushing them down the toilet rather than discarding in household trash, where children and pets may find them and ingest the remaining drug. The FDA has issued guidance on residual drug for transdermal systems (Guidance for Industry, Residual Drug in Transdermal and Related Drug Delivery Systems, August 2011)[15].

There are two major types of passive transdermal systems approved by the FDA (see Figure 13.2).

The common structural elements of TDDS include the following: 1) backing layer; 2) drug layer or reservoir; 3) adhesive layer; and 4) protective or release liner. A distinct drug layer or reservoir exists in the type I systems (Figure 13.1). In type II systems, the skin contact adhesive layer may also serve as the drug layer or reservoir. Other components such as permeation enhancers, viscosity inducing agents, etc., may also be included in this layer. Besides the four common structural elements

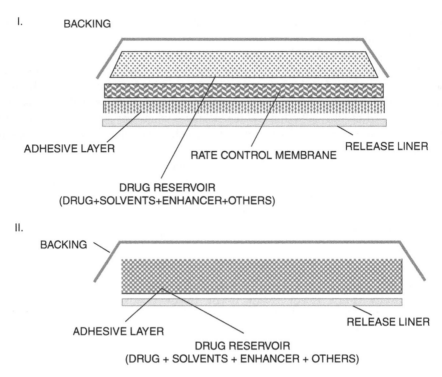

**FIGURE 13.2** Passive transdermal drug delivery systems.

mentioned at the start of this paragraph, some systems (generally the form-fill and seal TDS) include a microporous or a dense polymeric membrane between the drug reservoir and the skin contact adhesive layer. This layer may be designed to modulate/control the rate of drug release from the system (System type I, Figure 13.1) or form only a boundary to the drug reservoir compartment without acting to control the rate of drug release. There are several variations of the two systems that have been approved by the FDA in recent years.

### 13.4.2 TRANSDERMAL IN VIVO BIOAVAILABILITY TESTING – GENERAL DESIGN FACTORS

Since transdermal products are designed to deliver systemically active amounts of drug, direct in vivo bioavailability testing is usually quite straightforward and is generally analogous to oral drug development. Typical transdermal drug development program has single dose, multiple dose, dose proportionality studies, and where an oral or IV formulation is available, relative or absolute bioavailability studies are conducted. Normally, transdermal drug development is a line extension for a product available via alternative routes. Examples of such line extension would be fentanyl (IV), nicotine (inhalational) and methylphenidate (oral). In doing so, the developer can leverage the vast amount of information from these original approvals to support the transdermal development program.

In general, the pharmacokinetic parameters to be determined in such studies are identical to those used in the assessment of oral bioavailability. That is, AUC, $C_{max}$, Css, $T_{max}$, clearance (Cl) and peak-trough fluctuation (fluctuation index, FI). These latter parameters are consistent with the normally chronic nature of the disease. Due to the differences in stratum corneum thickness, site of application studies are necessary, especially so for those transdermal systems that are skin controlled, that is they lack a rate controlling membrane and rely on the skin permeability to regulate drug permeation. Studies focused on adhesion, the use of overlays and the consequences of product detachment need to be considered and tracked during the clinical development program. Often times during development, adhesives change due to problems seen in the clinical studies. In such instances, bridging studies to demonstrate the impact of the change in adhesive are necessary. While transdermal products do not have such a paradigm, they do have unique features to their Clinical Pharmacology development, which will be further discussed in this chapter.

## 13.5 SPECIAL CONSIDERATIONS FOR TOPICAL AND TRANSDERMAL SYSTEMS – AGE, GENDER AND RACE

Skin, like other organ systems, age and as it ages it loses some of its structure and function including its ability to regulate body heat and maintain fluid balance. The skin becomes wrinkled and furrowed making application of a topical product difficult and adhesion of TDDS complicated. In general, in vivo pharmacokinetic studies, be it for oral or topical products, are to be conducted in the population of interest, including the elderly.

In contrast in the pediatric population, especially in the neonate, differences in skin maturation can be profound in relation to disease severity. In adults the skin represents, on average, only 3% of total body weight while in neonates it can go as high as 13%. This, coupled with the fact that the ratio of surface area to body weight in neonates is four times that of adults, suggests that the relationship between surface area and volume need to re-considered. While full-term infants are born with and acquire all the characteristics of an intact skin barrier relatively soon after birth, these high ratios of surface area to weight would only tend to enhance the potential for circulating levels of topically applied drugs to occur after application. This is especially the case in diseases that are primarily pediatric in nature such as atopic dermatitis.

In the pediatric patient, atopic dermatitis represents the extreme of topical involvement and drug use where it is not uncommon to have 90% body surface area involvement. Unlike adults where the practicality of topical administration beyond 30% body surface area is rare, due to clothing, these considerations are not relevant in the infant population as they are often clothed only in a diaper or a diaper-shirt combination. Additionally, it is common in these infants to use moisturizers and other emollient agents that can temporarily hydrate the skin and can either enhance or retard drug absorption in this population. Because of these factors and under the Pediatric Research Equity Act[16], either topical or transdermal agents intended for use in the pediatric population must be studied in the relevant population. In general, to obtain approval of a pediatric dosing regimen, one has to study the age range in question with adequate numbers of subjects being present at the lowest desired age ranges. The protocol for such studies should pre-specify the numbers of children at each age group to be studied and steps should be taken to ensure that the enrolled subjects are distributed throughout the age range to prevent clustering at the upper age limits of each bracket. Extrapolations down from adult data to pediatric populations are to be discouraged and used only to plan an appropriate pediatric program.

With regards to race and gender, to date no new differences have been shown in the bioavailability of drugs from either topical or transdermal systems that were not previously observed with oral or other routes of administration. That is not to say that such differences cannot or do not exist. As with clinical studies conducted with other routes of administration, the subjects enrolled in these studies should reflect the US population in ethnicity. Ideally, the studies for each formulation or delivery system should include sufficient numbers of subjects to allow for a secondary pharmacokinetic analysis using demographic factors such as race, gender and age as covariates.

## 13.6 SPECIAL CONSIDERATIONS FOR TOPICAL AND TRANSDERMAL SYSTEMS – IRRITATION AND SENSITIZATION

As part of the development of any topically applied product or transdermal system, there is the need for dermal sensitization and irritation testing in both humans and animals. For topically applied products, as they are applied to diseased (irritated) skin, care must be taken to ensure that proper observation and scoring is done during the clinical trials to differentiate between the disease process itself and any induced irritation or sensitization.

For transdermal systems, the combination of adhesives and the administration of the drug itself under the occlusive nature of TDDS for a prolonged duration can raise the potential for local reactions. To mitigate effects of local trauma following system removal and to allow for the reversal of occlusion related changes in the skin, the site of application for a transdermal product should be rotated to allow for skin recovery following use[17]. The clinical observations must differentiate between true irritation and a demonstration of the pharmacologic effect of the drug itself. For example, vasodilatory substances such as nitroglycerin and nicotine can cause reactive hyperemia and can be mis-identified as a rash or allergic reaction. Proper training of clinical staff and a consulting dermatologist can be very helpful in adjudicating these types of reactions (see Table 13.2).

---

**TABLE 13.2**
**Irritant versus Allergic Reactions General Differential[a]**

| Irritant Reactions | Allergic Reactions |
|---|---|
| -Greatest at time of removal | -Severity MAY increase following removal |
| -No reaction at previous sites | -Reactions at previous sites possible |
| -Localized to the site of application | -May extend beyond the site of application |
| | -Vesicles possible |

a Table 13.2 modified from Murphy M, et al. Am J Clin Dermatol, 2000;6:361–68. Copyright Adis International Limited, used with permission of SPRINGER.

---

## 13.7 SPECIAL SITUATIONS – TOPICAL APPLICATION TO A MAXIMUM SURFACE AREA

Dermatologic conditions range in surface area involvement from almost total involvement (atopic dermatitis) to lesional in nature (atopic keratosis). These latter disease states range in severity from squamous and basal cell carcinoma to warts. They are generally confined to a specific area and are distinct from normal skin. Treatment of these lesions can include surgical removal via cuttage or laser ablation and the use of locally applied caustic agents such as levulinic acid. In this situation, the Maximum Usage Trial (MUsT) paradigm must be modified to reflect that wide sections of skin are not going to be treated at a simultaneous time. The study should, however, include the maximum number of lesions to be treated at one time that is conducted in both the phase III study program and as proposed for marketing. In such a situation, it may be possible to accomplish the MUsT evaluation as part of a phase III trial rather than as a separate trial. Both approaches have been used and are acceptable, provided that the objectives of evaluating absorption are achieved.

## 13.8 DEVELOPMENT PATH OF BOTH TOPICAL AND TRANSDERMAL AGENTS

Once a drug has been selected, a route of delivery (topical vs transdermal) and a formulation has been developed, clinical development can begin. Although often demonstrated as a linear process, with development neatly progressing from phase I to phase III and thus to approval (Figure 13.3), the reality is somewhat different[18].

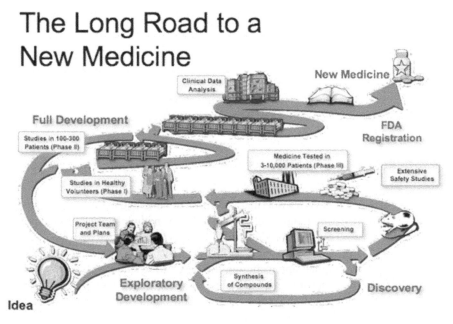

**FIGURE 13.3** Illustration of the drug development path[20].

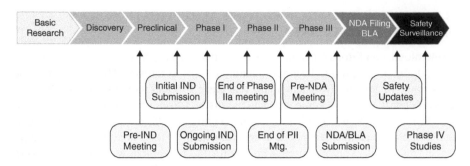

**FIGURE 13.4**  Key milestones in the drug development path.

The process is in fact a parallel one with many activities existing at the same time as the chemistry, preclinical (long-term animal safety and teratology studies), clinical pharmacology and clinical program progress in a real-time fashion with all elements of the program feeding results to each other. At all steps in the development program the sponsor should seek out and avail themselves of meetings with the FDA or the appropriate regulatory body. Using the FDA as an example, the key milestone meetings are the Pre-IND meeting, the End of Phase II meeting and the pre-NDA meeting. These are the decisional meetings and the sponsor should seek the opportunity to engage the FDA as a partner in drug development at these key milestones (Figure 13.4)[19].

Beyond that, the FDA does strive to be responsive to requests for information and guidance. That is not to say that the FDA has unlimited resources, but well formulated questions and protocols submitted to the FDA with a clear request for response and a reasonable timeline for response are given full consideration. On the other hand, meeting packages with sparse details, or with last minute questions being appended at the time of the meeting, are not evidence of a well-designed development plan or regulatory strategy. The old adage that an "ounce of prevention saves a pound of cure" is just as true today in drug development. A hastily prepared, ill-considered meeting request with undefined questions is unlikely to yield the necessary information to speed up the development program.

### 13.8.1 REGULATORY APPROACHES FOR APPROVAL OF TOPICAL AND TRANSDERMAL PRODUCTS

As noted previously, most transdermal systems are "line extensions" to an existing approved product line. Examples of such would be methylphenidate, fentanyl and oxybutynin. That is, they are products that were originally approved for the same indication but with another route of administration. They would be approved as supplements to the original application in the case of the same sponsor. In the situation where another sponsor wanted to pursue the transdermal route of delivery independent of the innovator the application would be submitted under the Food Drug and Cosmetic (FDC) Act section 505(b)(2)[20].

A 505(b)(2) application is an application submitted under section 505(b)(1) for which:

- The investigations the applicant relied on for approval were not conducted by or for the applicant.
- The applicant has not obtained a right of reference or use for the investigations (21 U.S.C. 355(b)(2)).

Section 505(b)(2) expressly permits FDA to rely, for approval of an NDA, on data not developed by the applicant – such as published literature or the agency's finding of safety and/or effectiveness of a previously approved drug product.

Approval under this section focuses the development program and review on the differences between the two routes. For a transdermal product it is *highly* unlikely for the product to be bioequivalent to the original or "listed drug" product – nor must it be. What would need to be investigated is the difference between the two products, that is, if the levels of the drug following transdermal application were lower than that from the approved route of administration, then the clinical development program would focus on efficacy (as lower levels cannot be less safe – systemically). If the levels were higher, due to a reduced first pass metabolism effect, for example, then the program would focus on the safety of these increased drug levels (as higher levels in and of themselves cannot be associated with a lower efficacy – unless there was new dose limiting toxicity). In both cases, the dermal safety (irritation and sensitization) profile of the product would also be assessed in the clinical program, especially as the two formulations would more than likely differ in the type and ratio of excipients to the drug product.

From a clinical pharmacology perspective, the changes in route of delivery (from oral to transdermal/topical application) can have a significant impact on the information needed. Some of the issues that would need to be addressed would include, but not be limited to,

- Site of application
- Dose proportionality
- Effect of heat/exercise
- Effect of overlays and skin adhesion
- Residual amount of drug on the skin
- Transferability and washing (removal) studies
- Use in special populations (elderly, pediatric, etc.)

Studies of this nature, if possible, should be done in the patient population of interest, especially in cases where the disease being treated can affect the pharmacokinetics or metabolic activity of the body.

Where the transdermal system is in fact the first market presentation it would then be approved as a 505(b)(1) application which is an application that contains full reports of investigations of safety and effectiveness[21]. Here the investigations being relied on for approval were conducted by or for the applicant or the applicant has obtained a right of reference or use for the investigations. In this case, beyond the description of the performance of the transdermal system, the applicant would have the burden of proving the safety and efficacy of the drug above and beyond the effect of the transdermal system. This would include animal models of disease, in vitro metabolism studies, radiolabeled studies of drug disposition, among others. A full description of the potential informational need for a 505(b)(1) application is beyond the scope of this chapter and the reader is referred to the FDA website where ample guidance documents are available that describe the general drug development requirements and clinically specific requirements of different therapeutic areas[22,23,24].

The topical drug product development program, from a regulatory perspective, is similar to that of the transdermal route, with the exception that, most often, the topical route is the first route approved. Thus most topically applied drugs are approved (initially) under the provisions of 505(b)(1) with additional formulations approved either as supplemental applications or as new 505(b)(1) applications. It should be noted that for both topical or transdermal products (or any other route of administration), the 505(b)(2) route is not open to the innovator. The 505(b)(2) route is intended to spur innovation by allowing new sponsors to develop new products based on the previous finding of safety and efficacy of a drug substance. Most commonly under the (b)(2) regulations, the new sponsor is able to reference the pharmacology/toxicology data from the original application without repeating the animal and reproductive studies. This is only possible where the resulting in vivo exposure is equal to or less than that from the referenced product. In situations where the new formulation results in a higher exposure or a differential safety profile, an individual determination of the safety and efficacy will be needed and may include new pharmacology/toxicology studies.

### 13.8.2 Regulatory Guidance on Pharmaceutical Development

The principles described in the ICH Q8 guidelines[25] and a quality by design (QbD) approach to drug development are highly recommended. A detailed pharmaceutical development report is recommended to be submitted to the NDA outlining the justification for the chosen processing options, product and process development, critical quality attributes, critical process parameters and scientific approach to process scale-up based on product and process understanding. Pharmaceutical development information is submitted in Section P.2 of the CTD (Common Technical Document). Other information resulting from pharmaceutical development studies could be accommodated by the CTD format in a number of different ways and some specific suggestions are provided later. However, the applicant should clearly indicate where the different information is located. In addition to what is submitted in the application, certain aspects (e.g., product life cycle management, continual improvement) of this guideline are handled under the applicant's pharmaceutical quality system.

Pharmaceutical development should include, at a minimum, the following elements:

- Defining the quality target product profile (QTPP) as it relates to quality, safety and efficacy, considering, e.g., the route of administration, dosage form, bioavailability, strength and stability.

- Identifying potential critical quality attributes (CQA) of the drug product, so that those product characteristics having an impact on product quality can be studied and controlled.
- Determining the critical quality attributes of the drug substance, excipients, etc., and selecting the type and amount of excipients to deliver a drug product of the desired quality.
- Selecting an appropriate manufacturing process.
- Defining a control strategy.

Two critical factors affecting TDDS performance are skin adhesion and rate and extent of in vivo drug release. These quality attributes are particularly important for the delivery of highly potent drugs with narrow therapeutic range. It is known that poorly adhering products result in low drug permeation and lack of efficacy. Adhesive and cohesive failures can be related to product design or manufacturing defects, as well as to stability failures. Also, high serum levels and overdose could result from manufacturing defects, and from conditions such as heat, occlusion due to over-taping or compromised skin. Therefore, biorelevant in vitro test methods indicative of in vivo product performance are recommended.

The most critical formulation variables affecting adhesion in the development of TDDS are the type and concentration of additives used, the drug load, the thickness of the adhesive layer, the composition and thickness of the backing layer and the solvent residue. These should be considered when evaluating the pharmaceutical development report as discussed later. For in vivo skin adhesion studies, a five-point scale has been recommended in FDA draft guidances[26]. Recent EMA guidance described how the in vivo adhesion studies need to be conducted based on current science[27,28]. In general, the information gathered during clinical trial is documented in the label. Also, in-use study to simulate an actual wear is being recommended. For clinical purposes, it is more logical to take into consideration "natural" test conditions on the human skin such as applied heat and moisture on the skin. Furthermore, the influence of different types of skin should be taken into consideration.

In vitro skin permeation study is an excellent tool for transdermal product development and is generally predictive of in vivo characteristics. The skin permeation study refers to the diffusion of active ingredients including penetration enhancers (when present) across the skin. Usually, the lag time, steady state delivery rate and amount delivered in 24 hours and at end of use are reported results of the in vitro skin permeation studies. Formulation optimization with respect to the concentration of drug and penetration enhancer is typically conducted via skin penetration studies and an approach to modeling transdermal drug release is described by Kalia and Guy[29]. This test may also be useful to document that drug and enhancer (when present) delivery characteristics change when formulation, component, manufacturing or other factors are varied.

To increase the skin flux of drugs, supersaturation conditions are often employed (Pellett et al.)[30]. Supersaturation is a state at which the amount of drug solubilized in a vehicle is greater than its equilibrium solubility. This has the effect of increasing the thermodynamic activity of a drug, and enhances the flux. However, such systems are thermodynamically unstable and a supersaturated drug solution has a tendency to form crystals. Drug crystallization within a pressure sensitive adhesive matrix may cause a reduction in skin permeation and/or tack of TDDS. Therefore, the control of drug crystallization is of particular interest for the efficiency and quality of TDDS application as evaluated by Ma et al.[31]. Developmental studies are recommended to include investigations of the effects of polymeric additives and solvents on the crystallization of drugs within the adhesive matrix. Conventional polymorph mining studies using different solvents and different crystallization conditions may not always predict whether new polymorphs can be formed inside a patch. It is possible that the drug may crystallize into a known or new polymorph inside TDDS on storage. Similarly, information on solubility of drugs in individual components of the TDDS should be used carefully because the inhibitory effect of a solvent on the crystallization of a drug may not be predicted simply from the solubility of the drug within that solvent.

### 13.8.3 Preparing and Organizing the Common Technical Document

The common technical document format for marketing applications is depicted in the ICH M4 – Organization of the Common Technical Document for the Registration of Pharmaceuticals for Human Use guidance (www.ich.org).

For the transdermal drug product section, the component/composition section differs from the conventional dosage forms. In a passive transdermal system components including the drug substance are typically: (1) Release liner; (2) Backing film; (3) Membrane (optional); (4) Pressure sensitive adhesive; (5) Penetration enhancers/solvents (optional). The typical container/closure system for a transdermal drug product is a foil pouch.

The release liners are generally polyester based. The chemistry, manufacturing and controls (CMC) information of the release liner should be documented in DMF (Drug Master Files). If that information is not available in the form of a DMF, the CMC information should be provided by the sponsor of a submission. Usually, specification with the following attributes is adopted: ID, thickness, weight/area, release, rub off test, tensile and elongation. The release test, i.e., release force necessary to remove a specific tape with adhesive of known chemistry from the liner without cohesive failure, is an important practical test for measuring surface characteristics of a release liner.

The CMC information of the backing materials should be documented in DMFs along with dermal safety information. If the information is not available, the CMC information should be provided by the sponsor of the submission. The backings may be classified as occlusive or non-occlusive when used in a transdermal system. The occlusiveness may be determined by transmission of moisture vapor or oxygen. Based on the non-occlusive or occlusive nature of the film, in vitro or in vivo overlay study may be requested or waived by the review division. The occlusiveness of the backing may increase the skin penetration rate. The backing film surfaces are non-porous and may be of low surface tension causing them to be non-receptive to bonding with substrates such as printing inks, adhesives or adhesive-based formulations. Therefore, the backings may need surface treatment to improve bonding characteristics.

The chemical penetration enhancers have functional characteristics of increasing skin permeation rate; therefore, they are controlled by ID, assay, purity, melting point, etc. On rare occasions, novel penetration enhancers are used. The novel penetration enhancers are treated in a manner similar to that of a new molecular entity. Therefore, complete characterization and toxicity information may be required. Applicants are recommended to contact the respective clinical divisions for the specific requirements for the novel penetration enhancers. Compendial chemical penetration enhancers are most common since once a pharmaceutical use of the penetration enhancer is identified by the manufacturer of the penetration enhancer, the company facilitates the compendial monograph process for this specific chemical.

The membranes, either dense or microporous, have been used in Type I transdermal systems depicted in Figure 13.1. The dense membranes or polymeric films usually constituted of high-polymer density and void space in these membranes are rare. These membranes are usually manufactured by solvent casting, melt extrusion or by membrane formation during polymerization process. Similarly, microporous membranes are manufactured using dry, wet, phase inversion and various other techniques. The CMC information of the membranes is usually documented in DMFs and is usually manufacturers' proprietary information. The common specifications for solid membranes are: ID, membrane thickness, tensile, elongation, weight/meter. For a microporous membrane, ID, membrane thickness, porosity, gurley, tensile, elongation, weight/meter specifications are usually adopted.

Skin adhesion is a critical quality attribute of TDDS that assures desired drug delivery. The adhesion of TDDS to the skin is obtained by using pressure sensitive adhesives (PSAs), which are defined as adhesives capable of bonding to surfaces with the application of light pressure. Typically, a PSA is cured at the time of use, permanently tacky and removable. It is *soft* under the conditions of *bond formation* (smaller strain) and becomes *strong* during *bond rupture* (higher strain). As a part of the pharmaceutical development, the applicants may develop data on rheological measurements of chosen adhesive in its native form as well as in the adhesive formulation prototypes containing all components. A design of experiments (DoE) approach may be used in selecting various formulations for this study. Based on the analysis of the viscoelastic properties, a justification may be provided for the chosen adhesive and the chosen transdermal formulation.

The adhesive properties of TDDS are directly related to three tape properties of PSAs; those are: (1) Tack: The property that enables an adhesive to wet and form a bond with the surface of another material upon brief contact and under light pressure; (2) Creep resistance or shear: The resistance to flow that could be considered as an expression of the cohesiveness of the adhesive in the system. Increased shear strength may sacrifice tack and peel or adhesion strength; (3) Adhesion strength: The force required to peel away the TDDS from a substrate surface.

Three major groups of adhesives are usually used in transdermal products. Those are: Polyisobutylene/polybutylene, acrylic and silicone. On rare occasions, hydrophilic adhesives and block copolymer based hot-melt pressure sensitive adhesives have been used. Polyisobutylene is a synthetic polymer produced by the low-temperature polymerization of isobutylene in liquid ethylene, methylene chloride or hexane, using an aluminum-chloride or boron-trifluoride catalyst and may contain a suitable stabilizer. Tackifiers provide tack and specific adhesion qualities to the adhesive mass. Plasticizers soften the adhesive mass. Both tackifiers and plasticizers act as viscosity enhancers and modify the flow properties of the polyisobutylene. The modifiers such as hydrocarbon resins and low molecular weight polyisobutylenes may also be used to improve adhesion/flow properties[32].

Soft skin adhesives are two-part silicone adhesive gels that may provide adequate creep resistance when formulated for transdermal applications. They can be loaded with drugs and excipients. In terms of chemistry, the silicone adhesive gels are two-part systems based on a vinyl functional polydimethylsiloxane and a hydrogen cross-linker, reacted in the presence of a platinum catalyst.

The pharmaceutical acrylic PSAs are usually copolymers of a soft monomer (low $T_g$), hard monomer (high $T_g$) and functional monomer. These copolymers are random polymers of monomers of different functionality usually manufactured using a solution polymerization technique by slow addition where molecular weight is determined by stoichiometry and the amount of initiator used. The residual monomers present at the end of the reaction can be reduced by the use of a scavenger. These copolymers may also be cross-linked by the addition of a cross-linker. The emulsion polymerization technique is also used to manufacture acrylic adhesives. The characterization of a typical PSA could be achieved by the following attributes: molecular weight and its distribution, spectroscopy, thermal analysis and rheology.

A typical specification for a PSA could be as follows: appearance, ID, viscosity, intrinsic viscosity, solid content, residual monomer on a dried basis, adhesion to a substrate, tack, shear, release from a substrate. The PSA CMC information is usually provided in a DMF by the manufacturers of PSAs.

The pouch components are purchased as laminates of several films by the drug product manufacturers. They are either laminated together by the use of adhesives or, in the case of thermoplastic materials, are laminated by heat. An aluminum foil component is used in most laminates for its low permeability. Some products are susceptible to moisture and some contain volatile components. Therefore, the moisture vapor transmission properties and barrier properties are important when selecting a pouch component. A special child resistance feature is needed for some drugs such as narcotics. Pouches usually have a printable surface. The pouch CMC information is usually provided in a DMF by the vendors of the pouch materials.

The manufacturing operations, validation and process control considerations for drug-in-adhesive matrix (DIA) or reservoir systems are documented in workshop reports[33]. For the reservoir systems (type 1), the following process steps have been identified: drug/gel/penetration enhancer manufacturing; dispensing and sealing; manufacturing of adhesive solution; coating and drying; lamination of membrane; system formation; die cutting; pouching. For DIA systems (type 2), the following process steps are considered: drug/pressure sensitive adhesive/penetration enhancer mixing, coating and drying, lamination, die cutting and pouching.

The following attributes are recommended to be considered during the drug product stability studies: (1) Description/appearance, the presence of crystals should be monitored; (2) Cold flow; (3) Content of drug; (4) Impurities including related substances; (5) Drug release; (6) Content of enhancer; (7) Adhesion to a substrate; (8) Release liner peel force; (9) Tack; (10) Shear; (11) Burst strength (for type 1 formulation, reservoir); (11) Pouch integrity; (12) Microbial limits. The content uniformity and residual monomers are tested at the initial testing point and it is usually not tested during stability studies.

Several test methods for adhesion, peel, shear and tack are available in ASTM or PSTC standards[34,35,36,37,38,39]. The USP test apparatus are available for testing in vitro release properties of the transdermal systems. The other test methods, such as cold flow, appearance, burst strength, pouch integrity, are developed by individual sponsors and submitted in the regulatory submissions. The remaining test methods are standard test methods for non-complex dosage forms and, therefore, they are not repeated here.

There are some other considerations with regard to transdermals that are currently of interest. In 2011 the FDA issued the Guidance for Industry: Residual Drug in Transdermal and Related Drug Delivery Systems which recommends "that sufficient scientific justification to support the amount of residual drug in TDDS, transmucosal delivery systems, or topical patches be included in an application"[40]. The development factors associated with TDDS are discussed in other chapters in this book.

## 13.9 GOING FORWARD

Both the FDA and the European Medicines Evaluation Authority (EMEA) publish guidance documents on drug development and make them available at their respective websites. In addition the FDA makes available at the Drugs@FDA website the approval packages for all NDAs either at the time of approval or shortly thereafter. These packages include copies of the relevant Medical, Chemistry, Pharmacology, Statistical, and Clinical Pharmacology reviews along with the approval memos. These documents, redacted when necessary to protect individual patient privacy and commercial confidential information (CCI), provide an overview of successful drug development programs and a detailed examination of these documents should be the first step on initiating a development plan. While it is true that the data represents a "historical perspective" on drug development, drug development and regulatory policy is evolutionary in nature. Thus, an examination of the last three approved NDAs in a therapeutic area or with a particular type of release mechanism (e.g., topical or transdermal) will give an insight into the current Agency thought and direction.

This, along with the FDA's use of external meeting presentations, working groups and Advisory Committee meetings, allows the developer/clinician opportunities to engage the FDA on general developmental topics in an open setting. These activities are very important to the FDA as they allow the Agency to get input on policies and procedures prior to adoption. These are not, however, a substitute for communication with the FDA (or other regulatory body) directly on a development project but can be used to refine questions and development strategy to make the most of the meeting opportunities one has.

In conclusion, the development of a successful topical or transdermal product is the result of the interplay between the formulator, the skin and the pharmacologic goal. All drug development shares a similar regulatory framework and an informational need focused on the demonstration of safety and efficacy. As the globalization of pharmaceutical development continues, the overriding concern of regulators and drug developers remains the promotion of health.

## REFERENCES

1. Jacob SW and Francone CC. Structure and Function of Man, 2nd Edition, W.B. Saunders Co., Philadelphia (1970), Chapter 4.
2. Chandrasekhar S, Iyer LK, Panchal JP, Topp EM, Cannon JB, Ranade VV. "Microarrays and microneedle arrays for delivery of peptides, proteins, vaccines and other applications." Expert Opin Drug Deliv. 2013 Aug;10(8):1155–70.
3. www.clinicalresolution.com/main/whatismts.html
4. 3M. Drug Delivery Systems. About 3M Microneedle Drug Delivery Systems. http://solutions.3m.com/wps/portal/3M/en_WW/3M-DDSD/Drug-Delivery-Systems/transdermal/microneedle/
5. Lebwohl M, Herrmann LG. "Impaired skin barrier function in dermatologic disease and repair with moisturization." Cutis. 2005 Dec;76(6 Suppl):7–12.
6. Farahmand S, Maibach H. "Estimating skin permeability from physicochemical characteristics of drugs: a comparison between conventional models and an in vivo-based approach." Int J Pharm. 2009 Jun 22;375(1–2):41–7.
7. Huang S, Gupta S, Bashaw E. "Pharmacokinetic and pharmacodynamic modeling of transdermal products" In: Shah and Maibach (eds) Topical Drug Bioavailability, Bioequivalence, and Penetration., 1st Edition. (1993). Boston, MA: Springer.
8. Anderson DT, Muto JJ "Duragesic transdermal patch: postmortem tissue distribution of fentanyl in 25 cases" J Anal Toxicol 2000 Oct;24(7):627–34.
9. Sindall K, Sherry K, Dheansa B. "Life threatening coma and full thickness sunburn in a patient treated with transdermal fentanyl patches: a case report" J Med Case Rep. 2012 Jul 26;6(1):220.
10. Cabrera SM, Rogol AD "Testosterone exposure in childhood: discerning pathology from physiology" Expert Opin Drug Saf. 2013 May;12(3):375–88.
11. Martinez-Pajares JD, Diaz-Morales O, Ramos-Diaz JC, Gomez-Fernandez E. "Peripheral precocious puberty due to inadvertent exposure to testosterone: case report and review of the literature" J Pediatr Endocrinol Metab. 2012;25(9–10):1007–12.
12. Stahlman J, Britto M, Fitzpatrick S, McWhirter C, Testino SA, Brennan JJ, Zumbrunnen TL. "Effects of skin washing on systemic absorption of testosterone in hypogonadal males after administration of 1.62% testosterone gel." Curr Med Res Opin. 2012 Feb;28(2):271–9.
13. Stahlman J, Britto M, Fitzpatrick S, McWhirter C, Testino SA, Brennan JJ, Zumbrunnen TL. "Effect of application site, clothing barrier, and application site washing on testosterone transfer with a 1.62% testosterone gel." Curr Med Res Opin. 2012 Feb;28(2):281–90.
14. Bashaw ED, Tran DC, Shukla CG, Liu X. "Maximal usage trial: an overview of the design of systemic bioavailability trial for topical dermatological products" Therapeutic Innovation & Regulatory Science. 2015;49(1):108–15.
15. www.fda.gov/media/79401/download
16. www.fda.gov/drugs/development-resources/pediatric-research-equity-act-prea
17. Fang JY. "In vitro and in vivo evaluations of the efficacy and safety of skin permeation enhancers using flurbiprofen as a model drug", International Journal of Pharmaceutics. 2003; 255:153–66.
18. https://en.wikipedia.org/wiki/Drug_development
19. Yetter P. "PDUFA activities in drug development" FDA. www.fda.gov/media/78711/download

20. FDA. Applications Covered by Section 505(b)(2). 1999. www.fda.gov/regulatory-information/search-fda-guidance-documents/applications-covered-section-505b2
21. General Considerations for the Clinical Evaluation of Drugs, February 1997. www.fda.gov/regulatory-information/search-fda-guidance-documents/general-considerations-clinical-evaluation-drugs
22. Guideline for the Clinical Evaluation of Antianxiety Drugs, September 1997. www.fda.gov/media/71189/download
23. Establishing Effectiveness for Drugs Intended to Treat Male Hypogonadotropic Hypogonadism Attributed to Nonstructural Disorders, Guidance for Industry, U.S. Department of Health and Human Services, Food and Drug Administration, Center for Drug Evaluation and Research (CDER), May 2018. www.fda.gov/media/110004/download
24. Guideline for the Clinical Evaluation of Antidepressant Drugs, 1997. www.fda.gov/media/71189/download.
25. International Conference on Harmonisation of Technical Requirements for Registration of Pharmaceuticals for Human Use, ICH Harmonised Tripatrite Guideline, Pharmaceutical Development Q8(R2).
26. Assessing Adhesion with Transdermal and Topical Delivery Systems for ANDAs Guidance for Industry, Draft Guidance, 2018. www.fda.gov/media/98634/download
27. EMA. Guideline on the Pharmacokinetic and Clinical Evaluation of Modified Release Dosage Forms. 2014. www.ema.europa.eu/docs/en_GB/document_library/Scientific_guideline/2014/11/WC500177884.pdf
28. EMA. Guideline on Guality of Transdermal Patches, 2014. www.ema.europa.eu/docs/en_GB/document_library/Scientific_guideline/2014/12/WC500179071.pdf
29. Kalia YN, Guy RH. "Modeling transdermal drug release", Adv. Drug Delivery Reviews, 2001;48:159–72.
30. Pellett MA, Davis AF, Hadgraft J. "Effect of supersaturation on membrane transport: 2. Piroxicam", Int. J. Pharm, 1994;111:1–6.
31. Ma X, Taw J, Chiang C-M. "Control of drug crystallization in transdermal matrix system", Int. J. Pharm, 1996;142:115–19.
32. Handbook of Pressure Adhesives and Products, Fundamental of Pressure Sensitivity, Edited by Istavan Benedek and Mikhail M. Feldstein, CRC Press, 2009.
33. Workshop Report, Scale-up of Adhesive Transdermal Drug Delivery Systems; Pharmaceutical Research, Vol. 14, No. 7, 1997.
34. American Society for Testing and Materials, ASTM D2979: Pressure Sensitive Tack of Adhesives Using an Inverted Probe Machine.
35. American Society for Testing and Materials, ASTM D3121-94: Rolling Ball Test for Surface Tack.
36. American Society for Testing and Materials, ASTM D3330: Standard Test Method for Peel Adhesion of Pressure-Sensitive Tapes.
37. American Society for Testing and Materials, ASTM D3654: Shear Adhesion of Pressure Sensitive Tape.
38. Pressure Sensitive Tape Council, PSTC 101: Peel Adhesion of Pressure Sensitive Tape.
39. Pressure Sensitive Tape Council, PSTC 107: Shear Adhesion of Pressure Sensitive Tape.
40. www.fda.gov/media/79401/download

## DISCLAIMER

This book chapter reflects the views of the authors and should not be construed to represent FDA's views or policies.

# 14 Innovations and Future Prospects of Dermal Delivery Systems

*Rashmi Upasani, Anushree Herwadkar, Neha Singh and Ajay K. Banga*

## CONTENTS

## 14.1   INTRODUCTION

Dermal drug delivery systems comprise of products which use transdermal and topical routes of administration. Transdermal administration implies delivery of drugs across skin into systemic circulation. Topical administration implies delivery of drugs to various layers of skin and is typically intended to treat local skin conditions. The estimated worth of the transdermal market is about $32 billion and this can be attributed to the advances in transdermal formulations and drug delivery systems (Paudel et al. 2010). Topical drug delivery systems still largely comprise of creams, ointments and gels. However, there have been several recent developments in topical formulations and drug delivery systems including aerosol products like foams and sprays and other novel delivery systems such as microsponges and organogels. This chapter aims to summarize recent advances in transdermal and topical drug delivery systems.

## 14.2   INNOVATIONS IN TOPICAL DERMATOLOGICAL DOSAGE FORMS

Developing a product for topical application involves a challenge of controlling the distribution of the active within the skin. The physicochemical properties of an active pharmaceutical ingredient (API) and vehicle are key factors in determining the amount of drug that reaches different skin layers. Recent advances in topical formulations and drug delivery systems, such as aerosols, Microsponge® technology and lecithin organogels, have been developed with an aim of achieving controlled and enhanced topical drug delivery.

### 14.2.1   PHARMACEUTICAL AEROSOLS

Pharmaceutical aerosols are dynamic systems which have gained popularity as topical vehicles. These are formulations comprising of a gas dispersed in liquid phase. The basic components of the aerosol system are container, propellant, formulation concentrate, valve and actuator. The formulation is typically an emulsion containing one or more actives, surfactants, co-solvents and a propellant. Upon valve actuation, the propellant evaporates to produce foam or a spray. If the propellant is in the internal phase of the emulsion, stable foam is discharged, and if the propellant is in the external phase, a spray or quick-breaking foam is discharged. The nature of these device and formulation components determine foam/spray characteristics such as particle size distribution, dose uniformity (for metered valves), delivery rate, spray pattern, foam density, etc. The propellant plays a pivotal role in the delivery of foam/spray on to the skin. It supplies the necessary pressure within the aerosol system to expel material from the container. A variety of propellants are included in formulations, including compressed gases (carbon dioxide, nitrogen), hydrocarbons (butanes, pentanes) and hydrofluroalkanes.

Foams for dermal delivery offer remarkable advantages over traditional vehicles such as creams, gels, ointments, lotions and solutions. Ointments are composed of viscous, oily vehicles that are unpleasant to apply. Their tacky properties can result in patient discomfort and they can be difficult to remove from clothing. Similarly, creams and gels can leave a residue after application, which can stain clothing. Topically applied solutions may flow away readily from the site of application. The main attribute of foams is their exemplary cosmetic appeal. Foams, following expansion, can easily spread onto target areas, especially areas that are difficult to access such as behind the ear and neck. They are less sticky than cream formulations, easy to apply, leave fewer residues and hence are less likely to soil clothes and other parts of the body. They do not require rubbing during application and hence avoid the pain or irritation experienced during application of ointments, making them a dosage form of choice to treat highly inflamed skin conditions such as sunburn, eczema and psoriasis. Moreover, due to the evaporation of the propellant, they are likely to be cooler than ambient air, producing a cooling effect to the inflamed skin. Though there is no clinical evidence for foams to be superior to other formulations, their ease of application results in a high consumer appeal (Arzhavitina et al. 2010).

Recent patents on foam technologies can be further classified into four areas: (a) novel formulations for delivery of specific drug molecules; (b) advances in formulations and devices used to generate foam; (c) advances in foam technologies aimed for enhancement of cosmetic appeal; and (d) advances in foam technologies aimed for enhancement of skin permeation. An example of this is a foam for delivery of minoxidil containing chemical permeation enhancers such as oleic acid, isopropyl amine, triethyl amine and propylene glycol. Other examples include foams for delivery of water soluble vitamins containing flavonoids as a stabilizing agent and foams containing vitamin D and corticosteroid for synergistic psoriatic treatment (Jacques et al. 2005; Peck et al. 1988; Tamarkin et al. 2008). Novel foam generating compositions include the use of HFA propellants instead of hydrocarbons, compositions containing high concentrations of solids to stabilize foams and novel devices for application of foam.

The Airpsray® pump foam dispenser is a breakthrough technology that creates foam without the use of gas propellant. This technology allows mixing of liquid and air, resulting in foam generation. The foam quality generated by this patented technology is fine, porous and more viscous than the propellant-based product (Van der et al. 2013) Other innovations to enhance the cosmetic appeal include alcohol free foams to reduce skin irritation, ultrafine foaming emulsions containing nanosized droplets with improved cosmetic appearance and water resistant topical foams to eliminate the need of reapplication following water exposure. Penetration enhancing foams are compositions with skin permeation enhancers, e.g., alcohols and fatty acids.

Foams offer an alternative means of product presentation that has a greater consumer appeal compared to traditional topical dosage forms, which has resulted in a number of existing gel and cream products being reformulated as a foam product. Currently there are more than 20 commercially available topical foam products and a number of products under development. Representative examples of commercially available products are Extina® foam (Ketacanazole) for treatment of seborrheic dermatitis and Evoclin (clindamycin phosphate) for treatment of acne vulgaris.

Typical agents delivered via foam are corticosteroids, nonsteroidal anti-inflammatory drugs, antibacterial agents, antifungal agents and local anesthetic agents. At present, even though the number of foam products on the market compared to conventional topical dosage forms are less, this scenario is expected to change as foams have shown to deliver agents with a range of lipophilicities from log P of $-2.1$ (urea) to 4.75 (pipernyl butoxide).

Additionally, the dynamic nature of foam vehicles provides potential benefits for dermal delivery of nanoparticles. Nanoparticles are included for a variety of reasons in topicals, e.g., for improving the formulation's aesthetics, protecting chemically unstable agents from degradation and prolonging the drug release. However, the ability of nanoparticles to release the therapeutic agent upon application to the skin remains uncertain. Foam formulations have significant phase transformations occurring during their discharge, which triggers the breakdown of nanoparticles, resulting in ensured drug release and drug delivery (Zhao et al. 2010).

Dermal sprays like foams minimize pain and irritation experienced during application of conventional dosage forms, thereby offering superior patient compliance. Dermal sprays are commercially available mainly for application to wound sites, treatment of fungal infections and as anti-itch products for veterinary use (Kapadia et al. 2012).

### 14.2.2 MICROSPONGE®

Microsponge® is a proprietary drug delivery system which enables controlled delivery of topical agents. It consists of macroporous microspheres, typically 10 to 25 µ in diameter, loaded with an active agent. These microspheres are interconnected by a myriad of interconnecting voids in a single microsponge, making them amenable to accept a wide variety of substances. When applied to the skin, they release drug in a controlled fashion. Drug release may also occur in response to stimuli, such as rubbing or friction, exposure to skin temperature, pH and moisture (Patel et al. 2012). Traditional dosage forms typically release API in a high concentration over a short duration, which may lead to undesirable side effects such as irritation and rashes. The microsponge delivery technology is designed to release drug gradually over a period of time, thereby providing efficacy with minimal irritation for drugs such as benzoyl peroxide. Improved stability for actives and aesthetic elegance are other benefits conferred by these delivery systems. Also the subcomponents of these systems are non-irritating, non-toxic and non-allergenic. Products based on the Microsponge® delivery system are formulated as gels, liquid, creams or powders and are currently being used in cosmetics, sunscreens, over-the-counter skin care and prescription products to address a variety of skin therapies such as rejuvenation, acne, hyperpigmentation, dark circles and moisturization.

### 14.2.3 LECITHIN ORGANOGELS

Lecithin organogel vehicle is another delivery system that is regarded to have potential for its ability to facilitate topical delivery for dermal and transdermal effects. These vehicles have a "jelly like" appearance and are composed of phospholipids (lecithin), organic solvent (e.g., isorpropyl myristate and isopropylpalmitate) and water. The "bio-friendly" lecithin functions as gelator molecule with the non-polar organic solvent as external phase and water as internal phase. When lecithin comes in contact with the external organic phase they self-assemble into reverse micellar structures, which go on to form elongated tubular micelles with the addition of water. These structures subsequently entangle to form a three-dimensional network leading to the formation of a lecithin organogel (Kumar et al. 2005). These vehicles can incorporate a wide array of substances with diverse physicochemical properties (e.g., size, molecular weight, solubility). Their well-balanced hydrophilic and lipophilic character and supersolubilizing capacity make them suitable vehicles for effectively transporting drug molecules (both hydrophilic and lipophilic actives) into and across the skin. They are thermodynamically stable and insensitive to moisture attack due to their organic nature. As they form spontaneously, their processing is very simple. While the excipients included in these formulations are non-immunogenic and bio-compatible, they contain high levels of surfactant and organic solvent. Therefore, it is important to consider the safety and irritancy of the formulation for prolonged use. Lecithin organogels entail the use of high purity lecithin for gelling, which is expensive. Inclusion of pluronics as co-surfactants in these formulations makes organogelling possible with a less purity lecithin. Several antiemetics, muscle relaxants, neuropathy drugs, nonsteroidal anti-inflammatory drugs (NSAIDs) and systemic analgesics and hormones are commercially available as pluronic organogels. Bhatia et al. carried out a formulation optimization study for incorporating tamoxifen in lecithin organogels. The outcomes of the study demonstrated that properties of the tamoxifen loaded lecithin organogels were dependent on the type and amount of phospholipid, auxiliary gelators, organic solvents and Poloxamer™ used in the for-mulation. Figure 14.1 is a pictorial description of the procedure followed for prepar-ation of lecithin organogels used in this study (Bhatia et al. 2013). Organogels have emerged to be a potential carrier system and offer an edge over other vesicular-based delivery systems (e.g., liposomes) in terms of efficacy, stability and technological simplicity. Additionally, their potential for the topical delivery of biotechnology-based molecules, e.g., peptides, makes them attractive.

Apart from the aforementioned innovations, several advancements have been documented in the nanotechnology sector, which are discussed in Section 14.7 in this chapter.

## 14.3 INNOVATIONS IN THE SOLID TRANSDERMAL DOSAGE FORM

### 14.3.1 CRYSTAL RESERVOIR TECHNOLOGY

In order to improve the performance and patient compliance of the solid transdermal (patch) dosage form, several new technologies have been investigated in recent years. Aveva DDS novel Crystal Reservoir Technology has been able to provide con-trolled, sustained release of drugs having a consistent supply of drug in each patch. This technology is based on the concept of oversaturation of the adhesive polymer in the patch with the drug resulting in partial drug crystallization. The patch thus

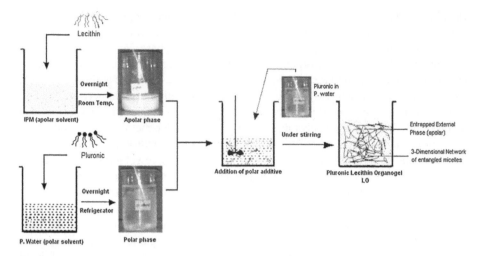

**FIGURE 14.1** Pictorial description of a procedure used for preparation of lecithin organogels. (Reprinted with permission from reference: Bhatia et al., 2013.)

contains dissolved drug molecules as well as drug crystals in the adhesive layer. As drug delivery progresses, the drug crystals would re-dissolve to maintain saturation conditions in the patch ensuring consistent and maximum thermodynamic activity for percutaneous drug permeation. This technology could thus translate into production of aesthetic – smaller and thinner patches improving patient compliance (Hadgraft et al. 2006). An additional advantage of the Crystal Reservoir Technology includes the ability to attain various patterns of drug release. Sustained drug release can be obtained due to the presence of excess drug in the adhesive polymer. Nitto Denko has incorporated this technology into different types of release systems. Isosorbide dinitrate, an anti-anginal agent, has been formulated using this transdermal system by Nitto Denko which allows increased patient compliance, and the use of Lipo-gel adhesive reduces skin irritation. Similarly burst release (rapid release of drug on the surface of skin) and chrono-controlled release (release based on state of disease and need of the patient) have been achieved using the Crystal Reservoir Technology. Lidocaine and tulobuterol transdermal systems, developed by Nitto Denko, are burst and chrono-controlled release respectively as these release patterns help in exercising a better control over delivery of these local anesthetic agents meant to alleviate pain in patients (Pecha et al. 2000).

### 14.3.2 GEL-MATRIX ADHESIVE SYSTEM

Tolerability and wear properties of the solid transdermal dosage form are becoming important concerns for patient compliance. Conventionally, drug-in-adhesive (DIA) systems use acrylic, silicone or polyisobutylene polymers as adhesives depending on drug properties and delivery requirements. A novel gel-matrix adhesive system was developed by Aveva DDS (Apotex Inc.) having more gentle wear properties in comparison to conventional solid transdermal systems. The gel-matrix adhesive is composed of an acrylate-based polymer crosslinked in such a way that it retains its cohesive strength as well as maintains a low polymer density. This is achieved by incorporating a liquid component in the adhesive layer to an extent as high as 60% of the matrix weight. The liquid is typically lipophilic, functions as a drug solubilizer and may also function as a permeation enhancer. The high liquid content allows incorporation of substances at a high concentration. Also the high cohesive strength of the system prevents possible cold flow due to the high liquid content of the system. The softer adhesive matrix of this patch is able to conform to the contours of skin maximizing the contact surface of the adhesive with skin. This results in maximum adhesion being obtained immediately and retained over long periods of time. Thus, formation of strong adhesive bonds typically required for conventional adhesives is not a necessity for gel-matrix adhesives. In addition, significant reduction in skin irritation and lesser peeling of stratum corneum accompanying patch removal was achieved using this technology. In vitro permeation studies were carried out to test delivery profiles of compounds of different classes formulated using the gel-matrix technology. Compounds tested included lidocaine (high dose and high drug loading), nicotine (liquid drug) and estradiol (low dose, poorly soluble drug). Permeation profiles of these drugs formulated using the gel-matrix technology were comparable to marketed formulations. The gel-matrix technology thus seems to be effective, broadly applicable and highly patient compliant innovation in the patch dosage form (Adams 2007).

### 14.3.3 DOT SOLID TRANSDERMAL SYSTEM

The DOT (delivery optimized thermodynamic) solid transdermal system developed by Noven Pharmaceuticals Inc. helps achieve higher drug loading in a smaller patch size. In this case, the drug is loaded in acrylate adhesive and the drug/acrylate blend is dispersed through the silicone adhesive resulting in a semisolid suspension. This design eliminates the issue of compromised adhesive properties and improves patient compliance. These systems have also been formulated as suspensions of drugs in multilayer matrix systems to allow drug delivery at a pre-determined rate (Hadgraft et al. 2006).

### 14.3.4 "PATCHLESS PATCH" – METERED DOSE TRANSDERMAL SPRAY

The "patchless patch" technology or the metered dose transdermal spray (MTDS®) developed by Acrux Ltd (2013) is another innovation in transdermal technologies. The MTDS results in application of a defined quantity of liquid on the skin surface for transdermal delivery. This results in passive and non-occlusive delivery with minimum irritation. The MTDS is a rapid drying spray containing a solution of drug in a mixture of volatile and non-volatile solvents. The volatile component ensures uniform formulation distribution, reproducible dose delivery and defined volume and area of application. The non-volatile component prevents drug from precipitating on the surface of the skin and may assist partitioning of drug in the stratum corneum. The system forms an invisible depot of drug and enhancer. A single application of this spray can provide drug delivery for two–four days (Thomaset et al. 2004). The spray is now branded as Evamist® and distributed by Perrigo in the USA.

## 14.4 CHEMICAL PERMEATION ENHANCERS – HOW REALISTIC?

Over the past couple of decades, many molecules have been investigated as potential chemical permeation enhancers for transdermal delivery based on empirical screening as well as high throughput screening assays. However only a limited number of these molecules fall in the category of GRAS (Generally Regarded As Safe) substances, which are typically used in commercial transdermal and topical formulations. Some well-known and widely investigated enhancers can be chemically classified as alcohols, glycols, fatty acids, esters, terpenes, surfactants, sulfoxides, phospholipids and 1-dodecylazacycloheptan-2-one (Azone). Chemical enhancers assist transdermal and topical delivery via a variety of mechanisms. They may solubilize and extract the lipid components of the stratum corneum (e.g., alcohols), induce lipid fluidization or phase separation within the stratum corneum membrane (e.g., fatty acids) or simply act as cosolvents enhancing the solubility of the drug in the formulation and therefore increasing the concentration gradient and driving force for percutaneous penetration. The enhancement in percutaneous permeation also depends on the concentration of the enhancer in the formulation and the physicochemical properties of the drug to be delivered into/across skin. Ethanol, oleic acid and oleyl alcohol have been used in marketed estradiol systems as well as some combination drug systems. Ethanol has also been used in marketed fentanyl and testosterone systems. Dimethyl sulfoxide has been used in diclofenac sodium topical solution (approved in the USA for treatment of osteoarthritis) and in idoxuridine topical solution (approved in Europe for treatment of herpes zoster). Gattefosse (France) has developed a range of products acting as solubilizers/skin penetration enhancers. Although chemical permeation enhancers are promising for assisting transdermal/topical delivery of smaller molecules (< 500 Da), their application for enhancing the delivery of macromolecules is limited. A challenge in the use of chemical permeation enhancers for transdermal delivery is that the activity of these enhancers is closely related to their irritation potential. Enhancers, thus, have to be used in a concentration range in which they would be non-irritating and non-sensitizing to skin. Also, factors such as reversibility of skin barrier following the use of chemical enhancers and the possibility of long-term local and systemic toxicity must be taken into consideration before the inclusion of these molecules in a commercial formulation (Banga 2011).

## 14.5 PHYSICAL ENHANCEMENT TECHNOLOGIES – FUTURE PERSPECTIVES

The current transdermal market is limited to delivery of small (MW < 500 Da), potent (dose ~10 mg per day from a 10 $cm^2$ patch) and moderately lipophilic drugs (log P 1- 3.5), as they are able to cross the skin passively. In recent years, transdermal delivery has enjoyed significant innovations with respect to physical enhancement technologies such as iontophoresis, electroporation, sonophoresis, jet propelled particles and microporation, expanding its horizon to the delivery of biotherapeutic macromolecules and water soluble molecules. This section will focus on the most promising technologies, including iontophoresis, sonophoresis microporation and microneedles.

The use of physiologically acceptable iontophoretic current to facilitate localized drug delivery has been extensively used in physical therapy clinics for years. However, it is only within the past decade that the iontophoretic equipment and drug reservoir has been miniaturized into self-contained patches and has been approved and commercially marketed for systemic delivery. This technology facilitates transdermal delivery of charged as well as neutral drug molecules. Charged molecules are driven by electrorepulsion, i.e., when a charged drug molecule is placed under a like charged electrode; it is repelled by the electrode into skin upon application of current. Neutral molecules are transported by solvent drag or electroosmosis that occurs in the direction of anode to cathode. The ideal candidates for iontophoretic delivery are charged, water soluble molecules with a molecular weight not greater than 10–12KDa (Sachdeva et al. 2009).

An iontophoretic system (Ionsys™) for transdermal delivery of fentanyl to manage postoperative pain was approved by the FDA and European Medicines Agency in 2006. However, it was later withdrawn from market due to corrosion issues in one batch, and was later approved again for marketing, after improvement of the formulation/device. Also Wearable Electronic Disposable Drug Delivery (WEDD) technology adapted by the Travanti Medical unit of TapeMark is commercially available as IontoPatch. Recently, an iontophoretic transdermal system (Zecuity™) by NuPathe/Teva had received FDA clearance for delivery of sumatriptan intended for acute treatment of migraines, but the product has been withdrawn to investigate some reports of skin burns. A number of other former companies like Transport Pharmaceuticals, Iomed, etc., have worked on this technology but efforts are constrained due to device complexity and the gaining popularity of other relatively simple, inexpensive emerging technologies like microporation.

Microporation technology involves creation of temporary micron-sized pores or micro-channels in the skin to facilitate delivery of macromolecules and hydrophilic moieties. Microporation has gained significant attention in the last few years for delivery of biopharmaceuticals which are water soluble and often macromolecules. This technique is minimally invasive and painless as it creates micropores that superficially breach the stratum corneum, with no impact on the nerve endings that reside in the dermis. Several technologies have been explored to create these micropores such as mechanical microneedles, thermal or radiofrequency ablation and laser ablation (Banga 2009). A representative list of companies developing microporation-based products with a brief description of their technologies and product pipelines are presented in Table 14.1.

Microneedles have been explored since the 1990s when the microfabrication technology enabled the manufacture of a variety of microneedles for pharmaceutical application. The microneedle-based patch is very simple, inexpensive and does not require any power supply or advanced microelectronics or sophisticated devices, unlike other physical methods. Microneedles bear a close similarity to hypodermic delivery

**TABLE 14.1**
**Microporation Technologies**

| Microporation Technique | Company/Technology | Technology description | Product pipeline |
|---|---|---|---|
| Microneedles[1] | BD/Soluvia™ | • A single hollow microneedle that is 1.5mm long attached to the syringe prefilled with influenza vaccine | • Marketed worldwide as IDflu®, Itanza® and Fluzone Intradermal ® |
| | Nanopass/Micronjet® | • Four hollow silicon microneedles mounted on a plastic adapter which is used in conjunction with standard syringe | • Received FDA clearance |
| | Zosano/ Macroflux®technology | • Comprises of precision microprojections on thin titanium sheets | • PTH patch for osteoporosis has successfully completed phase II clinical trials, and Migraine Patch is in phase III trials |
| | 3M/ Microstructured Transdermal Systems | • Solid microneedles (sMTS) or hollow microneedles (hMTS) available in various shapes and sizes | • Preclinical studies on human growth hormone, naloxone, tetanus toxoid and ovalbumin |
| Thermal | Altea Therapeutics Technology now acquired by Nitto Dento Passport™ | • Thermal energy ablates the stratum corneum under an array of metallic filaments in patch to create micropores, followed by application of drug to microporated skin, | • Clinical studies were conducted for delivery of hydromorphone HCl, fentanyl citrate and apomorphine HCl |
| Laser | Pantec Biosolutions AG / P.L.E.A.S.E, | • Ablation of skin with erbium:YAG laser | • Preclinical studies in diabetes, pain and vaccines |
| Radiofrequency Ablation | Transpharma Medical Ltd. Technology now acquired by Syneron Medical Ltd/Viador™ (formerly known as Viaderm) | • Radiofrequency energy emitted from array of microelectrodes is used for creating micropores in the skin | • Successfully completed phase I clinical trials with calcitonin, human parathyroid hormone and GLP1 agonist. • Currently used for skin rejuvenation and delivery of cosmetic agents acting on skin |

[1] Other companies developing microneedle-based patches are Theraject, Corium, Nanopass jointly with Silex Microsystems, Apogee Technology, Becton Dickinson, Elegaphy, Imtek, ISSYS, Kumetrix, Norwood Abbey, Valeritas and Zeopane.

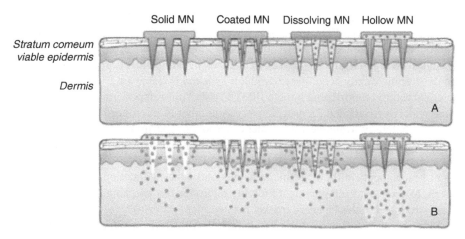

**FIGURE 14.2** Types of microneedles – using different methods to achieve dermal drug delivery. (Reprinted with permission from reference: Kim et al., 2012.)

systems with several advantages such as no risk of needle stick injuries and high patient compliance with no trauma. They are available in several configurations: (a) solid microneedles for skin pretreatment to enhance skin permeability of drug formulation; (b) drug coated microneedles from which the drug dissolves in the skin; (c) polymer or sugar microneedles that encapsulate the drug and dissolve in the skin; and (d) hollow microneedles for drug infusion into skin. Figure 14.2 demonstrates types of microneedles with these configurations using different methods to achieve dermal drug delivery (Kim et al. 2012). Coated microneedles are inexpensive, but can have about 1 mg of dose coated onto an array, making them suitable only for delivery of vaccines or other potent drugs. Injection of drugs through hollow microneedles is considered as a potential method of microneedle-based drug delivery that would enable precision over the amount and kinetics of drug delivery.

The geometry of microneedles is another important consideration determining the drug delivery profile. Typically microneedles are 100 to 750 μm in length and are available either as single entity or as an array. They can be applied using manual insertion in the skin with thumb or finger pressure or alternatively with the aid of an applicator. Historically, microneedle arrays were made of silicon, but due to their expensive microfabrication and propensity to break off in the skin, the current trend is to fabricate microneedles of metal, polymer and sugars. These microneedles can be manufactured at a low cost and may be more acceptable from a regulatory perspective (Banga 2009).

Literature has reported microneedles to deliver low molecular weight drugs (e.g., lidocaine, phenylephrine), therapeutic proteins (e.g., insulin, leuprolide acetate, desmopressin, human growth hormone) and vaccines (Influenza, BCG, HPV, etc.) in preclinical and human clinical studies (Banga 2011).

Microneedle-based products have already found their way in the commercial realm. Soluvia®, a single hollow microneedle, is 1.5mm long and is attached to the syringe prefilled with influenza vaccine and is marketed globally as IDflu®, and Fluzone Intradermal®. Additionally microneedle-based device, MicronJet®, has recently received FDA clearance. MicronJet® comprises of four hollow silicon microneedles mounted on a plastic adapter which is used in conjunction with a standard syringe (Kim et al. 2012). A number of companies are actively working on developing microneedle-based products as listed in Table 14.1. The 3M's hollow microstructured transdermal system (hMTS) with "mini-hypodermic" structures has been widely investigated for drug delivery. A number of microneedle-based products are commercially available for cosmetic purposes. The first commercial cosmetic product is the Dermaroller which is a cylindrical roller covered with solid, metal microneedles that are 0.2–0.25 mm in length. This device is used for skin pretreatment before application of cosmetic agents and acne medication. Recently a new patch, MicroHyala®, employing dissolving microneedles containing hyaluronic acid was introduced in the Japanese market for treatment of wrinkles.

Skin recovery following use of microneedles has been a subject of research as it is a determinant of safety and it is important from a regulatory perspective to show that creation of micropores in the skin does not pose safety/infection risks. Transepidermal water loss (TEWL) and tissue staining techniques have been used to show that the micropores remain open if they were occluded with an occlusive film or solution/buffer/water for 72 hours as opposed to closure within 15 hours if not occluded. This suggests that pores would remain open when a formulation/patch would be placed on microporated skin and start to close when the formulation/patch would be removed (Kalluri et al. 2011). Also, the kinetics of pore resealing was studied by electrical impedance measurements in human subjects, which showed that pores formed by microneedles sealed within two hours when the skin was not occluded, while it took three to 40 hours to recover when the skin was occluded, depending upon the geometry of the microneedles.

Patients and health care professionals have expressed a preference for microneedle products over hypodermic injections with negligible or no pain associated with these systems. The skin may show mild transient erythema following therapy, but there have been no reports of skin infection in the many human and clinical studies reported in the literature (Kim et al. 2012). The field of microneedles has rapidly progressed over the past 15 years and is geared to make a substantial impact in medicine in the coming years.

Apart from microneedles, other technologies involving thermal energy, laser or radiofrequency ablation and ultrasound are also being developed to enable microporation. Thermal microporation utilizes short high temperature pulses to cause structural disruption and vaporization of stratum corneum to create temporary micropores/micron-sized channels in the skin. A single disposable patch based on this patented technology (PassPort®) is being developed by Nitto Denko. Radiofrequency ablation is similar to thermal microporation technology; it utilizes electrical current in the radiofrequency range (100–500 KHz) applied to an array of microelectrodes to cause ionic vibration in the skin cells, leading to localized heating and cell ablation. A parathyroid hormone patch based on this technology was developed; but was not able to achieve the primary endpoint in phase II clinical trials.

Laser technology functions by specifically superheating water molecules on the skin surface causing them to flash evaporate and create microchannels. A handheld laser device termed as Painless Laser Epidermal system (P.L.E.A.S.E®) by Pantec Biosolutions is available in the Europeon market, which uses erbium:YAG laser to create micropores, typically 150 μm in diameter and 100–200 μm in depth.

Microporation is also being investigated in combination with iontophoresis to facilitate or enhance transdermal delivery. While iontophoresis is limited to delivery of molecules up to 12kDa, microporation enables transport of larger molecules by creating large transport pathways. These technologies have significant potential in combination, e.g., with the iontophoretic current driving ionized moieties along pathways created by microporation.

Sonophoresis utilizes ultrasonic energy to deliver drugs into or through the skin. While research studies with high frequency ultrasound (> 0.7MHz) have been documented since the 1950s, low frequency sonophoresis (20–100KHz) is a relatively newer field that has been investigated in the last two decades. These two technologies differ in the mechanism and extent of permeability enhancement and have varied applications.

Low frequency sonophoresis is associated with transient acoustic cavitation (i.e., formation or growth of gas bubbles in the bulk of liquid) above the skin membrane, which is considered to be the primary permeation enhancement mechanism. It has an ability to deliver a wide range of molecules through the skin (transdermal), including hydrophilic as well as hydrophobic molecules, small as well as macromolecules (proteins), hormones, vaccines and even nanoparticles. High frequency sonophoresis, on the other hand, causes cavitation within the skin appendages or adjacent to the keratinocytes of the stratum corneum, inducing disorder in the stratum corneum lipid bilayers. This technology does not cause significant changes in the skin barrier integrity, and thus has shown to be effective in enhancing the permeation of only small molecular weight compounds for localized (topical) delivery. It has been shown that acoustic cavitation (and hence enhancement in permeation) is inversely proportional to the frequency of ultrasound. Therefore, low frequency sonophoresis is now being investigated as a physical enhancement technique with a potential of expanding the scope of transdermal delivery to hydrophilic molecules/macromolecules. High frequency ultrasound technology has a proven track record of safety as it is utilized in physical therapy clinics and more amenable to use in human trials, as is evident from the large number of documented in vivo human studies. On the other hand, the clinical research with low frequency ultrasound is in its infancy with comparatively fewer in vivo studies performed (Chen et al. 2010).

The main hurdle for development of the sonophoresis technology is the difficulty in miniaturizing the technology into a self-contained patch achieved in case of iontophoretic.

Ultrasound has been investigated in combination with other enhancement techniques like microporation and iontophoresis. The SEMA (sonophoretic enhanced microneedle array) technology greatly enhances delivery rates by employing hollow microneedles in conjunction with a sonophoretic emitter. The emitter provides energy to the fluid media and induces acoustic cavitations to enhance the diffusion rate of large molecular weight compounds through microfluidic channels within the microneedles, bringing the drug in contact with the epidermis for deeper diffusion into the dermis (Polat et al. 2011). In combination with iontophoresis, the permeability enhancement results from sonic energy resulting in loosening of the stratum corneum connection followed by an enhanced electrosomotic flow by iontophoresis.

Each of the physical enhancement techniques discussed in this chapter has their own advantages. A number of factors such as physicochemical properties of drug molecules, desired degree of permeability enhancement, drug dose, desired onset of action and patient acceptability drive the choice of enhancement technique. While iontophoresis and microporation-based products for transdermal delivery have already been introduced in the market, investigative work with sonophoresis is still in the early stages.

## 14.6 COSMECEUTICALS AND DERMAL DELIVERY

Cosmeceuticals represent a rapidly evolving frontier in dermatology. They represent a category of products that lie on the fence between cosmetics that simply cleanse and beautify, and pharmaceuticals that cure and heal. Cosmeceuticals essentially are cosmetic products with biologically active ingredients professing to have medical or drug-like benefits. While pharmaceuticals are intended to alter, change or protect skin from abnormal or pathological conditions, cosmeceuticals are intended to enhance the health and beauty of skin and hence improve skin appearance but not function. They are considered to be hybrids of pharmaceuticals and cosmetics. The cosmeceutical term only applies to topically applied products such as creams, lotions and ointments. Though dermatological research implies these products have benefits, there are no requirements for them to be clinically tested to live up to their claims.

The rapid growth in the cosmeceuticals market is primarily attributed to consumer demand, discovery of new ingredients, improved understanding of skin physiology and the financial rewards associated with developing these products. The modern consumer has access to medical archives through internet resources and is constantly on the lookout for ingredients that will make the skin function better rather than just look better. The sophisticated genre of cosmeceutical consumers demand outstanding quality from the products and hence technological advances will have to keep up to meet consumer expectations (Draelos 2008).

In the USA and Europe, cosmeceuticals are sold as cosmetics, while in Japan they comprise a novel category of "quasi-drugs" that are sold directly to the consumer. In the USA, careful attention needs to be given to the claims made by these products. For example, these products can claim to improve the appearance of the wrinkles, which is a cosmetic claim, but not get rid of wrinkles, which is a drug claim. Similarly they can claim to brighten skin but not treat abnormal pigmentation. Most claims made by cosmeceuticals are moisturizing claims.

Cosmeceuticals employ over-the-counter (OTC) ingredients to serve as functional cosmetics. The ingredients used are derived from a list of raw materials that are generally recognized as safe. Botanic extracts obtained from plants form the basis of these functional cosmetics. Plant extracts are rich in endogenous antioxidants and meet the Food and Drug Administration criteria for substances that can be included in OTC formulations (Draelos 2011). Once a cosmeceutical active ingredient is identified, it is tested for activity in cell culture models and sometimes in a rodent model for confirmation of the desired skin benefits. These are followed by human clinical studies which if successful open the door for its introduction into the marketplace.

Since cosmeceuticals are unregulated, this category of products has unlimited potential uses such as improving skin radiance and luminosity, improving skin tone and texture, decreasing the appearance of skin wrinkling, providing antiaging benefits, decreasing facial pore appearance, minimizing acne, shining hair, decreasing nail brittleness, etc.

Representative ingredients used in cosmeceuticals for acne, antiaging, improving skin texture and skin lightening are presented in Table 14.2.

Acne cosmeceuticals are based upon acne inhibiting substances such as salicylic acid willow bark, elemental sulfur and tea tree oil. They have keratolytic, antiinfective and anti-inflammatory properties.

Cosmeceuticals for improving the appearance of aged skin have a significant place in the market. These preparations are mostly based upon peptides, but botanic extracts functioning as antioxidants and sunscreen actives are also used in antiaging cosmeceuticals.

Cosmeceutical peptides are sub classified into four categories: carrier, signal, neurotransmitter and enzyme modulating. The first commercial peptides were carrier peptides designed to bind to another ingredient, e.g., copper, and facilitate its penetration into wounded skin for healing purposes. This carrier concept was adapted to antiaging products, for example a peptide known as GHK-Cu was developed into

## TABLE 14.2
## Representative Ingredients in Cosmeceutical Preparations

| Acne | Antiaging | Anti-wrinkle | Pigment lightening | Exfoliants |
|---|---|---|---|---|
| • Willow bark | **Peptides** | *Occlusive*: | Liquorice extract | Glycolic acid |
| • Sulfur | • *Carrier*: GHK-Cu | Dimethicone | Kojic acid | Lactic acid |
| • Tea tree oil | • *Signal*: Pal-KTTKS | | Arbutin | Ferulic acid |
| | • *Neurotransmitter*: Acetyl hexapeptide-3 | | N-acetylglucosamine | Gluconolactone |
| | **Antioxidants** | | Aloeresin | |
| | • *Carotenoids*: Vitamin A derivatives, | *Humectant*: Honey | | |
| | • *Flavonoids*: Tetrahydrocurcumin, Gingko | *Hydrophilic matrix moisturizer*: Hyaluronic acid | | |
| | • *Polyphenols*: Sources are Green tea, Pomegranate juice and Grape seed | | | |
| | **Sunscreen** | | | |
| | • Avobenzene | | | |
| | • Benzophenone | | | |
| | • Ecamsule | | | |

a line of products to minimize the appearance of fine lines and wrinkles. Then the signal peptides were developed which were designed to mimic a natural body structure and regulate the production of endogenous protein. The most popular and widely distributed signal peptide is a palmitoyl pentapeptide (Pal-KTTKS), commercially known as Matrixyl (Sederma, Paris, France). This peptide is a procollagen fragment composed of amino acids Lysine, Threonine and Serine, that downregulates the production of collagenase, thereby increasing dermal collagen and minimizing the appearance of aging. Acetyl-hexapeptide-3, commercially known as Argireline, and pentapeptide-3, commercially known as VIALOX (Centerchem, Norwalk, CT, USA), are examples of neurotransmitter peptides that are suggested to topically relax the muscles and reduce the appearance of facial wrinkles. Enzyme modulating peptides are botanic extracts. An example is a peptide found in soy protein that inhibits the formation of proteases and is used as cosmeceutical facial moisturizers.

One of the primary causes of skin aging is oxidation of cutaneous structures due to highly reactive oxygen molecules present in the environment. Botanic extracts such as carotenoids, flavonoids and polyphenols are capable of quenching the singlet oxygen and reactive oxygen species. Examples of these ingredients are listed in Table 14.2.

Sunscreen actives that provide broad spectrum photoprotection in the UV-A wavelengths are very effective antiaging ingredients, as UV-A radiation is the prime driver of premature aging. These ingredients include benzophenone, benzophenone complexes, avobenzene and ecamsule. Ecamsule is a newer ingredient that is expected to find its way into antiaging cosmeceuticals to provide long lasting UV-A protection (Amer et al. 2009).

A commonly made claim by cosmeceuticals is decreased appearance of wrinkling. Traditional ingredients for this purpose include Occlusives (Dimethicone, mineral oil, etc.), Humectants (Glycerin, Honey, Propylene glcol, etc.) and hydrophilic matrix moisturizer. Hyaluronic acid is a newer hydrophilic matrix moisturizer present in many antiaging cosmeceutical moisturizers for wrinkle reduction.

Cosmeceuticals for pigmentation is another popular market. These products are based upon vitamins and botanicals that are able to interrupt melanin production at key steps. In recent years efforts have been focused on developing a hydroquinone alternative without the melanocyte toxicity associated with the oxidized version of hydroquinone. Hydroquinone is a recognized gold standard for its skin lightening properties. Till date, no single ingredient has been able to measure up to hydroquinone. Kojic acid (5 hydroxymethyl-4H pyrane 4-one) is one of the most popular skin lightening agents worldwide, however it has been removed from Japan due to its sensitizing properties (Reszko et al. 2009). The newer cosmeceutical skin lightening preparations contain multiple ingredients for optimal efficacy. For example, one cosmeceutical product contains Kojic acid in combination with embelica fruit extract and glycolic acid.

A subgroup of functional cosmetics has been recently termed as neurocosmeceuticals. These are topical agents applied to skin to induce a feeling of well-being, exploiting the physiological concept of mind–body interaction. These products are catered for consumers who believe that skin cannot appear healthy until the mind is at ease and the health of the mind can be improved through skin.

Neurocosmeceuticals claim to improve the well-being by altering neurotransmitters, for example inhibiting release of substance P and enhancing release of beta endorphin through topical application.

Numerous companies such as Dermelect Cosmeceuticals and Hale Cosmeceuticals sell products that bridge the gap between pharmaceutical and cosmetic products.

Over the next years, innovations in cosmeceutical products will most likely be in the areas of:

- Identification of efficacious ingredients, specifically natural products and extracts as well as synthetically engineered materials.
- Complex and effective delivery systems such as controlled, triggered delivery and nanostructured delivery.

The cosmeceutical realm will continue to combine the skills of a cosmetic formulator, knowledge of the dermatologist, the creativity of the marketing expert and wishes of the aging population into a "hope in a jar" that is sold to the consumer.

## 14.7 NANOTECHNOLOGY AND DERMAL DELIVERY

During the last two decades there has been an increasing excitement about nanotechnology in a number of fields ranging from information technology, biology to cosmetic and pharmaceutical products. The industry has been invigorated with breakthroughs in nanopharmaceuticals, due to the ability of the nano-sized compounds to localize, target drug delivery and surmount solubility and stability issues.

A variety of nanocarrier-based dosage forms, e.g., microemulsions, vesicular transport systems (Liposomes), nanoparticles and dendrimers, have been explored for dermal and transdermal delivery. The primary goal of these dosage forms is to overcome the formidable barrier of the stratum corneum (Neubert 2011).

### 14.7.1 MICROEMULSIONS

Microemulsions, also known as nano-sized emulsions, are defined as colloidal, transparent or slightly opalescent formulations comprising of oil, water, surfactant and co-surfactant. They can be classified as oil-in-water (o/w) and water-in-oil (w/o) systems, with the internal phase droplets embedded and stabilized in an external phase with the aid of surfactant rich layers separating the two phases. The internal phase droplets range in size between 20 to 100nm (Zhao et al. 2011). These optically isotropic, thermodynamically stable dispersions have low viscosity and are formed spontaneously without any energy input.

This dosage form presents significant advantages to dermal and transdermal drug delivery such as providing a highly solubilizing milieu for poorly soluble drugs and enhancing the cutaneous absorption of both hydrophilic and lipophilic drugs (as compared to conventional vehicles). The amphiphilic components in microemulsions act as penetration enhancers. The drug exhibits a high internal mobility within the vehicle resulting in high permeation rates due to solvent drag effect. Till date much of the research in the microemulsion arena has been limited to in vitro studies and only a few in vivo studies have been reported for dermal delivery using these vehicles (Kreilgaard 2002).

The main drawback for these systems is the use of high quantities of surfactants with a potential for skin irritation (Heuschkel et al. 2008). A number of research studies have used medium chain alcohol as co-surfactants which are not suited for pharmaceutical purposes due to their propensity to irritate skin. The development of well-tolerated surfactant systems and their precedent use in approved product(s) will provide impetus to the growth of these nanocarrier-based delivery systems.

Reverse (w/o) microemulsions are being investigated for delivery of hydrophilic biopharmaceuticals like peptides and proteins. The use of nano-sized emulsions for follicular targeting has also been a research topic of interest (Wosicka et al. 2010).

### 14.7.2 Vesicular Delivery Systems

In the last 20 years, colloidal vesicles such as liposomes have emerged for localized dermal and transdermal drug delivery. These vesicular drug carrier systems are primarily composed of lipids such as phospholipids and cholesterol. In 1995, MIKA Pharma was the first company worldwide to introduce a stable topical liposomal product heparin-spray in the pharmaceutical market.

In recent years, it has become evident that liposomes remain mostly confined to the upper layers of the stratum corneum and hence are not suitable for transdermal drug delivery. Innovations have been related to including novel additives in the carriers resulting in the emergence of many new vesicle types – transfersomes, ethosomes, flexosomes, niosomes, vesosomes, polymerosomes, specifically designed to enable transdermal drug delivery (Neubert 2011).

Transfersomes®, also termed as deformable liposomes, are elastic vesicles that consist of phospholipids and an edge activator. Typically these edge activators are single chain surfactant molecules (e.g., sodium cholate, sodium deoxycholate, Span's and Tween's) that destabilize and deform the lipid bilayers of the stratum corneum. Studies have reported that deformable vesicles are able to penetrate intact skin in vivo and able to deliver therapeutic amounts of a number of actives including macromolecules. Some examples include lidocaine, cyclosporine A, insulin, diclofenac, triamcinolone acetonide, levonorgesterel, ethinylestradiol and zidovudine (Elsayed et al. 2007). The ability of transfersomes to squeeze between cells in the stratum corneum under the influence of an in vivo transcutaneous hydration gradient is one of the proposed mechanisms for their ability to facilitate transdermal delivery. Figure 14.3 shows pictomicrographs from a study by Chaudhary et al. demonstrating increased permeation of the transfersomes formulations in skin layers in comparison to control vehicle formulations (Chaudhary et al. 2013). Products based on this technology are under development by a biopharmaceutical company IDEA AG. Their transfersome-based gel product for ketoprofen is currently in phase III trials in Europe for treatment of peripheral pain.

Ethosomes are another novel lipid carrier comprising of phospholipids, water and ethanol (20–45%) that have reported to deliver molecules through the skin into the

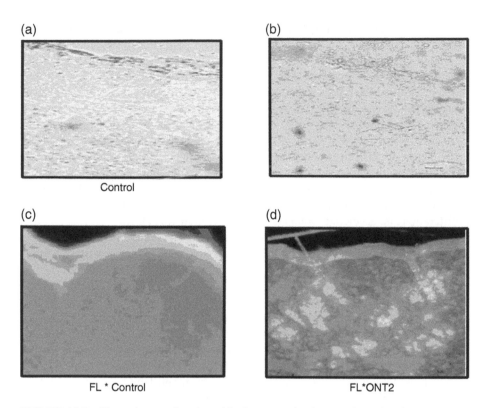

(a) Control
(b)
(c) FL * Control
(d) FL*ONT2

**FIGURE 14.3** Pictomicrographs of rat skin demonstrating increased uptake of transfersomes over control vehicle (A) vehicle treatment (B) optimized transfersome formulation treatment – 100X and fluorescent pictomicrographs of rat skin after application of rhodamine B in (C) vehicle (D) optimized transfersome formulation. (Reprinted with permission from reference: Chaudhary et al., 2013.)

systemic circulation. Ethanol is a well-known permeation enhancer. However lipid vesicles containing ethanol have shown to be superior to hydroethanolic solutions in enhancing percutaneous permeation, suggesting a synergistic mechanism between ethanol, skin lipids and vesicles. Novel Therapeutic Technology (NTT) Inc, has a portfolio of dermal products in development based on the ethosomes technology (Elsayed et al. 2007).

### 14.7.3 Nanoparticles

Nanoparticles are defined as particles having dimensions between 1–100nm as recognized by American National Standards (Prow et al. 2011). A number of nanotechnology platforms are currently being developed by several companies. The use of nanoparticles for dermal and follicular delivery has been of interest in the last decade. They provide the benefit of penetration into deeper layers of skin compared to microparticles. Very small particles (less than 10nm), such as functionalized fullerenes and quantum dots, have shown to penetrate in the viable layers of epidermis and dermis.

One of the main features of the nanoparticles is to increase the permeation of the encapsulated drug. Nanoparticles of 20nm and above have shown to penetrate deeply in the hair follicles and form a long-term reservoir for drug delivery. The corneocyte lining in the lower follicular tract is not well developed and provides a port of entry for the nanoparticles into the viable layers of the epidermis. Nanoparticles (40nm in size) have shown to deliver vaccines transcutaneously into human-antigen presenting cells. Nanoparticles can interact with skin on a cellular level and exert an adjuvant effect in topically applied vaccines (by enhancing the immune reactivity). Their skin interaction can also be exploited for controlled delivery of actives, e.g., slow release of silver ions from nanoparticles residing on the skin has shown to inhibit microbial proliferation and accelerate wound healing (Prow et al. 2011).

Several types of nanoparticles have been investigated for dermal delivery. Examples include micellar nanoparticles, solid lipid nanoparticles, nanostructured lipid carriers, fullerenes, quantum dots.

### 14.7.3.1  Micellar Nanoparticles

Micellar nanoparticle technology (MNP) was invented and patented by Novavax in mid-1990s, with the first nano-engineered-based transdermal lotion product, Estrasorb (for 17b-estratidol), being launched in 2003. The basic components of the MNP system are oil, water, stabilizer and solvent. The MNP-based nano emulsion system presents the API in a more bioavailable form and facilitates systemic drug delivery via topical application. It allows for high concentration of drug to penetrate the skin and create a depot in the stratum corneum and epidermis, resulting in a constant and controlled systemic delivery. With the MNP technology, it is possible to tailor drug disposition and permeation kinetics by changing drug loading, droplet size of the nano-emulsion and other formulation parameters.

Another MNP-based formulation (Androsorb™) has successfully completed the phase I clinical trials. The MNP technology can be applied to other drugs and offers a fresh outlook to the field of topical drug delivery, for the delivery of NSAIDS, antifungals, antibacterials, antivirals, antispasmodic and vasodilatory drugs (Chaudhari 2012).

### 14.7.3.2  Solid Lipid Nanoparticles and Nanostructured Lipid Carriers

Solid lipid nanoparticles (SLN) and nanostructured lipid carriers (NLC) have been explored in cosmetic and dermatological preparations. SLNs are composed of 0.1% to 30% w/w solid lipid entrapping the active dispersed in aqueous media with the aid of stabilizing surfactant (Pardeike et al. 2009). The particles range in size between 50 to 1000nm and can be considered more as microparticles than nanoparticles.

Nanostructured lipids are similar to SLN carriers with a difference that they contain a blend of solid and liquid lipids (oils). NLCs have shown to possess a higher drug loading capacity and an improved stability (i.e., reduced drug expulsion) during storage as compared to SLNs. SLNs and NLCs offer several features such as controlled drug release, protection of encapsulated drug from degradation and low skin irritation that make them attractive candidates for dermal application. These nanoparticles also demonstrate occlusive properties thereby helping to maintain skin hydration. Due to their small size, they provide intimate contact with the stratum corneum and thereby have shown to increase permeation for a number of drugs, e.g., clotrimazole, prednicarbate, glucocorticoids, podophyllotoxin and isotretinoin. SLNs and NLCs have also been shown to be effective in targeting drug delivery to certain layers of skin. SLN formulations have demonstrated localized delivery of triptolide in the epidermis, which is the site of action for this drug. The localization further helps to reduce the dosing frequency and hence reducing dose dependent side effects such as irritation. These nanoparticles also act as physical UV blockers and are reported to be an appealing carrier for a number of sunscreen agents.

SLNs are rightfully referred to as "nanosafe" carriers as they are only nanoparticulate delivery systems composed of natural compounds found in the body (e.g., non-hydroxy fatty acids, cholesterol, stearic acid, cholesterol, etc.) and are degraded by processes in the body resulting in excellent tolerability.

The first product on the market utilizing lipid nanoparticles was a cosmetic. Since its introduction in 2005 more than 30 cosmetic products based on this technology have been introduced (Pardeike et al. 2009). Till date there haven't been any pharmaceutical products containing lipid nanoparticles. Nevertheless, due to their outstanding features and high benefit/risk ratio as evidenced in a number of studies, their commercial introduction as a pharmaceutical dermal product is expected to be in the near future

### 14.7.3.3 Fullerenes

Fullerenes are carbon-based molecules that resemble a hollow sphere. In contact with the skin, they migrate through the skin intercellularly rather than transcellularly. They can be used to encapsulate and transport active moieties which get released into epidermis. There is literature evidence of these molecules acting as antioxidants. Studies performed so far have shown fullerenes to be well tolerated and hold a considerable promise for future dermatological and cosmetic formulations (Kato et al. 2010).

### 14.7.3.4 Quantum Dots

Quantum dots are nanostructures made of semiconductor materials having unique optical and electronic properties. Research studies have revealed their ability to permeate through the stratum corneum of human skin equivalent models (Epiderm™). Their ability to accumulate in the epidermis may have implications on transdermal delivery upon long-term dermal exposure (Jeong et al. 2010).

### 14.7.4 Dendrimers

Dendrimers are a unique class of polymers, which are an integral part of the new nanotechnology era. They are hyperbranched, monodisperse, three-dimensional macromolecules having a high surface charge density and ability to entrap active moieties. Due to the presence of multiple ionizable groups at the periphery, each dendrimer molecule can attach to a number of drug molecules electrostatically. This configuration allows for enhancement in solubility for hydrophobic drugs presenting the drug in a more diffusible form for transdermal delivery. Dendrimers have been shown to enhance transdermal delivery of nonsteroidal anti-inflammatory drugs (NSAIDs) (Cheng et al. 2007). The propensity of the dendrimers to enhance the solubility of hydrophobic drugs may offer a viable alternative for their iontophoretic delivery (Chauhan et al. 2003).

A vast body of literature has been published regarding "nano"-based delivery systems for dermal delivery. Numerous nanotechnology related products for cosmetics are already on the market. With regards to the pharmaceutical sector, these technologies are in various stages of development ranging from early feasibility assessment to late stage development and/or commercialization. Products based on the liposome technology and micellar nanoparticles have reached commercialization, while products based on the ultradeformable liposome technology are likely to be on the market soon. The microemulsions with their ease of formulation and infinite stability are very promising vehicles for future topical formulations, provided well-tolerated surfactant systems are developed. Nanoparticles have potential for follicular targeting while SLNs/NLCs by virtue of their excellent tolerability are attractive delivery candidates of the future. Research efforts are being directed towards gaining a mechanistic understanding of the interaction of the nano delivery systems with the skin components, which will guide development of the most efficient carriers/delivery systems causing least damage to the stratum corneum barrier.

## 14.8  SUMMARY

Transdermal delivery offers a promising alternative route of administration overcoming caveats associated with conventional oral drug administration such as gastrointestinal side effects as well as avoiding patient compliance concerns associated with parenteral administration. Topical drug delivery is widely being investigated for treatment of localized skin conditions. Recent developments in formulation and drug delivery systems have enhanced the scope of transdermal and topical drug delivery. Innovations in topical formulations such as foams, sprays and lecithin organogels have resulted in the availability of cosmetically elegant formulations which can be used for molecules having diverse physicochemical properties, Similarly, recent innovations in patch dosage forms such as crystal reservoir technology have allowed a better control over a desired pattern of drug release. The gel-matrix adhesive system offers improvements in tolerability and wear properties of transdermal patches. Physical enhancement techniques such as iontophoresis, microporation, sonophoresis and microneedles have expanded the scope of transdermal delivery to hydrophilic molecules as well as macromolecules. The growth of cosmeceutical industry has offered a variety of products to cleanse and beautify skin. Various nanocarriers are also being widely investigated for enhancing dermal permeation of molecules and stabilizing drugs during transdermal and topical delivery.

## REFERENCES

Acrux Ltd. 2013. www.acrux.com.au/irm/content/technology-overview.aspx?RID=275& RedirectCount=1. [cited April 2013].

Adams, C. 2007. Exploring properties of gel matrix technology. *Drug Delivery Technology* 7 (9):36–41.

Amer, M., and M. Maged. 2009. Cosmeceuticals versus pharmaceuticals. *Clin Dermatol* 27 (5):428–30.

Arzhavitina, A., and H. Steckel. 2010. Foams for pharmaceutical and cosmetic application. *Int J Pharm* 394 (1–2):1–17.

Banga, A. K. 2009. Microporation applications for enhancing drug delivery. *Expert Opin Drug Deliv* 6 (4):343–54.

Banga, Ajay K. 2011. *Transdermal and intradermal delivery of therapeutic agents: Application of Physical Technologies.* London: Taylor & Francis Inc.

Bhatia, A., Singh, B., Raza, K., Wadhwa, S. and Katara, O. P. 2013. Tamoxifen-loaded lecithin organogel (LO) for topical application: Development, optimization and characterization. *International Journal of Pharmaceutics* 444:47–59.

Chaudhari, Y. S. 2012. Nanoparticles – A paradigm for topical drug delivery. *Chronicles of Young Scientists* 3 (1):82–85.

Chaudhary, H., Kohli, K. and Kumar, V. 2013. Nano-transfersomes as a novel carrier for transdermal delivery. *International Journal of Pharmaceutics* 454:367–80.

Chauhan, A. S., Sridevi, S., Chalasani, K. B. et al. 2003. Dendrimer-mediated transdermal delivery: enhanced bioavailability of indomethacin. *J Control Release* 90 (3):335–43.

Chen, B., Wei, J. and Iliescu, C. 2010. Sonophoretic enhanced microneedles array (SEMA)—Improving the efficiency of transdermal drug delivery. *Sensors and Actuators B: Chemical* 145 (1):54–60.

Cheng, Y., Man, N., Xu, T. et al. 2007. Transdermal delivery of nonsteroidal anti-inflammatory drugs mediated by polyamidoamine (PAMAM) dendrimers. *J Pharm Sci* 96 (3):595–602.

Draelos, Z. 2008. The cosmeceutical realm. *Clinics in Dermatology* 26 (6):627–32.

Draelos, Z. D. 2011. The art and science of new advances in cosmeceuticals. *Clin Plast Surg* 38 (3):397–407, vi.

Elsayed, M. M., Abdallah, O. Y., Naggar, V. F. and Khalafallah, N. M. 2007. Lipid vesicles for skin delivery of drugs: reviewing three decades of research. *Int J Pharm* 332 (1–2):1–16.

Hadgraft, J., and Lane, M. E. 2006. Passive transdermal drug delivery systems: Recent considerations and advances. *Am.J.Drug Deliv* 4 (3):153–60.

Heuschkel, S., Goebel, A. and Neubert, R. H. 2008. Microemulsions—modern colloidal carrier for dermal and transdermal drug delivery. *J Pharm Sci* 97 (2):603–31.

Jacques, E., and Tickle, S. 2005. Minoxidil pharmaceutical foam formulation. In *United Stated Patent US 20050079139 A1.*

Jeong, S. H., Kim, J. H., Yi, S. M. et al. 2010. Assessment of penetration of quantum dots through in vitro and in vivo human skin using the human skin equivalent model and the tape stripping method. *Biochem Biophys Res Commun* 394 (3):612–5.

Kalluri, H., and Banga, A. K. 2011. Formation and closure of microchannels in skin following microporation. *Pharm Res* 28 (1):82–94.

Kapadia, M., Thosar, M. and Pancholi, S. 2012. *Formulation and Evaluation of Econazole Nitrate Topical Spray: Topical Antifungal Treatment* LAP LAMBERT Academic Publishing

Kato, S., Aoshima, H., Saitoh, Y. and Miwa, N. 2010. Fullerene-C60/liposome complex: Defensive effects against UVA-induced damages in skin structure, nucleus and collagen type I/IV fibrils, and the permeability into human skin tissue. *J Photochem Photobiol B* 98 (1):99–105.

Kim, Y. C., Park, J. H. and Prausnitz, M. R. 2012. Microneedles for drug and vaccine delivery. *Adv Drug Deliv Rev* 64 (14):1547–68.

Kreilgaard, M. 2002. Influence of microemulsions on cutaneous drug delivery. *Adv Drug Deliv Rev* 54 Suppl 1:S77–98.

Kumar, R., and Katare, O. P. 2005. Lecithin organogels as a potential phospholipid-structured system for topical drug delivery: a review. *AAPS PharmSciTech* 6 (2):E298–310.

Neubert, R. H. 2011. Potentials of new nanocarriers for dermal and transdermal drug delivery. *Eur J Pharm Biopharm* 77 (1):1–2.

Pardeike, J., Hommoss, A. and Muller, R. H. 2009. Lipid nanoparticles (SLN, NLC) in cosmetic and pharmaceutical dermal products. *Int J Pharm* 366 (1–2):170–84.

Patel, E. K., and Oswal, R. J. 2012. Nanosponge and micro sponges: a novel drug delivery system. *International Journal of Research in Pharmacy and Chemistry* 2 (2):237–244.

Paudel, K. S., Milewski, M., Swadley, C. L. et al. 2010. Challenges and opportunities in dermal/transdermal delivery. *Ther Deliv* 1 (1):109–31.

Pecha, R., and Gompf, B. 2000. Microimplosions: cavitation collapse and shock wave emission on a nanosecond time scale. *Phys Rev Lett* 84 (6):1328–30.

Peck, M. S., Pena, E. L., Thoennes, J. C. and Valvani, C. S. 1988. Foams for delivery of minoxidil. In *WO1988001863 A1*, edited by T. U. Company.

Polat, B. E., Hart, D., Langer, R. and Blankschtein, D. 2011. Ultrasound-mediated transdermal drug delivery: mechanisms, scope, and emerging trends. *J Control Release* 152 (3):330–48.

Prow, T. W., Grice, J. E., Lin, L. L. et al. 2011. Nanoparticles and microparticles for skin drug delivery. *Adv Drug Deliv Rev* 63 (6):470–91.

Reszko, A. E., Berson, D. and Lupo, M. P. 2009. Cosmeceuticals: practical applications. *Dermatol Clin* 27 (4):401–16, v.

Sachdeva, V., and Banga, A. K. Autumn 2009. Skin deep. *Drug Delivery and Dosage Forms, PMPS*, 17–24.

Tamarkin, D., Eini, M., Friedman, D. et al. 2008. Sensation modifying topical composition foam. In *United States Patent US 20080253973 A1*, edited by F. Ltd.

Thomas, B. J., and Finnin, B. C. 2004. The transdermal revolution. *Drug Discov Today* 9 (16):697–703.

Van der, H., and Edgar, I. M. 2013. Foam-forming assembly, squeeze foamer and dispensing device. In *United States Patent US 8360282 B2*, edited by R. A. N.V.

Wosicka, H., and Cal, K. 2010. Targeting to the hair follicles: current status and potential. *J Dermatol Sci* 57 (2):83–9.

Zhao, J. H., Ji, L., Wang, H. et al. 2011. Microemulsion-based novel transdermal delivery system of tetramethylpyrazine: preparation and evaluation in vitro and in vivo. *Int J Nanomedicine* 6:1611–9.

Zhao, Y., Brown, M. B. and Jones, S. A. 2010. Pharmaceutical foams: are they the answer to the dilemma of topical nanoparticles? *Nanomedicine* 6 (2):227–36.

# Index

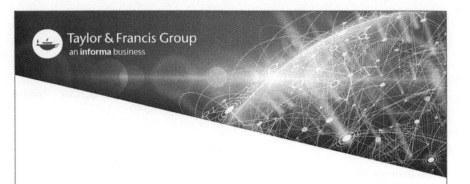

Milton Keynes UK
Ingram Content Group UK Ltd.
UKHW031138141024
449569UK00024B/1238

9 781032 337418